Ritual Retellings

Series: Epistemologies of Healing

General Editors: David Parkin and Elisabeth Hsu: both are at ISCA, Oxford

This series publishes monographs and edited volumes on indigenous (so-called traditional) medical knowledge and practice, alternative and complementary medicine, and ethnobiological studies that relate to health and illness. The emphasis of the series is on the way indigenous epistemologies inform healing, against a background of comparison with other practices, and in recognition of the fluidity between them.

Ritual Retellings
Luangan Healing Performances through Practice

Isabell Herrmans

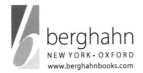

berghahn
NEW YORK · OXFORD
www.berghahnbooks.com

First published in 2015 by
Berghahn Books
www.berghahnbooks.com

Library of Congress Cataloging-in-Publication Data
Herrmans, Isabell, author.
Ritual retellings: Luangan healing performances through practice / Isabell
Herrmans.
pages cm. — (Epistemologies of healing; volume 16)
Includes bibliographical references and index.
ISBN 978-1-78238-564-6 (hardback) — ISBN 978-1-78238-565-3
(ebook)   1. Dayak (Indonesian people)–Rites and ceremonies.
2. Healing–Indonesia–Kalimantan.   3. Traditional medicine–Indonesia–
Kalimantan.   4. Ethnology–Indonesia–Kalimantan. I. Title.
DS646.32.D9H47 2015
305.8009598'3–dc23   2014033540

British Library Cataloguing in Publication Data
A catalogue record for this book is available from the British Library

ISBN: 978-1-78238-564-6 (hardback)
EISBN: 978-1-78238-565-3 (institutional ebook)

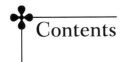

Contents

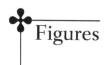

Figures

All images by the author or by her fieldwork partner Kenneth Sillander

✤ Acknowledgments

This book has been long in the making. Like the journey of *belian* curing which it is about, the process toward its completion has followed a meandering and often ramifying path. Along the way significant political and environmental changes have occurred: Indonesia has left the New Order era behind and entered an era of reformation and democratization; the narrow forest trails along which I first walked in 1992 to reach what later was to become my field site are now roads, some even paved, and recently large parts of the rainforests encircling central Luangan villages have, to both my regret and that of many Luangans, been converted into oil palm plantations.

Writing the book would not have been possible if it was not for the advice and inspiration received from numerous people that I have encountered at different steps of this journey, or the financial support of many foundations. I would like to thank them all here. I have shared all parts of the journey, from fieldwork through the process of writing the book, with my partner, fellow anthropologist Kenneth Sillander. Sometimes it is hard to say where his input ends and mine begins and my gratitude to him is beyond words.

Many of the people to whom my greatest thanks are due sadly passed away before this book was completed. I would like to dedicate the book to them, and especially the many *belian* curers who so generously shared their knowledge with me. Without the late *belian* Kakah Ramat, who seemed to enjoy telling us myths and chants as much as we enjoyed listening to them, this book would not have been the same. The near-daily discussions with him during fieldwork on all things ritual have served as my basic guide to *belian* curing and Luangan tradition. Besides Kakah Ramat I would also like to thank all other ritual specialists who shared their knowledge with us, among them especially Tak Ramat, Ma Buno, Ma Putup, Ma Sarakang, Mancan, Ma Dengu, Nen Bai, Tak Dinas, Ma Lombang,

Ma Kerudot, Ma Joke, Nen Tampung, Nen Bola, and Ma Beliai. Besides them, I am especially indebted to the late Tak Ningin and Ma Bari who took us into their family, allowed us to live in the village longhouse and shared their sparse resources with us throughout our fieldwork. Special thanks are also due to the schoolteacher Thomas who helped us with translating myths and chants whenever we visited Benangin on the Teweh River. Lemanius, a death ritual specialist from the village of Lawarang in the upper Teweh region, was also a major source of information on Luangan life and ritual, and he generously allowed me to copy his manuscript (1996) on Luangan myth and religion. The late *kepala adat besar* and *wara* of Lambing, Mas Arsa Muda Idjau Duk, allowed us to stay in his house whenever we passed by on our way to or from Samarinda, and shared his countless stories and knowledge of Benuaq ritual, myth, and history with us. In Palangkaraya, capital of Central Kalimantan, the members of the Hindu Kaharingan Council, and Mantikei R. Hanyi in particular, welcomed us with utmost hospitality, guided us around, and allowed us to participate in their ceremonies.

Financial support for our fieldwork was provided by the Nordic Institute of Asian Studies and the Finnish Cultural Foundation. I am grateful to the Sasakawa Young Leaders' Fellowship Fund, the Oskar Öflund Foundation, the Ella and Georg Ehrnrooth Foundation, the Alfred Kordelin Foundation, the Nordenskiöld Foundation, Vetenskapsstiftelsen för kvinnor, and the University of Helsinki, for supporting my writing.

The Indonesian Institute of Sciences (LIPI) provided me with a research permit. Professor Parsudi Suparlan at Universitas Indonesia acted as local sponsor of the research. For practical assistance in helping me to obtain the research permit and for encouragement as well as valuable information on Borneo, I am greatly indebted to Bernard Sellato. Joseph Weinstock likewise generously shared his knowledge on the Luangan region before I started my fieldwork.

The final form of this book was influenced by critiques and comments generously provided by several readers. I am especially grateful for the comments provided by Clifford Sather, Peter Metcalf, Marina Roseman, Timo Kaartinen, Karen Armstrong, Jukka Siikala, Jane Margold, Louise Klemperer Sather, Pascal Couderc, Elisabeth Hsu, an anonymous reader of the *Journal of Ritual Studies*, and the three anonymous reviewers of Berghahn Books. I am also grateful for comments and encouragement by colleagues and students from the Social and Cultural Anthropology department at the University of Helsinki.

Permission to reprint a revised version of my article "Representing Unpredictability: An Analysis of a Curing Ritual among the East Kalimantan Luangan," previously published in the *Journal of Ritual Studies* (vol. 18, 2004: 50–61), in chapter 2, has been granted by the co-editors of the *Journal*, Dr. Pamela J. Stewart and Prof. Andrew Strathern. A version of chapter 3, "Making Tactile: *Ganti Diri* Figures and the Magic of Concreteness among the Luangan Dayaks," appeared in the *Journal of the Finnish Anthropological Society* (vol. 30, 2005: 44–67), as well as in the *Borneo Research Bulletin* (vol. 36, 2005: 108–138).

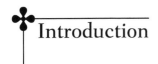

Introduction

And yet, can the knowledge deriving from reason even begin to compare with knowledge perceptible by sense?

—Louis Aragon (1994: 9)

This book is a study of the emergent and variable character of ritual performances for healing and how they enable ongoing negotiation of participants' life conditions. It is an ethnography of *belian*, a lively and unobjectified tradition of shamanistic curing rituals which are performed by the Luangans, an indigenous population of shifting cultivators of Indonesian Borneo. In *belian* rituals one or several shamans negotiate with and present offerings to a variety of spirits in order to cure illness and improve well-being more generally. Ranging from sleepy low-key affairs involving small circles of close kin and neighbors to festive crowd-seizing community rituals, these events interpunctuate work and other activities on an almost daily basis and provide principal occasions during which the generally dispersed swidden-cultivating communities gather.

The principal purpose of the book is to investigate the formation and significance of these highly popular rituals in practice. It explores how *belian* rituals concretely operate in the variable contexts of their performance, and what they do for particular people in particular circumstances. Departing from conventional conceptions of rituals as ethereal liminal or insulated traditional domains, the book demonstrates the importance of understanding rituals as emergent within their specific historical and social settings, and highlights the irreducibility of lived reality to epistemological certainty. Focusing on how the *belian* rituals unfold in everyday life, it explores how different aspects of Luangan "reality"—social relationships, existential and political concerns, ontology, cosmology, etc.— are portrayed and shaped through ritual representations—in chants

1

and visual imagery—and how the rituals' objectives and capacity to influence are enabled by what I call the "openness between reality and representations," the dialectical, two-way relationship between these aspects of reality, and their expression in ritual media.

I will begin my exploration of *belian* rituals by presenting a short vignette which illustrates some of their prominent characteristics, such as their frequency, integration with everyday life, and what might perhaps be called their "everydayness"—their informal and habitual nature. This vignette also serves to illustrate that the principal strategy through which I have chosen to approach my topic is by way of providing concrete examples. Each chapter in the book presents a case study in the form of a narrative account of a particular ritual performance and some related life events, and describes the importance of these performances and events for the particular people who were most centrally involved in them. This strategy of approaching my material through concrete, situationally contextualized examples and concomitant analysis is motivated by a fundamental fieldwork experience, namely, that the *belian* rituals were thoroughly shaped by their organization and significance in practice: by the form and circumstances of their enactment, and by their role in the personal lives of the participants. In particular, it serves to evoke the rituals' situationally emergent character, as well as other associated characteristics such as their loosely framed and open-ended nature, and to explore how these qualities affect the appropriation of ritual representations and facilitate the rituals' capacity to influence people's life conditions.

* * *

Navigating the darkness of a moonless night in March 1996, lighting my way with a flickering torch, watchful of water buffaloes roaming free in the village, I follow the sound of drums (*tuung*) to Ma Kelamo's house. As I get closer, the sound of drums gets louder and is accompanied by the reverberating sound of a xylophone (*kelentangen*), the melody revealing that a *belian* ritual in the *sentiu* style is being performed. As I enter the small modern-style house, I am met by the sharp light of a kerosene lamp and the pungent scent of *gaharu* incense (*Aquilaria* sp.), emerging from among the porcelain bowls of offerings arranged on the floor in the middle of the room. Next to the offerings, Mancan, a *belian* curer in his mid-thirties, is dancing with a small bowl on his head, containing rice and a lighted candle, chanting to invoke his spirit familiars. Lida, an eight-year-old girl suffering from flu, is lying on a rattan mat in a corner of the room, half-asleep. She is surrounded by her father and mother, who play the drums, her older sister Ena and her sister's newly wed husband Mohar, as well as Nen Bai, a female neighbor, who is playing the xylophone. Lida, a much loved daughter who usually lives with an aunt in the neighboring village where she attends her first year at school, has been brought home for the ritual, a rather small event, arranged to maintain her well-being as much as to cure illness.

As I sit down on the floor, joining in the small talk of those present, distractedly observing Mancan's movements as he dances, trying to grasp the words of his chant, there is suddenly a sound of another drumbeat, emerging from Kakah Unsir's house which is situated opposite Ma Kelamo's, just a few meters away, across the village path. Apparently, and to the surprise of at least some of us, another *belian* ritual is being performed there. Jokingly, Ma Kelamo, Nen Lida and Nen Bai join in the rhythm coming from next door, playing the drums and the xylophone faster and louder, laughing as the beat from the other house increases in pace and force in response to their own. The penetrating voice of Ma Putup, the shaman next door, can be discerned through the drumming, causing Nen Lida and Nen Bai to declare that they are frightened of his strange and curious spirit familiars, called in a language unintelligible to them.

Mancan finishes early, and as he blows on his bear-tooth whistle as a sign of closing up, I excuse myself and rush over to Kakah Unsir's house. Ma Putup, a man in his sixties who has just married into the village and who is known for his peculiar style of curing in which he summons a variety of spirits from all over the island and beyond, often in foreign sounding names and words, stops in the middle of a sentence to welcome me. He points out that he is pleased about my presence, the presence of an anthropologist somehow adding to the authority of the occasion, along with the strange and powerful assemblage of spirit beings congregated. He then resumes his chanting, continuing from where he just left off. The people present in Kakah Unsir's extended-family house (*lou*) sit scattered around the room, plaiting rattan baskets, chewing betel, smoking, playing cards, chatting about everyday affairs, with some people taking a nap on the floor. The objective of this ritual, eclectically combining

3

the *belian sentiu* and *belian bawo* shamanic traditions, is to cure Kakah Unsir, who is said to be tired due to old age, and Milu, his granddaughter, who suffers from a stomach-ache. Ma Putup takes turns attending to the two patients, and addressing the various spirit familiars (*mulung*) and malevolent spirits (*blis*) invoked with offerings and requests of either assistance or withdrawal. As this is the first evening of a several-day long ritual, and as word of it has not yet been spread widely, people being away on their swidden fields as it is harvest time, the event draws only a rather small audience, mostly consisting of members of Kakah Unsir's extended family. A couple of hours later, as the ritual finishes for the evening, I join the other participants in eating the variety of rice flour cakes (*okan penyewaka*) and small pieces of grilled chicken that are offered as rewards to the spirits during the ritual, before returning home to sleep in the village longhouse (*lou solai*), my principal residence during my fieldwork.

The Frequency of *Belian*

Attending *belian* rituals was a major experience of my fieldwork, conducted intermittently between 1993 and 2011, and, after a while, an unexceptional and rather mundane occurrence, part of the expected course of events. In fact, it was *belian* rituals, and the popularity of these rituals, that first attracted me to do fieldwork in Kalimantan (Indonesian Borneo), and to do it among the Luangans rather than among some other Dayak (indigenous non-Muslim) group, so in a respect this was not unexpected, but anticipated.[1] My initial interest for the subject arose during a holiday trip to the middle Mahakam region in the province of East Kalimantan in 1991, which I made with my partner, fellow anthropologist Kenneth Sillander. Visiting a predominantly Christian Luangan village, we stumbled upon a *belian* curing ritual late one night as we were about to go to sleep. No one had mentioned that there would be a ritual in the village that evening. In fact, the village head had spent much of the day emphasizing how devoted they were as Protestant Christians, how they even had stopped smoking as a consequence. Thus I was utterly surprised as the sound of drums led our way to a house filled to the brim with people, with a shaman chanting and dancing in their midst, spinning around rapidly while shaking heavy brass bracelets. I was immediately drawn in by the music, the scent of incense, and the simultaneously dramatic and laid-back atmosphere. Providing a vivid expression of a vital shamanistic tradition, maintained, in this particular case, despite an apparently strong commitment to Christianity, the event continued to fascinate me long after and motivated me to start exploring the ethnographic literature on Borneo.

As a result, Kenneth and I set out the next summer on a two-month trip to southeast Borneo, with the objective of possibly finding a future field site (Kenneth was at that time attracted to Borneo primarily by its ethnic complexity). During this trip we visited several Dayak groups—among them the Siang, Murung, Ot Danum, and Luangan—on the upper Barito River and the eastern part of the mountainous area of the Barito-Mahakam watershed that forms the boundary between the provinces of East and Central Kalimantan. This time again it was our encounter with Luangan rituals that made the strongest impression on us, and it provided a decisive incentive for us to choose the Luangan area as a field site.[2] As we traveled through the central Luangan area, walking from village to village on a long-used footpath connecting Central and East Kalimantan, starting from the village of Lampeong in the subdistrict of Gunung Purei in Central Kalimantan, and leading into the Bentian Besar subdistrict in East Kalimantan, there were *belian* rituals performed in almost every village we stayed in, most of them small family affairs, curing rituals sponsored by individual households, but also, in one case, a large community ritual (*nalin taun*), at the time reaching its finale after weeks of ritual activity.

This rather extraordinary ritual activity continued during our main fieldwork in 1993 and 1996–1997. In broad statistical terms, there was a *belian* ritual going on every second night of the fieldwork, and sometimes, as in the event recounted earlier, several at the same time. As the rituals typically lasted into the middle of the night or even until morning, and larger *belian* rituals also featured activities in the daytime, I spent a large proportion of my time in the field observing *belian* rituals. Most Luangans also took part in rituals very frequently, although no one, of course, attended every ritual arranged, and few as many as Kenneth and I did. Remarkably many Luangans were also trained shamans themselves. In the small village of about ninety inhabitants in which the rituals performed by Mancan and Ma Putup recounted in the vignette above took place—where we did the larger part of our fieldwork—there were fifteen practicing *belian* (the person officiating for these rituals is referred to by the same term that designates the ritual), most of whom performed on a regular basis. In addition to these shamans, others were invited as guest performers from neighboring villages, and occasionally from more faraway places. Although ritual activity and the number of practicing *belian* relative to the total population may have been extraordinarily high in this village at this particular time, it was very high in many other upriver non-Christian Luangan villages as well. Providing a characterization of one such village, a woman who introduced me to it told me in Indonesian that they had "*belian terus*," arranged *belian* rituals incessantly. She did so expressing mixed feelings of pride and embarrassment, as the frequency of rituals, from an outsider's perspective, could be seen as an expression of both backwardness and spiritual power.

My most recent follow-up visits to the field area in 2007 and 2011 have showed that the popularity of *belian* curing has remained nearly undiminished so far among central Luangans. In the village where I did most of my fieldwork in the late 1990s, however, most of the older shamans have died (and, regrettably, quite a few younger ones as well), creating heavy pressure on those left behind. During a *belian buntang* family ritual performed in the late Kakah Unsir's house in 2011, the shaman Ma Kerudot held a speech in which he complained that he had been performing as *belian* for forty days in a row, officiating for four different rituals without any rest in between. He needed to tend to his fields as well, he pointed out, urging people to appoint other shamans besides him. It seems that there are currently less people willing to become shamans, even though the demand for *belian* still persists pretty much undiminished. The *belian* rituals themselves have also remained basically unchanged in terms of style, purpose, and duration during the twenty years I have experience of them, at least in those villages which I know the best. Exemplifying this continuity, both the format of, and the composition of the participants in the particular ritual performed by Ma Kerudot were virtually identical to another *buntang* ritual that I witnessed in 1996, as were the reasons for arranging it (listlessness and persistent minor illness among the core members of the sponsoring extended family, and concern with its standing relative to those of others in the village).

Even though central Luangan ritual activity may be uncommonly high in comparative perspective—a condition enabled by an unusually low degree of conversion to Christianity and a relative remoteness from larger government centers—there are indications that such a popularity of shamanic curing rituals may not have been exceptional in Borneo in a historical perspective. Indeed, similar rituals seem to have been fairly common among several groups of Dayaks, before many of them converted to Christianity a few decades ago. Douglas Miles (1966: 3) notes that there were seances arranged nearly every week among the Ngaju during the time of his fieldwork, one ceremony giving rise to another, while H.S. Morris (1997: 6) observes that "almost every night there were ceremonies held to cure illness" among the Melanau in the 1950s. Peter Metcalf (2010: 237) points out that among the Berawan in the 1970s "there were half a dozen active [shamans] at Long Teru, and when the house was full, there were sessions on many evenings, and occasionally, two or three going on simultaneously." In the same vein, Anna Tsing (1988: 830) notes that "rarely a week goes by in a Meratus community without a shamanic curing ceremony."

The persisting frequency of curing rituals among the Luangans—remarked on both by their neighbors and themselves—intrigued me from early on, all the more so as the literature on those Borneo peoples who, like the Luangans, practice secondary mortuary rituals, has paid considerable attention to these practices, while largely neglecting curing rituals.[3] Certain aspects related to the performance of *belian* rituals, such as their openness and flexibility—eclectically combining the new with the old and the local with the foreign—as well as the ease with which rituals tended to blend with each other and with everyday life, questioning conventional conceptions of ritual, only served to trigger my interest in *belian* and eventually came to define the theme of my research.

The question of why *belian* rituals are so frequent is important for this study. However, rather than being concerned with the somewhat unproductive question of whether or not their importance among the Luangans is unique—which the available evidence indeed seems to suggest it is not—I am interested in what prompts their indisputable Luangan appeal, in what motivates the Luangans to practice these rituals, even while they simultaneously, in some respects, work to marginalize them. In other words, I am interested in the significance of the *belian* rituals from the Luangan perspective and, more particularly, in how their form and content reflect or reproduce this

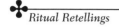

significance and thus contribute to their appeal and frequency. As with Sherry Ortner's study of Nepalese Sherpa rituals, this entails an interest in "what ritual does ... as a certain sort of event and experience for the society and the people" (1978: 4). How does the *belian* ritual, as a specific configuration of social practice and symbolic representation, influence Luangans in their life-worlds and social environment? How does the distinctive manner in which *belian* is typically performed and experienced by ritual participants potentially contribute to this? In particular, how do such prominent features of Luangan rituals as their often situationally emergent and open-ended, negotiable qualities and their practical constitution affect this process? And, on the other hand, what is the role of their "everydayness"—their habitual, tactile appropriation, and their non-objectified character—in this connection?

Ritualization, Practice, and Framing

Modern health care was still largely absent in the area where I did fieldwork—and, until recently, in much of Kalimantan—so this is obviously an important factor contributing to the popularity of *belian* curing. For this reason, among other things, infant mortality was high, and during my fieldwork people often died of what, from the viewpoint of modern medicine, could appear as unnecessary causes, including malaria, tuberculosis, gastrointestinal diseases, and bacterial skin infections. But taking into account the fact that *belian* rituals were often arranged even when no direct medical need appeared to be present, and notwithstanding, in some cases, concurrent medicinal treatment—or neglect of such treatment despite its availability—this explanation is clearly insufficient (cf. Hoskins 1996). Even more basically, it is insufficient for the reason that illness is defined very broadly among Luangans, and the field of application of these rituals even more broadly.

A principal way in which I will approach the above-mentioned concerns of this study is by presenting an ethnography of ritualization. This is to say that I intend to account for the popularity and distinctive characteristics of *belian* rituals by analyzing them in the context of their initiation, in terms of how they represent responses to specific or general concerns in the Luangans' social and cultural environment and how they as creative strategies act upon and reshape this environment. I use the term "ritualization" loosely in the sense that it has been developed by Catherine Bell (1992). Ritualization, in her practice theory-based understanding, refers to a special form of strategic action which "people engage in ... as a practical way of dealing with some specific circumstances" (1992: 92). Bell prefers to talk about ritualization, as opposed to ritual, to emphasize that it should not be studied as a separate reality, apart from the concrete social settings in which it is articulated and juxtaposed with other forms of action and various everyday and political concerns. In her view, "ritual should be analyzed and understood in its real context, which is the full spectrum of ways of acting within any given culture, not as some a priori category of action" (1997: 81). In this view, understanding rituals requires looking at what they *mean* in terms of how they are perceived and function in *practice*, that is, in terms of how the sponsors, officiants, and other participants experience, understand, and are affected by them, prior to, during, and after arranging them, and with a view to how this complex relationship between rituals and ritual participants is influenced by the latter's social relations, cultural understandings, and material life conditions.

However, at the same time as the ritualization concept highlights the fact that ritual is indissolubly linked with everyday life, it also stresses, like most approaches to ritual before it, that ritual is intrinsically differentiated from other forms of action in some fundamental respects. As Bell notes, ritualization refers to "a way of acting that distinguishes itself from other ways of acting in the very way it does what it does" (1997: 81), thereby "differentiating itself as more important or powerful" (1992: 90). It indeed represents a special form of strategic action, which is associated with culturally variable special properties whereby it is distinguished from "everyday," non-ritual action, and attributed special authority. By forming a "cultural strategy of differentiation" in this way, ritualization also entails "a translation of immediate concerns into the dominant terms of ritual" (Bell 1992: 8, 106), meaning that it restates the concerns it responds to in a profoundly different, ritual mode of representation. In acting upon social reality, ritualization thus at the same time distances itself from it, in terms of content as well as form.

In the Luangan case presented in this study, ritualization entails invoking an unseen world of spirits and souls, of hidden forces and processes, and doing so in a special register of "ancestral language" (*basa tuha one*) and symbolically encoded ritual action. Through an analysis of ritual chants and the use of material objects in ritual, this study explores the representational practices of *belian* curing, in order to better understand what constitutes their particularity. Following Webb Keane (1997: 8), I examine how representations exist "as things and acts in the world." This entails conceiving representations as "entities with their own, particular, formal properties (such as poetic structure and material qualities) and as kinds of practice, distinct and yet inseparable from the full range of people's projects and everyday activities" (ibid.). Since this unseen world—and the conventionalized symbolic mediation of it—is relatively rarely invoked outside ritual, ritualization also plays a crucial role in reproducing it, indeed, in bringing it into being for the Luangans, I claim. Thus ritualization not only represents reality but actively creates some dimensions of it.

My interest in *belian* as action not only involves an interest in how it reflects and responds to extra-ritual concerns—such as something which people want to do—but also in *how* it does so *as ritual*, largely by means of precisely those characteristics which distinguish it from non-ritualized action. In this respect, my approach to *belian* entails recognizing a complex two-way dialectic between ritual, on the one hand, and society and "everyday life," on the other. In fact, it allows for a view of *belian* as genuinely productive or creative, and thus not simply reflective, but transcendent, of extra-ritual reality. Thereby it mitigates a criticism of Bell's theory by Don Handelman (2005: 217) and Bruce Kapferer (2005: 39), according to whom it is characteristic of a tendency to reduce ritual to representations of a social, political, or other extra-ritual realm, and amounts to a failure to address "ritual in its own right."

The approach to *belian* applied in this study indeed involves an interest in what Kapferer calls the "virtuality" of rituals, referring to their quality of forming a "dynamic process in and of itself" or "a kind of phantasmagoric space ... in which participants can reimagine (and redirect or reorient) themselves into the everyday circumstances of life," although without a similar stress on rituals as lacking "essential representational relation to external realities" or forming "a self-contained imaginal space" (2005: 46–47). Inspired by Victor Turner's (1969) theory of ritual as process, and its stress on the generative and transformative, as opposed to representational and reproductive, dimensions of ritual—evident especially in its liminal stages—Kapferer regards ritual "as a crucible for the emergence of original meaning, of new ways of structuring relations and for reorienting experience" (2008: 5). Like Kapferer, and Turner before him, I perceive that the inner dynamics of *belian* do have a creative and transformative potential. Based on my field experience, however, I suggest that *belian* rituals are not closed to what goes on outside their boundaries, or unambiguously aimed at "holding at bay the chaotic qualities of reality" (Kapferer 2005: 48). In fact, I hypothesize that the chaotic, uncontrollable qualities of reality may form an intrinsic part of the ritual process itself in *belian*. This is so especially if *belian* is understood as a complex of activities—including both those of the shamans and those of the other participants—that go on during the progression of the ritual, but even, to an extent, if it is considered to be restricted to the more "structural" elements of the performance, such as the shamans' chants. An interest in how *belian* rituals are open, or responsive, to the contingencies of life, even while they serve to overcome their effects, occupies my interest especially in chapter 2 and chapter 4, which explicitly deal with unpredictability, including both the unpredictability of events, and that of representation.

For the Luangans, the frequency of *belian* curing means that rituals at times constitute "the everyday" as much as any other activity. What is more, the distinction between the ritual and the non-ritual realm—or between one ritual and another, as the example that I presented in the beginning of this introduction suggests—is not always clear-cut or absolute, but elastic, transgressed, and occasionally purposively played with. Indicating this, the word most often used to describe rituals among Luangans is *awing*, "work," expressing an understanding which places ritual on a par with other work, such as farming, pointing to its nature as an instrumental *activity*.[4] In an SMS message that I received after a short field visit in 2007, a young Luangan man referred to an upcoming large ritual as *aur*, a word meaning "obstacle" or "impediment," which may be used for any task or occupation which hinders one from performing other activities, thus separating ritual from other activities as it juxtaposes it with them.

The critique Handelman (2006: 582) has presented of what he calls "lineal framings" of rituals, "premised on hierarchical ordering and surgical incising of outside from inside," and his advocation of a "fuzzier," more "Moebius-like" framing instead, is thus highly relevant for my exploration of Luangan curing practices. Framing is a concept that has been used to describe how a social activity (e.g., ritual) is set apart from other activities (e.g., non-ritual activities) (see Bateson 1955; Goffman 1974). A frame is a schema of activity that also serves as a schema for the interpretation of that activity (T. Turner 2006: 235) and thus forms a sort of meta-commentary of it (Handelman 2006: 572). Contrary to "monothetic ideas of ritual organization" which, according to Handelman, "limit, skew, and reduce our comprehension of how change in ritual emerges from ritual practice itself, and draw attention away from complexities of the interpenetration of the interior and exterior of ritual" (2006: 582), I set out to examine how *belian* rituals constitute creative strategies that may be interactive with, occasionally inseparable from, and yet in some respects autonomous from non-ritual reality.

An issue of special interest in this connection is how ritual representation in *belian* involves both creation and recreation in that the shaman sensuously (through words, sound, movement, and objects) brings the world into being for his human and spirit audience as he tries to transform it. The process whereby the Luangans, through *belian*, "not only express but manipulate reality by means of its image," a process constitutive of what Michael Taussig calls "the magic of mimesis" (1993: 57), forms a leading theme of this study. In his book *Mimesis and Alterity*, Taussig describes his concern with mimesis as a concern "with the prospects for a sensuous knowledge in our time" (1993: 44). Mimesis, misjudged as "realist copying," is, as he sees it, essentially about "sensate actualization," about bringing something into being through tactile re-presentation. Instead of viewing mimesis primarily as an act of representation, as a naive form of realism, he focuses on its transformative and creative properties which he understands as being intimately associated with the representation's—or "copy's"—concrete and sensuous character by virtue of which it creates as much as it represents its referent. By treating the copy as a sensate actualization—rather than a representation—of the original, and by perceiving mimesis as what he calls "active yielding," as an act involving the subject's embodiment, or concrete emulation, of the object, he develops a view of mimesis as a productive practice in which the importance of its aspect of representation is subordinate (ibid.: 44–46).

How sensate actualization, in Taussig's understanding, may form an essential element of the curative properties in *belian* represents an important inquiry in my study. This is explored, for instance, through *pejiak pejiau*, an elementary activity in *belian* rituals, which consists of a two-phased process of "undoing and redoing," whereby a dramatized transformation of something bad into something good is evoked concretely, through words, acts, and objects illustrating the two phases. This process is part of a more general process in which the *belian* conjures a world of disturbed, and restored, human-spirit relations by sensuously bringing them into being. By giving concrete material form to his representations, the *belian* makes human-spirit relations objects of corporeal reality and experience, and thus enables their reorganization. This exemplifies one way in which ritualization forms what Michael Jackson (2005: 95) has called "a strategy for transforming our *experience* of the world."

The aspect of active yielding constitutive of mimesis according to Taussig, expresses an epistemology predicated upon a subject-object relationship based on continuity as opposed to discontinuity, a quality commonly attributed to animism in the recent theoretical revision of this long-devalued anthropological concept, which I will use to shed light on some aspects of Luangan world views and cosmology (see Bird-David 1999; Descola 2006; Ingold 2000; Viveiros de Castro 1998). *Belian* rituals are essentially about human-spirit relations, and Luangan human-spirit relations basically conform to the pattern which characterizes relations with the non-human environment according to this theoretical tradition, constituting, for example, in Nurit Bird-David's words, "an open-ended web of local connections and mutualities" (2006: 44). Important aspects of this pattern, which I will highlight especially in chapter 6, include what Tim Ingold (2006) has talked about in terms of "the primacy of movement" and a "relational constitution of being" with reference to how in "animic societies" the world and the identities of its inhabitants are in "perpetual flux" and humans and other beings are defined and continually shaped in the interactive field of their relations. These aspects illuminate, among other things, a "spiritual empiricism," a cosmological feature identified for traditional Austronesian religion already earlier by James Fox (1987:

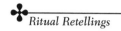

524), whereby the ever-differentiating, transitory, and never fully known manifestations of life and spirits of an immanent cosmos are made sense of through a pragmatic stance "in which various ritual procedures are employed as experiments to see what occurs."

Emergence and Tradition

> Reality is an active verb
>
> —Donna Haraway (2003: 6)

In the late twentieth century, a diverse approach to ritual as performance gradually gained momentum to become something of a major paradigm in anthropological studies of ritual (see, e.g., Atkinson 1989; Bloch 1974; Csordas 1996; Drewal 1992; Handelman 1990; Kapferer 1991; Roseman 1991; Schechner 1985; Schieffelin 1985; Singer 1958; Tambiah 1985; V. Turner 1969). Concurrent with a more general performative turn in the social and cultural sciences, this development reflected the influence of various strands of theory within and beyond anthropology, among which two stand out. First, a "dramaturgical approach" associated most prominently with Erving Goffman's sociology of ritualized everyday encounters (1959, 1974) and Victor Turner's (1969) theory of ritual as transformative social drama, and the interdisciplinary field of "performance studies" which they encouraged (Schechner 2002). Second, a linguistic tradition originating with John Austin's concept of "performative utterances" and the so-called "speech-act theory" (Austin 1962; Searle 1969), and subsequent developments in sociolinguistics and linguistic anthropology such as the "ethnography of speaking" (Bauman 1984; Hymes 1975).

Reflecting these influences, performance approaches to ritual have highlighted two distinct aspects of ritual which correspond to two different connotations of the word "perform": to stage or enact, and to accomplish or achieve. They have looked at how rituals represent performances in the sense of staged and distinctly framed events presented before an audience, which are organized by specific genre conventions and in interaction between the participants, and on how they represent performative or constitutive action, in Austin's sense, which do things "simply by virtue of being enacted" (Tambiah 1985: 135).

14

Like practice theory, performance theory essentially views rituals as action as opposed to representation, as creative activities which act upon the world rather than describe it, and they stress the presence, active role and creativity of the participants and the formative importance of the ritual event in itself over the formal, structural properties of rituals. In this respect it is obviously relevant to the present study and represents a complement to practice theory. An additional asset of this approach is the common stress on the sensory qualities and phenomenology of rituals, and on what Thomas Csordas (1996: 94) calls the "experiential specificity of participants." Beyond the emphasis on rituals as performative action and a distinct type of staged events, what is most distinctively valuable to me about this approach is largely summed up in Edward Schieffelin's understanding of performances as "emergent," which highlights their situational organization and historical contingency.

Echoing Dell Hymes' call to understand structure as "emergent in action" (1975: 71), Schieffelin (1985; 1996) has emphasized the ephemeral character of ritual performances. "While the form of a performance may recapitulate the forms of performances in the past and presage those of the future, the performance itself is of the particular moment, articulating cultural symbols and ritual genre at that particular time and submitting them to particular circumstances" (Schieffelin 1996: 66). Even though the aim of a performance may be formulated in advance, its outcome cannot be predetermined (see also Atkinson 1989: 13; Rao 2006: 147). This means that the success of a ritual performance is dependent on the performer's ability to respond, in a culturally appropriate way, to the circumstances in which it is performed (even if this may include distantiation from these circumstances, see Kapferer 2006: 671; also chapter 5 of this book). The authority of a ritual performance is thus, as Schieffelin (1996: 81) points out, "a fundamental condition of *emergence*."

One implication of this, which Schieffelin among others draws attention to, is that rituals involve "risk." For example, they entail the risk of failure and, even more momentously, can pose danger to the life and social status of those involved by attracting powerful and unpredictable forces or by provoking competition between sponsors (Howe 2000: 67–69). The correct performance of a ritual is thus not as straightforward a business as the common scholarly emphasis on their characteristic as rule-governed behavior might make them appear. Rules are not, for example, always well known by the participants, or agreed upon by them, or easy to implement even when they are known (Howe 2000: 69). In some instances it is precisely the aura of danger and risk encompassing rituals that endow them with much of their powerfulness (L. Pedersen 2006).

By analyzing *belian* as a fundamentally situated practice, an "emergent social construction" (Schieffelin 1985: 721), my aim is to draw attention to the indeterminacy and the uncertainties that are typically part of not only the Luangans' life-world but also their curing rituals. I want to investigate the risks involved in *belian* curing and how these risks and other conditions beyond the control of participants are reflected in the ritual form as well as in the enactment of particular rituals that never conform perfectly to the mold in which they are cast. At the same time, I seek to highlight the power of action "to bring the new into being" (Jackson 2007: 24). Rituals change, as we all know. They do so in response to happenings in the wider context of their implementation, but also as a result of developments arising out of their internal dynamic, such as in response to inspiration received during the ritual, or out of the interaction between human participants and between humans and unseen non-human actors. Thus I will examine the creative potential of *belian* rituals, how they are "not out-of-time but utterly full of time, bursting-with-time, with all of the possibilities (of becoming, being, existing) that time potentially enables" (Handelman 2005: 216; cf. Drewal 1992: xv). "Natality," as Hannah Arendt (1958) has labeled the human faculty to initiate something new, is something that cannot be ruled out from rituals, even when they are perceived as highly conservative by their participants.

However, at the same time it should be emphasized that for the Luangans the authority of *belian* rituals is considered to spring ultimately from ancestral tradition, and that *belian* rituals, like other rituals, are always performed in a world already pre-constituted in some respects. It is through a connection to what was done in the past, and especially in the ancestral past, that *belian* rituals are thought to gain their efficacy. However innovative they may be in practice, they must in some ways be incorporated within a tradition of *belian* curing in order to obtain legitimacy. In this sense, *belian* curers are always both "authors" and "not authors" of events (Humphrey and Laidlaw 1994; cf. Keane 1997: 24). The actions of *belian* curers are based on prior action and they are committed to the enactment of a certain kind of tradition, consisting of a set of performative codes, stylistic forms and genres. The following is a very concrete example of the importance of this connection: every *belian* ritual establishes a link with ancestral tradition through the enumeration and summoning of *belian* predecessors, including both mythical ancestors as well as more recent mentors, who are engaged as spirit familiars (*mulung*) in the ritual. The use of ancestral language, including archaic words and metaphors, serves as another example, as does explicit reference in ritual chants to how what one is doing is a repetition of what has been done in the past. But even to the extent that this connection may be left implicit, *belian* rituals minimally presuppose their own history through allusion and by taking certain things for granted. *Belian* rituals seem to an important extent to require integration with lived tradition in that they presuppose "habituation," an embodied appropriation of the ritual on the part of the rituals' participants acquired through repeated participation in *belian* rituals, which allows for the often conspicuous level of distraction that characterizes this participation.

"Tradition," in Alasdair MacIntyre's (1988: 12) words, is "an argument extended through time in which certain fundamental agreements are defined and redefined." This definition illuminates the negotiated character and the simultaneously reiterative and regenerative qualities of *belian* curing. Tradition, in this sense, is something that comes into being through practice at the same time as it constrains practice. It fundamentally involves both construction and reproduction. The tradition of *belian* curing necessitates, to borrow an expression by Jackson (2005: xxiii), "the presence of the past as the condition for the possibility of the future." By bringing the emergent and variable character of *belian* curing to the fore in this study, I do not want to downplay the conventional or structurally determining aspects of *belian*, but to emphasize how these aspects come into being through acts of production. One way in which I examine this dialectic is through a study of how different styles or genres of *belian* rituals constitute "orienting frameworks" for the production and reception of discourse (Hanks 1987: 670; cf. Bauman 1986). William Hanks proposes an approach to the study of linguistic genres based on Bakhtin's "sociological poetics" combined with Pierre Bourdieu's theory of practice in which "the idea of

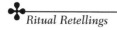

objectivist rules is replaced by schemes and strategies, leading one to view genre as a set of focal or prototypical elements, which actors use variously and which never become fixed in a unitary structure" (1987: 681). This is a view which corresponds to my experience of *belian* curing, in which different styles or genres of *belian*, addressing different spirit audiences through distinct performative codes and in different languages, are often performed in conjunction with each other, and thus, in some sense, always "remain partial and transitional" (ibid.).

In Ortner's (1989: 12) words, practice theory is a theory of "action considered in relation to structure." Studying *belian* as practice involves studying those cultural forms, social relations, and historical processes that move people to act in ways that produce those effects (ibid.). Structure in this sense is "doubly practiced: it is both lived in, in the sense of being a public world of ordered substantives, and embodied, in the sense of being an enduring framework of dispositions that are stamped on actors' beings" (Ortner 1989: 13). Like Bourdieu's notion of *habitus*, it implies "the active presence of the whole past of which it is the product" (Bourdieu 1980: 56), formed as a set of habitual dispositions through which people give shape and form to social conventions. The ritualized body, the production of which Bell (1992: 98) recognizes as the "implicit dynamic" and "end" of ritualization, thus comes into being through "interaction with a structured and structuring environment." Reflecting these understandings, this study is situated in the conjunction of a world already made and one constantly in the making.

Writing Strategies

Following Dorinne Kondo (1990: 304), I assert that theory lies in "enactment" and in "writing strategies," as much as in "the citation and analysis of canonical texts." In writing this book, I have tried to pay particular attention to the relation between what I present and how I present it. Since the focus of my interest is on the practice of *belian* curing, I have put concrete practices at the center of the analysis. Hence, every chapter of the book revolves around an account of an actual *belian* ritual (in some cases several). Trying to evoke the rituals in their particularity, I base my analysis of them on what these accounts bring out. By proceeding from particulars,

18

I have attempted to conjure the emergent quality of *belian* rituals and to let some central quality of the event direct the analysis of it. I have often chosen to use the "ethnographic present" in narrating particular ritual events. This strategy admittedly carries with it the risk that the presentation, against my intentions, may create what Tsing (1993: xiv) has called a "timeless scene of action." On the other hand, as Tsing (ibid.) also points out, the use of the past tense in describing people inhabiting "out-of-the-way" places, such as the Meratus or the Luangan, holds the opposite risk of suggesting not that these people *have* history, but that they *are* history, which in regard to a study of *belian* would be equally unfortunate.

The aim of this book is to present, not a generalized synthesis of Luangan curing rituals as such, but a situated study of their local significance focused on what the particular people who initiated or participated in them did and said, and how this was articulated within the wider context of local social life and culture. An important reason in choosing to talk about ritualization rather than just rituals is to emphasize *belian*'s quality as an ongoing process, subject to the interests, understandings, and interpretations of ritual participants in different contexts and at different stages of their lives (see Ortner 1978: 3). Focusing on real events as they unfold in time, I strive to put the people that carry out these rituals in the foreground. The same persons appear in several chapters of the study, sometimes as main characters, at other times in the background of events. Through these multiple references I want to conjure the complexity of agendas involved in *belian* curing, while simultaneously illustrating the interconnectedness of events. My intention has been to show the range of possibilities that *belian* may contain, its characteristically multilayered, variable, and even paradoxical character. Thus the different rituals analyzed exemplify very different and sometimes seemingly contradictory themes. Some illustrate the importance of invention while other conform to convention; some demonstrate the importance of government and other "outside" influence and political aspirations, while others turn inward to local concerns and inter-personal or spirit-related issues. My interest is not so much in "the obligatory" or "the orderly routine" of ritual (Rosaldo 1989: 13–15)—although I do hope that some picture of routine or common ground will emerge from my description as well—but rather in what makes the routines and the obligatory meaningful for those involved, in how it is made a dynamic part of the "actuality" of events.[5]

The general approach of the study is exploratory rather than explanatory. It follows multiple directions, trying to avoid totalizing explanations in order to enable description of the multiple possibilities inherent in ritual representation. Its technique can be described as "essayistic," in Theodor Adorno's (1991) conceptualization. In essays, according to Adorno's ideals, "thought does not progress in a single direction; instead, the moments are interwoven as in a carpet. The fruitfulness of the thought depends on the density of the texture" (1991: 13). Somewhat like Mancan's and Ma Putup's curing efforts which interact through the merging of sound, evoked in the example presented at the beginning of this introduction, I have purposively allowed different rituals described in the study to stand in contrast to each other, in order to add a dimension to the understanding of each of them.

It is through acts, things, and ritual language that I explore *belian* curing. As many observers of ritual have noted, "ritual practice, in its very nature, lies on the periphery of what can be thought and said" (Jackson 2005: 95; see also Lewis 1980: 24; Metcalf 1991: 262–263). Or, somewhat differently put, "ritual is not simply an alternative way to express any manner of thing," but perhaps the only way to express some things and achieve some intended effects (Rappaport 1999: 30). The resistance of ritual to translation is something that I experienced time after time during my fieldwork, as questions about ritual content or meaning were answered through the recitation of ritual chants, for example. These chants were not only provided as a key to the rituals' meaning but were, in their materiality and form—exemplified by their auditory qualities, their choice of words, their poetics, etc.—the meaning. Similarly, Luangans, like many other peoples (see, for example, Keane 2008: 113; Lindquist 2008: 117; Metcalf 1991: 242; Rousseau 1998: 118), have quite vague conceptions of spirits apart from those communicated through the practice of ritual. There are no consistent or very detailed perceptions of exactly who or where these spirits are or how they are connected to each other (although there are quite a number of studies by outsiders trying to figure this out). "Their existence is not a matter of belief, [but] of social practice" (Lindquist 2008: 117); hence, to study *belian* for me means to study its practices, and while translating these into written text necessarily means losing much of their tactile qualities, it is only through these chants, objects, and acts that these qualities can be textually mediated at all.

This book consists of five main chapters which are preceded by an ethnographic account of the Luangans, describing their local milieu, regional and national connections, and the role of ritual and religion in these contexts. All these chapters basically form independent units, which can be read as separate entities, although joined by a common, underlying theme. In the first of these chapters, chapter 2, I describe a rather eclectic and highly experimental ritual in which aspects of tradition and the exigencies of contemporary life were invoked by a female shaman, a ritual which formed a major social event and a forum for the negotiation of a variety of concerns in addition to curing, including shamanic authority, religious identity, and gender relations. Chapter 3 forms a contrast to chapter 2 in that it invokes a highly "traditional" and, in comparison, uneventful ritual, in which it is the conventional, corporeally mediated, and habitual aspects of the ritual that are at the center of the analysis (analyzed through material objects and a ritual chant). Chapter 4 deals with a prolonged curing *buntang* (a combined curing and thanksgiving ritual) in which the certainty of authority and authorship was called into question and tested as a local leader fell critically ill. Central questions dealt with in this chapter are how the uncertainty of life takes expression in the ritual form and content and how unpredictability influences the decisions made in *belian* curing. Chapter 5 juxtaposes three bathing rituals with the intention of showing how personal and social history is embedded in ritual practice and how ritualization works to diminish personal suffering by integrating participants with a collective past. The subject of the sixth and last chapter is the relation between myth and ritual and how Luangan mythmaking works to demarcate the identity and sphere of human beings, both in opposition to and in concert with spirits. Through an analysis of a *ngeraya* ritual, a ritual staged to ask for dry weather from the celestial *seniang* spirits in order to enable the burning of swidden fields, this chapter examines Luangan attempts at negotiating powers that regulate conditions in nature and the fates of human beings, powers which are ultimately beyond human control.

Notes

1. Borneo is divided into Indonesian Borneo (Kalimantan, further divided into the five provinces of West, South, Central, East, and North Kalimantan), which covers the southern two-thirds of the island, and the two northerly Malaysian provinces of Sarawak and Sabah, and the independent Sultanate of Brunei, located between them. "Dayak" is a generic designation for the various indigenous non-Muslim populations of the island, most of who used to be shifting dry rice cultivators. The term originated as an exonym adopted by early ethnographers and administrators, and was long perceived as derogatory, but has gradually become accepted and is now widely embraced as a self-designation by the increasingly politically conscious indigenous population, especially in Kalimantan. It is often contrasted with the term "Malay," which refers to the island's Malay-speaking Muslim populations.

2. Other factors also contributed to our decision; for example, the fact that due to weather and river water-level conditions we could not reach the Punan Murung on the upper Barito, while the distinct, Ot Danum-related Murung living downriver had all converted to Islam. These were groups that had been recommended to us as possible subjects of study by the Borneo ethnographer Bernard Sellato.

3. Since the publication of Rodney Needham's translation of Robert Hertz's (1960) famous essay on the collective representation of death, which was largely based on two-staged mortuary ceremonies in Borneo, death rituals have received considerable ethnographical and theoretical attention (Hudson 1966; Metcalf and Huntington 1976; Metcalf 1991; Miles 1965; Schiller 1997; Schärer 1966; Stöhr 1959; Wilder 2003). At the same time, the curing rituals of the peoples practicing secondary burial have received relatively little attention and even less theoretical consideration, especially in the south of the island. This state of discrepancy has also probably been influenced by the way in which some of these peoples themselves emphasize their death rituals in discourse, assigning them the status of "religion" (*agama*), while downplaying the importance of curing rituals and relegating them to the realm of "tradition" or "custom" (*adat*) (see Schiller 1997). In contrast, and as is the case also among the Kayan (Rousseau 1998: 269), all rituals are in a sense seen as curing rituals among the Luangans, even death rituals, in which it is the souls or spirits of the deceased that are said to undergo *belian* (*benelian*), rather than those of living persons.

4. The Luangans are far from unique in using "work" as a designation for ritual. For example, the Iban also use the word "work," *gawa,* to stand for rituals (see Sather 2001: 134; however, Sather also emphasizes the aspect of play, *main,* inherent in Iban curing and Iban talk about curing). Similarly, the Tikopians call their ritual cycle "the work of the Gods" (Firth 1967), while the Tewa Indians refer to their rituals as "works" (Ortiz 1969: 98ff; for more examples, see Rappaport 1999: 47). By conceptualizing ritual as work the Luangans emphasize its quality as action, as a means through

which one seeks to achieve something, a way of doing certain things. Of central importance in this definition of ritual as work is the fact that rituals demand a lot of physical work from their participants, primarily from the *belian* who perform the ritual, often chanting for days without much rest, and from their assistants, *penyempatung*, who stay by their side throughout it, but also, and not unimportantly, from those arranging the ritual, who are assigned roles as *pengeruye*, "makers of ritual paraphernalia," *pemasak*, "cooks," etc. The fact that it is not only the work of the *belian* that is of importance for a ritual's implementation can be seen in how delays in manufacturing ritual paraphernalia, for example, can often obstruct and delay the ritual work performed by *belian*.

5. This does not mean that questions of what constitutes the obligatory or the routine are not at times important for Luangans. Questions of right performance may rise to the fore, especially when a shaman comes from a different area than his audience. Still, performances are seldom judged as failures because of wrong procedure as such, even if they may cause discussion behind the shaman's back. Also, such discussion is, in my experience, often as much an expression of personal antipathies against a particular shaman, or the family organizing the ritual, as concern with right performance.

Chapter One
Luangan Lives
The Order and Disorder of Improvisation and Practice

Twilight is setting in when Ma Bari emerges from the forest on the other side of the river, returning from a day's work on his rice field in May 1996. As it has been raining, the water in the river is too high for wading so he fetches a canoe which is tied to a tree to cross the river. Standing up in the shallow canoe, which has been carved from a tree trunk, he punts himself across the river with the help of a long stick. Ignoring the people who are taking a bath on some rocks nearby, he climbs the muddy path up to the village. Slowly he walks through the village on his way to the longhouse, his back stiff from a life of hard work, his head held straight. His son Ma Kelamo is stacking rattan canes along the way but Ma Bari passes without any greetings being said between them. Entering the house through the back door he silently leaves some greens in the kitchen, washes his muddy feet with water kept in a jar, and heads for his sleeping mat for a rest. After a while, as dinner is served by his wife Tak Ningin, he utters his first words since he entered the village: "ayo man," let's eat, he calls out to the rest of us.

This chapter presents the people who are the main characters of this study: the Luangans. It gives an overview of who they are, where they live, and how they live, with special reference to the role of ritual and religion in their lives. Beyond representing an ethnographic sketch of the Luangans, the chapter also aspires to convey something of the distinctive tone and cadence of their being-in-the-world, and to give a picture of their patterns of interaction and ways of conduct (through short, descriptive passages, based on

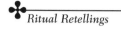

modified field notes, providing glimpses of everyday events, which are interspersed in between the principal, synthesizing paragraphs of the chapter). A central theme running through the chapter is how different fields or areas of Luangan society and culture—ethnicity, geography, social organization, politics, kinship, and religion—are constructed through practice according to a fluid and flexible pattern, commonly interpreted by Indonesian authorities as expressions of a disordered backwardness. Rather than implying a lack of organization or an undeveloped social order, however, I argue that this pattern possesses a coherence and order of its own, which reflects active adaptation to the contingencies and exigencies in a complex social, natural, and cosmological environment. Like Renato Rosaldo for the Ilongots of the Philippines, I am concerned with describing how Luangan lives form "a series of improvisations on certain social forms and cultural patterns," and with how tradition is "an active force in the lived-in present" (1980: 23–24). Various characteristics of Luangan social life, such as the lack of an objectified ethnic identity, a dispersed and shifting settlement pattern, a weakly codified customary law, the absence of a calendric ritual schedule etc., may all be seen as expressions of a generalized Luangan cultural dynamic, which has long persisted precariously in tension with hegemonic outsider visions of order.

Who are the Luangans?

An elderly man enters the longhouse at dusk one evening in September 1996, a stranger to most of us. He walks in with his back bent, politely marking his way with his hands. He hangs up his jungle knife on a nail on the wall and sits down on a rattan mat. He sits there, quietly. No one says anything or pays him any apparent attention. Only after quite a while Ma Bari comes forward and puts a pack of cigarettes and a basket with betel quid ingredients in front of the guest. The visitor mixes some betel leaves, areca nuts, and lime and starts chewing while Ma Bari lights a cigarette, in silence. Then the man starts talking. He is heading upriver and on his way to the upper Teweh area where he was born, to visit relatives he has not seen in twenty-eight years, having lived his adult life among the Benuaq. He gives an account of his journey, where he has stayed, where he is going. More people gather around him, asking questions, requesting stories and myths as they learn that he is quite a famous death shaman. "What is the origin story of ironwood?" they ask. "What is the origin of honey?"

As is so often the case when it comes to ethnic classifications on Borneo, the question of who the Luangans are is far from easy to answer (see, e.g., Babcock 1974; King 1979; Metcalf 2002: 93; Sillander 1995, 2004: 43–44; Wadley 2000). In fact, my use of the term "Luangan" as a designation for the people studied is in itself not unproblematic or straightforward. The fact that my fieldwork companion, Kenneth Sillander, has chosen to use another ethnic marker, "Bentian," the name of a Luangan subgroup, in his work only proves this fact. As Metcalf (2002: 93) notes for another area of Borneo: "In the earnest pursuit of autonyms, the first problem is usually that they are not used at all." In terms of indigenous notions and practices, whether cultural or political, there is no Luangan nation, no Luangan tribe. In this respect, the Luangans conform to a typical historical pattern in Borneo, which today has undergone various degrees of transformation, but to a comparatively low degree in the Luangan case. It seems that many of the ethnonyms designating major categories of Dayaks—like the term Dayak itself—were imposed by administrators, while "traditionally," and in some cases still today, people only identified with localized groups encompassing the members of a community or, at most, a particular river basin (Babcock 1974; King 1979). Up until the late nineteenth century, the Luangans consisted of a large number of such subgroups who had only vague conceptions of a common identity, and even today many members of the category do not know the term "Luangan" itself, nor the cognate term "Lawangan" by which they were more commonly known in the older ethnography.[1] The processes of political mobilization and ethnic awakening that gradually led to the formation of "the Iban," and "the Ngaju," to mention the two most famous and largest groups of Dayaks in Borneo, are developments that have not yet occurred, and may never occur in the Luangan case.[2]

In choosing to use the Luangan term, I am following the lead of some previous scholars and administrators who have classified the Luangan as an ethnic unit, although my application of and motivation for using the term differs in some important respects from theirs. Jacob Mallinckrodt (1928), a Dutch colonial officer who tried to codify the *adat* (customary law) of all the Dayaks of southeast Borneo, was the first to identify the Luangan, or "Lawangan," as an entity; he designated them the "Stammengroep der Lawangan," the Lawangan tribal group. According to his definition, this entity consisted of more than twenty culturally related subgroups that inhabited an area located between the middle reaches of the Barito and Mahakam Rivers, in the present-day Indonesian provinces of Central and East Kalimantan. Later, slight modifications as to which subgroups should be included in this category were made by the famous first governor of the province of Central Kalimantan, Tjilik Riwut (1958), who based most of his data on Mallinckrodt's. In addition to sharing cultural similarities (Mallinckrodt's *adat* law), some of which I will return to in a moment, these subgroups have also been shown to be linguistically related. According to Alfred Hudson's lexico-statistical investigation of the languages of South Borneo (1967a), they belong, with a couple of exceptions, to what he calls the "northeastern division of the Barito language family." They are also linguistically and culturally related to the three other major Dayak groups of south Borneo, the Ngaju, Ot Danum, and Ma'anyan, who roughly make up the other three divisions of the Barito family.

The next scholar who made an attempt to define the Luangan as an ethnic unit, and the first to call them "Luangan" as opposed to "Lawangan," was Joseph Weinstock, an American anthropologist who did fieldwork on the upper Teweh River in the period 1979–1981. Beyond linguistic and cultural affinities, what, in his view, most importantly set the Luangan apart from their neighbors were a common origin and a common religious tradition, Kaharingan (1983: 81–82). According to Weinstock, all the different Luangan subgroups (with the exception of the originally unrelated Tunjung, who have adopted Luangan identity on religious grounds alone) trace their origins to the source of the Luang River at the upper Teweh, an area located close to the famous Mount Lumut, where the souls of the dead (*liau*) reside. During secondary mortuary rituals, the souls or spirits of the newly dead are guided by death shamans and their previously deceased relatives to Mount Lumut. According to Weinstock, the journey of the souls to the mountain follows, in reverse, the routes of migration that the various Luangan subgroups followed when they left their ancestral homeland (1983: 73).

According to my information, however, which was obtained from informants of several Luangan subgroups, this hypothesis does not seem correct. In the first place, the remembered routes of migration are much more circuitous than the routes followed by the spirits of the dead, which tend to lead directly to Mount Lumut (cf. Sillander 2004: 40). In the second place, the different subgroups were in the past differentiated into numerous smaller groups, all of which have complex and different histories of migration and intermarriage of their own. Moreover, the claim that the Luangans ultimately originate from the Luang River, and that the term "Luangan," as Weinstock suggested, is etymologically derived from the word for the river, was not substantiated by the Luangans I knew. According to my information, the Luangans regard the upper Teweh area as their ancestral homeland in a more general and "mythological" sense, as an area where the mythological heroes used to live and where many of the Luangans' ritual practices are considered to have originated.

Whereas Weinstock's theory of the geographical origination of the Luangans is untenable upon closer examination, his identification of "religion" as a key criterion (1983: 85) for Luangan identity comes closer to how many of the Luangans I talked to used the term. As Sillander (2004: 40) has observed, it is primarily as a concept signifying identification with a "religious" tradition, rather than as an ethnonym, that the Luangan concept should be understood.[3] In autonymic usage, to be Luangan is to eat pork (which implies Dayak identity in contrast to Malay or other Muslim identity) and to practice *belian* curing and *gombok* secondary mortuary rituals, both considered essential parts of a tradition originating on the upper Teweh River. This is also an important reason why I have chosen to use the Luangan concept as a designation for the people studied in this book, even though most of my examples come from a particular Luangan subgroup, the Bentian, and, to a lesser extent, their Taboyan and Benuaq neighbors. This concept allows me to approach these people, for whom ethnic identity generally is of little concern, in a non-exclusive way, at the same time as it connotes some important aspects of their being-in-the-world.

What I refer to when I speak about "the Luangans" then is less a particular ethnic or geographic field, than, following James Clifford (1997: 69), "a field as a habitus … a cluster of embodied dispositions and practices." The Luangan region is less a "place" than a "space" in the sense that "a space is a practiced place" (de Certeau 1984: 117), something never "ontologically given," but "discursively mapped and corporeally practiced" (Clifford 1997: 54). To be Luangan, as I use the term, is to engage in certain practices and discourses (mainly of a "religious" character) that allow a Luangan to experience that he or she has something essential in common with other Luangans, despite having a different subgroup identity, for example. An advantage with the concept used in this way is that it enables me to include people with different subgroup identities in my description, without having to stake out boundaries between them where none are deemed to exist, or are considered unimportant. At the same time, my use of the concept helps to facilitate my more specific agenda of exploring the importance of ritual representations in shaping Luangan life-worlds.

However, in order to more precisely map the people I am talking about geographically and culturally, I have often chosen to talk about the central Luangans as opposed to the Luangans in general. This category includes Luangans from an area that stretches approximately from Benangin on the middle reaches of the Teweh River in the province of Central Kalimantan, to Dilang Puti on the middle reaches of the Lawa River in the province of East Kalimantan (see Figure 1.1). In terms of subgroup identities, the central Luangans mostly consist of upper Teweh Taboyans (Tewoyans) and Bentians. The central Luangan area is one I traveled through several times during my fieldwork and came to know quite well, but my use of the concept is not only motivated by my own field experience. It is also motivated by an indigenous notion of this area (and especially the upper Teweh River region) as a cultural and cosmological center, the importance of which is recognized throughout, and even beyond, the Luangan area.[4] It is in this area that Mount Lumut is situated and where many events described in Luangan mythology took place and its protagonists lived, and from where many ritual practices are said to originate (especially the *belian luangan* tradition, but also the mortuary rituals). Besides constituting a cosmological center, this upland area also forms a kind of geographical center in that many large rivers running out in different directions have their headwaters there, a fact which might have made it expedient to think of this area as a place of origin (Sillander 2004: 42; cf. Metcalf 1991: 25; and Rousseau 1990: 71, for examples of similar upland

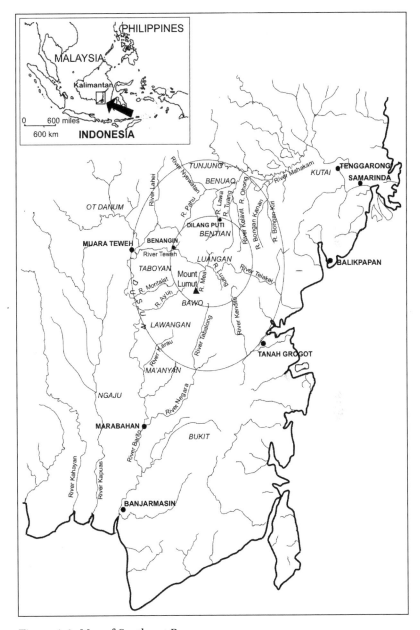

Figure 1.1. Map of Southeast Borneo

31

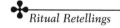

areas serving as similar geopolitical and conceptual origin-centers in Central Borneo).

The central Luangan category is moreover a category corresponding to what Lemanius, an indigenous author and ritual specialist on whose unpublished manuscript on Luangan history and mythology I will draw on a number of occasions in this study, calls *"suku bangsa jumben Tewoyan barung Lewangan."*[5] This is, according to Lemanius, a category including people precisely between Benangin in the west and south to the Bentian region in the east and north. These people share what could be called a fundamental feeling of sameness, a feeling of being, as an informant stated it, *mengkaben* ("related"), and not *ulun* ("people," "strangers"). In addition to essentially following the same ritual tradition (with minor local alterations and with the exception of *belian sentiu*, a curing style which is practiced mostly in East Kalimantan), they speak mutually understandable dialects. They also frequently intermarry and regularly travel to visit relatives within the area. However, this does not mean that contacts outside the area are not locally relevant and, at times, as frequent as inside it, nor that the outer boundaries of this region would be clearly demarcated or unambiguous. Still, Lemanius' concept, which is used by other ritual specialists as well, especially in ritual language, highlights an important perceived likeness and a feeling of sameness which comes to the fore especially in ritual practice, and which indeed largely results from ritual practice and interaction.

Field Work and Field Site

Everyone is asleep in the longhouse when Ma Denia and Ma Kelamo return from a hunting trip in the middle of a night in September 1996. The hunting dogs rush in, running around the large undivided space that makes up the longhouse, one of them urinating on a house post, while some drowsy inhabitants shout angrily at them, chasing the dogs away. The hunters have been successful and have caught a large wild boar. Everyone sits up, lighting the oil lamps as the hunters start to tell their stories. Every stream passed during the hunt is named, the large trees, the hills climbed. As Ma Denia and Ma Kelamo describe the hunt, the scent trail picked up by the dogs, the chase, the seizure and stabbing of the boar, Ma Dengu, who joined them on the trip, enters the house as well, and the story is told again, the details repeated. At the same time Tak Ningin and Nen Ena start to chop up the meat, sorting out the different pieces. A fire is lit at the hearth in the kitchen, some water is put to a boil. Rice is washed and cooked, and slowly a meat sauce is prepared, while some chili is pounded. Around two o'clock in the morning everyone then sits down to eat together, enjoying the fresh meat, the abundance of it.

My fieldwork among the central Luangans was mainly carried out in two stages: during six months in 1993 and during twelve months in 1996–1997. Three shorter visits to the area were also conducted in 1998, 2007 and 2011. All periods of fieldwork were carried out together with Kenneth Sillander. During these two major periods we approached the field in two different ways: by mainly traveling around in 1993 and by mostly staying in place in 1996–1997. Both approaches have influenced my view of the Luangans, and both had their advantages as well as their disadvantages.

The decision to move around between villages and farmsteads during the first period of fieldwork was a result both of Kenneth's interest in ethnicity at the time and of the Luangans' relatively mobile lifestyle. By traveling around we got a sense of the space inhabited and practiced by the people studied, both geographically as we learned to know forests and trails, rivers and old house sites, fruit and honey trees, and socially, as we met the same people in different contexts: visiting relatives, attending rituals, or just wandering about, looking for a chance to earn some money, or to find a spouse. Meeting an acquaintance on a forest trail, somewhere midway between two villages, perhaps in the rain, with leeches crawling up our tired legs, or in a "foreign" village while attending a major ritual, provided a ground for a particular kind of intimacy: beyond the ears of fellow villagers and the constraints of everyday life. Traveling around, visiting some fifteen villages in the upper Teweh and Bentian area, we also became aware of local differences and consequently grew wary of generalizations about *the* Luangan or *the* Bentian—a reason why I mostly prefer to speak about the Luangans in the plural in this study. On the other hand, it was hard to form long-term relationships with people and to understand the sometimes intricate ways in which they were related to each other during these shorter visits. Exhaustive travel and occasional poor food also made us prone to illness (or poisoning as many Luangans would have it, always weary of poisoning when visiting non-relatives).

The advantages and disadvantages of staying in place were pretty much the opposite of those of moving around, and the decision to stay mostly in one village for the second part of the fieldwork was basically a result of what we experienced as the negative aspects of this kind of "walking fieldwork" (cf. Tsing 1993: 65). It gave us the opportunity to get to know people more thoroughly and gain their trust, and to explore their everyday interaction over a longer time span, which is perhaps also why it has been so much easier for me to write about the rituals performed in the village in which we spent the greater part of our second fieldwork period, than about the rituals performed in any of the other communities we visited. On the other hand, many Luangans spent much of their time out of the village, hunting, gathering forest products such as resins or rattan, visiting relatives, participating in rituals, and, most importantly, tending to their fields, which meant that villages could become practically deserted at times. Even while staying in place we subsequently moved around quite a bit, just to be where the people were, instead of spending time in empty villages.

Of the villages we visited during our first period of fieldwork we stayed for the longest time (about a month) in Sembulan, a small village of about ninety inhabitants located in the sub-district (*kecamatan*) of Bentian Besar within what is today the district (*kabupaten*) of Kutai Barat, in East Kalimantan. For several purposes we found this village to represent the best option for extended field research, therefore we returned to it for our second period of fieldwork in 1996, and stayed there for most of this period. This was a village where almost one hundred percent of the population claimed adherence to Kaharingan (a designation used today for the local religion), in contrast to most other villages, which usually had a mixed Christian and Kaharingan population. Kaharingan adherence was not our primary criterion for choosing Sembulan as a field site, however. The picturesque village, at the time consisting of one village longhouse (*lou solai*), two traditional extended family houses (*lou*), and eleven single-family houses, is situated by a rocky part of the shallow Kenamai River, a tributary of the Lawa, providing relatively clear drinking and bathing water, in contrast to many of the other villages in the area. The fact that the longhouse was permanently inhabited and in active use by villagers, especially during rituals and public meetings, also contributed to our decision to stay in Sembulan, as did the comparatively welcoming attitude of its inhabitants. There was no electricity in Sembulan, only a privately owned gasoline generator which was used sporadically when someone could afford to buy the gasoline. There was no primary school either, which meant that children attended school in the nearby village of Jelmu Sibak, some three kilometers away, and often stayed there with relatives during weekdays. In fact, Sembulan did not have the status of an official village (*desa*), although it had been an independent village in the past, but was now officially a "sub-village" or hamlet (*dusun*) of this neighboring village, much to the indignation of its inhabitants, who felt marginalized and robbed of a voice of their own in government contacts.

In Sembulan we stayed in the longhouse, which, like most Luangan examples of its kind, was a rather small building (about 30 meters long) if compared to the famous massive longhouses of some other Borneo peoples (e.g., the Iban or the Kayan). In contrast to these longhouses, which normally consist of a long row of family compartments with a common veranda in front, the longhouse of Sembulan was composed of only one large undivided room, with an attached kitchen at the back. As is typical for central Luangan longhouses (*lou solai*), most of the principal room consisted of an empty unfurnished space, where rattan mats, used for seating, covered part of the slatted bamboo floor. Along the walls were the rolled-up sleeping mattresses and mosquito nets of the inhabitants of the house, which were rolled out at night when their owners slept there. Interspersed between them were large brass gongs (*gendring*) and wooden drums (*tuung*), musical instruments used to accompany the chanting of shamans during life or death rituals. Next to the back wall, in the middle of the rectangular interior space, was the village's only *longan*, a wooden construction composed of eight upright ironwood (*teluyen, Eusideroxylon zwageri*) poles holding up a shelf with small ancestral objects, and above it, in the rafters, a box of ancestor skulls was stored, both objects representing storehouses of spiritual potency that were anointed with blood of sacrificed domestic animals during major community rituals. Skulls of water buffaloes sacrificed during previous rituals were attached to the house posts and used to store skewers of meat or to hang up the jungle knives of visitors. During daytime the front door of the house usually stayed open if there was someone at home, providing daylight in the rather dark, windowless space. Dogs walked in and out, trying to steal some food, or take a nap in the ashes of the hearth in the kitchen. Beneath the house, chickens and pigs dwelled, usually waking up the inhabitants in the early hours of the morning.

During the time of our fieldwork the longhouse was permanently inhabited by Ma Bari and Tak Ningin, an elderly couple who owned two-thirds of the house. Ma Bari was a quiet, serious-minded, hard-working man who held the unofficial position of *kepala adat*, head of customary law, and radiated an unquestioned but soft-spoken air of authority. Tak Ningin was the village midwife, a restrained but kind-hearted woman who prepared most of our meals during fieldwork. The other third of the house was owned by Ma Buno and Tak Hai, a middle-aged couple who stayed in the house sporadically (spending much time in their field house) together with their young adopted son Buno, their grown-up daughter Kiding, her husband Karim, and Kiding's and Karim's three children, two of whom were born in the longhouse during our fieldwork. Ma Buno was a knowledgeable and popular *belian* who conducted many rituals in the house during our stay. Mompun, a mentally disabled woman whom Tak Ningin took care of, also stayed permanently in the house. In addition to these persons, there were a number of people moving in and out of the longhouse, including Tak Ningin's and Ma Bari's three grown-up children with their respective families, and Ma Bari's widowed sister Tak Rosa and her extended family. People passing by the village or visiting it often stopped by or stayed over in the longhouse as well. During busy periods of the agricultural year the house was often deserted in the daytime, but there was always someone returning to it at nightfall, at the very least Tak Ningin and Ma Bari, who saw it as their responsibility to watch over the house and protect the valuables stored in it (and who because of their advanced age made their swidden field close to the village).

Our choice to stay in the longhouse was in part motivated by its central role as a ritual arena. Usually, when someone related to those living in the longhouse fell ill, they moved into the house and a curing ritual, typically lasting two to three nights, would be staged there. During larger rituals in particular, which were often arranged in the longhouse, it would become rather crowded, with up to a hundred guests. Many children were born in the longhouse, or rather at a separate, temporary platform (*blai sawo*) constructed behind it, since Tak Ningin was the village's only midwife. Birth rituals were consequently often held in the longhouse, as were larger family and community rituals (*buntang, nalin taun*), which attracted a large audience. Similarly, lawsuits and village meetings were usually arranged there. By staying in the longhouse we were able to observe these rituals and events during both day and night and to overhear the discussions and decisions leading up to them. It also allowed us to observe a wide spectrum of everyday life activities of a varying number of inhabitants, even if sometimes at the cost of our sense of privacy and peace of work.

Mobility and Social Landscape

A small group of women has decided to make a trip to Sigei's swidden to bring home some vegetables. None of them make a swidden of their own this year (Milu being pregnant, Tak Ningin because of her husband's recent illness, Neti because she still attends school, Nen Bai because her husband currently works for a logging company, Tak Lodot because of ill health) and thus they depend on relatives for fresh vegetables. Located in primary forest, a couple of hours walk from the village, there are plentiful crops at Sigei's swidden. The women ask me and Kenneth to join them, so that Kenneth can help with carrying back the heavy load. As we set off an early November morning in 1996, first wading over the shallow river, then entering the barely recognizable forest path, Neti slashing away the thorny rattan canes that seem to grow almost overnight, a mood of exhilaration besets the women. Leaving the village behind, entering farther into the forest, Tak Ningin soon starts to sing, and before long Tak Lodot and Nen Bai join in. These usually quiet and reserved women change almost beyond recognition, becoming joyful, playful, as they leave village life behind. Walking, often complained about as a hard and exhausting part of Luangan life, here still brings with it a sense of freedom or release.

The central Luangans live in an undulating, hilly territory covered with secondary and, to an ever decreasing extent, primary rainforest. Timber and forest plantation companies started to operate in the area in the 1980s, destroying vast areas of land, including rattan gardens from which most central Luangans received their principal cash income, triggering, especially among the Bentian subgroup, a wave of protests and lawsuits against the companies in the 1990s (see Fried 2001, 2003), as well as some internal fraction between those who wanted to profit from selling land and those who wanted to preserve their rights to it. Until the mid-1990s, there was no road connecting the villages on the upper Teweh River in Central Kalimantan with those in the Bentian region in East Kalimantan. Because most rivers are shallow and unnavigable, travel was generally only possible by foot along forest paths. Today most villages are connected by an interprovincial road, which, at least until recently when part of it was paved, has been poorly maintained and frequently impassable, bridges crossing minor watercourses often being broken.

No public transport was available in the area during the time of our main fieldwork, although there were a small number of privately owned motorcycles and, on rare occasions, a few cars that could be hired. Travel between villages was thus still mostly by foot and the condition of the road was a constant source of irritation among the local population, who felt that the lack of transportation put them in a marginal position, both economically and socially, compared to people in other regions. Travel out of the area was similarly difficult, whether by outboard engine-equipped boats down the Lawa or the Teweh rivers, both of which were unnavigable when the water level was low (for at least half of the year), or, when weather conditions and company policies allowed, at the back of logging trucks along logging roads.

The fact that there are virtually no larger, navigable rivers in the central Luangan area implies that the central Luangans, unlike most Dayaks, cannot be described as riverine peoples (Sillander 2004: 29). This also affects their self-understanding and certain important aspects of their way of life. They identify, and are identified by Malays and other Dayaks, as an upriver, hill, or inland population. They indeed inhabit an ecological zone which in many other areas of Borneo is often inhabited by hunter-gatherers (Punan, Penan, Basap) or then, as in their own case, by comparatively small and dispersed groups of shifting cultivators (such as the Meratus, or some Bidayuh of Western Sarawak). However, although their remoteness and low population numbers are today an often-lamented condition, their locality and settlement pattern has been intentionally maintained despite a consciousness of alternatives and overt government pressure to change this situation, and it has, until recently, enabled certain characteristic features of their lifestyle and economy, such as their extensive rattan gardens, their husbandry of exceptionally large numbers of semi-wild water buffalos, and their residential mobility and relative political autonomy.

The central Luangan way of life can, like that of the Meratus Dayaks described by Tsing (1993), and many other Southeast Asian upland shifting cultivators (see, e.g., Scott 2009), be characterized by a high degree of mobility. As swidden cultivators of rice, vegetables, and rattan which is grown for commercial purposes (as well as oil palm and rubber in recent years), complemented with hunting and gathering, the central Luangans practice a dual pattern of residence, the majority of them spending approximately half of their time in villages, and the other half in swidden huts close to their fields, situated between half an hour and up to three or more hours of walking distance from the village. Individual settlement arrangements vary considerably and normally change several times during a lifetime. During my fieldwork, some people, like Ma Bari and Tak Ningin, seldom spent the night in their field hut but returned to the village at nightfall, while others spent almost all their time at their swidden and did not even own or share a house in the village. Still others, like Ma Buno's family, stayed for months in the longhouse, then moved to their swidden house for an indefinite period. In 2007, when we revisited Sembulan after a nine-year break, the longhouse was abandoned because a number of deaths had occurred there, causing Ma Isa, Ma Bari's eldest son, who was the new custodian of the house since his parents' death a few years earlier, to move into another house in fear of his wife's poor health. During our fieldwork, smaller villages were occasionally almost abandoned and houses were in disrepair as owners stayed in their swiddens or had moved to other villages, a state of affair already observed by early Dutch observers (Knappert 1905: 627).

Historically, the mobility of individuals in south Borneo was high and the control of movements of people limited. As Han Knapen (2001: 85) has observed, "not only individuals were very mobile, but villages as well showed a very fluid pattern of construction and movement." Small groups of Dayaks regularly broke away from one village to found another, often out of economical opportunism

(Knapen 2001: 85; Maks 1861: 481–482), but also as an escape strategy. In southeast Borneo groups of both Dayaks and Malays commonly fled or moved upriver to escape government control, taxation, and attempts at labor extraction (see, e.g., Hudson 1967b: 15; *Struktur Bahasa Bawo* 1989). In times of war people sometimes gathered in large fortified villages (*benteng*), at other times chose to escape enemies, or epidemics, through dispersion in the forest (Müller 1857: 226; Schwaner 1853: 219). There are many instances of use of both strategies to confront both types of danger in central Luangan oral history.

The central Luangans did not, in fact, stay in nucleated villages until the latter part of the nineteenth century, but alternated residence between swidden huts and extended family houses (*lou*), which were situated in the forest, close to swidden fields. These extended family *lou* were smaller than the "village longhouses" (*lou solai*) that they gradually started to build in response to government orders in the late nineteenth century. They were usually inhabited by a set of closely related families, often centered on a set of siblings, their spouses and children, and perhaps their children's families, one of the founding siblings often acting as the "house leader" (*manti lou*). In the past, like today, most people stayed for much of the time in their individual swidden houses (*blai ume*)—a variable number of such houses (usually between two and seven) frequently forming a "cluster" (*teming*)—and it was mainly at times of ritual that their members congregated in any larger numbers and that friends and relatives from neighboring *lou* came together. The forest *lou* were relatively short-lived constructions built, unlike the villages longhouses, of impermanent building materials and they were usually moved and rebuilt within a couple of decades, whereas the similarly lightly constructed swidden huts were ordinarily moved every two to four years, as they still are today. The members of a swidden cluster could choose to move to a new site altogether or to form a new cluster with other people, depending both on what sort of land they preferred and on personal relations.

In the latter part of the nineteenth century, and especially in the early twentieth century, the central Luangans started to build what were intended to become permanent villages along the largest rivers in the area. This was a result of pressure from the Dutch, who had assumed political and economic control over the coastal sul-

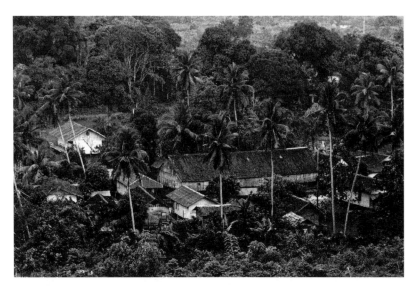

Figure 1.2. Village longhouse surrounded by "development houses." Sambung Village

tanates, and wanted to concentrate the Dayaks in more accessible locations to restrict mobility and enable taxation. In parts of South and Central Kalimantan this process had started already in the late eighteenth century (see Knapen 2001: 88), although it began only about a century later on the Teweh River, and still later over the border in the Bentian area in present-day East Kalimantan, where it was initiated under the administration of the Kutai Sultanate, which retained (partial) sovereignty much longer than the other sultanates in the region. In these permanent villages the members of several forest *lou* typically first joined together in one large village longhouse (*lou solai*), around which a number of extended family houses (*lou*) and, later, smaller single-family village houses (*blai*), were then constructed. After Indonesian independence in 1945, and in particular during President Suharto's New Order regime (1967–1998), the single-family village houses, or "development houses" (*rumah pembangunan*) as they were often called in the 1990s, gradually became more common, initially largely as a result of government pressure (longhouse residence was said to be disordered and unhygienic and thus was discouraged). Today there are only a few Luangan village longhouses or extended family houses left in Central Kalimantan (where both pre- and post-independence government influence was more extensive), while in East Kalimantan, one or a few of either or both categories typically remain in most villages. Although several of these are now deserted, many of them continue to be used for ritual purposes, and some of the so-called development houses accommodate almost as many people as the traditional extended family houses, and appear to function much like the latter did in the past. Even when residing in separate houses, groups of families, corresponding to the extended families of the past, still often collectively own certain ancestral valuables (*pusaka*), a soul search ship (*sampan benawa*), as well as a soul house (*blai juus*), and come together during *buntang* family rituals when this ritual paraphernalia is used.

Like other so-called Dayaks, the Luangans reckon kinship bilaterally. Ideally, and usually in practice as well, affinal and cognatic kin are treated equally. The Luangan kinship system is characterized simultaneously by a high degree of inclusiveness and a pragmatic attitude, by which I mean that the people interacted with either are kin or are made kin—through marriage or classificatory kinship—whereas relatives with whom one has no active relationship can be forgotten, at least temporarily (see Sillander 2004: 142). There is, however, a strong incentive to keep up at least some kin relations, and the practice of visiting one's relatives (*koteu*), often in quite faraway places, is important. Adoption is common, especially among childless or better-off couples, but also, for example, in cases when a child has suffered from prolonged illness. Polygamy, both polyandry and polygyny, occurred during my fieldwork, even if rather infrequently. Divorce and remarriage is very common, especially among young couples. In the past, there was a strong preference for village and even *lou* endogamy, but today more and more young people marry outside their own community (partly as a result of new educational and work opportunities). Still, even today there is an inclination to marry people with whom one already has some form of previous, direct or indirect, kin connection.

In Sembulan the great majority of the inhabitants were cognatically related to each other. Most people shared descent from the inhabitants of a few extended family houses who together had founded the village, and those who had married into the village mostly came from a couple of other villages in which they were cognatically related from before. Kin obligations were strong when

42

it came to sharing food (especially meat) and participation in work parties and rituals. People also frequently made requests on each other as kin, requests that were hard to ignore (except, to a certain extent, by staying in their swidden fields away from the village), and, in return, often received help from their relatives, both in the form of services and economic contributions.

In contrast to their Benuaq neighbors who have been described as possessing something of a class system in the past (see, e.g., Gönner 2002: 49), the central Luangans were never consistently stratified and social relations were and are generally rather egalitarian, both in the past and today. This is not to say, however, that there are no status differences. Age or seniority is an important source of status and authority among the central Luangans. The house leaders or *manti lou* of the past were usually elderly men (sometimes women) who through their seniority made claims and requests on the inhabitants. Some of these *manti* were also undoubtedly and recognizably more powerful than others, their authority expanding outside the immediate sphere of their own *lou*. Important attributes in forming such authority were, among other things, skill in oratory, knowledge of *adat* law, and accumulated wealth obtained through trade which allowed the staging of large rituals.

In the nineteenth and early twentieth century, the Sultans of Kutai and Banjarmasin started to distribute titles (*mangku, singa, temangung*) to inland tributary leaders (Sjamsuddin 1989: 312, 321; Wortmann 1971: 54), among them central Luangan *manti*, at the same time as trade relations intensified (Magenda 1991: 31; Tromp 1887) and allowed these leaders to increase their wealth. The power of these leaders was, however, quite restricted, not least since there was a number of such title-holding *manti* in each village, competing largely over the same followers.

Today, old men still exercise considerable authority over younger people and are in this capacity and in their role as community arbitrators referred to as *manti*. The highest positions attributed to villagers by the Indonesian authorities are those of *kepala desa* (village head) and *kepala adat* (head of customary law). The *kepala desa*, who mostly take care of village administration and bureaucracy, and provide the authorities with village statistics, for example, are usually younger men with some formal education, whereas the *kepala adat* hold a position more similar to that of the traditional *manti*, negotiating in matters of law and tradition. As Sembulan is not an official village there is no *kepala desa* there. During the time of my fieldwork Ma Bari was regarded as an (unofficial) *kepala adat* and he was the one who presided over disputes, lawsuits (*perkara*) and negotiations pertaining to land rights, marriage, and other interpersonal and public matters. An important capacity of a *manti* such as Ma Bari is the ability to integrate villagers and maintain village harmony. Whereas *belian* have considerable spiritual authority and are highly respected and valued for their curing skills, they rarely possess political power or strive for such, in contrast to what is reported for some similarly unstratified upland peoples such as the Wana or the Meratus (Atkinson 1989; Tsing 1993). *Wara*, or death shamans, seem to pursue political authority somewhat more often than *belian*, perhaps because they are less occupied with ritual duties as death rituals are much less frequent than life rituals. Death shamans are also considered to hold considerable knowledge about ancestral tradition and kin relations, as both the living and dead relatives of a deceased person are invited to participate in death rituals, a knowledge they may make use of for political purposes as well. In theory, women are considered equal to men and can become both *manti* and *belian* (although not *wara*, *kepala desa* or *kepala adat*), but in practice they did not occupy or aspire for such positions very often in the late 1990s (although in the past there were several examples of both great female *manti* and *belian*).

In short, the social landscape inhabited by the central Luangans during my fieldwork was characterized by a high degree of residential dispersal and individual autonomy, at the same time as it was marked by a strong ideological aspiration for communal harmony and social integration. There was, for example, a widely held sentiment that no one should have to stay alone, and should they become so, a great deal of improvisational effort was applied to attend to the situation (allowing marriage over generational gaps otherwise forbidden, promoting adoption or turning a blind eye to polygamy, etc.). Historically, and up until today, the Luangans have been less politically centralized and organized and lived in a more dispersed way than most other swidden cultivating Dayak groups of Borneo, often more closely resembling uncentralized upland peoples in other islands of the archipelago (such as the Wana, the Teduray, and the Ilongots). As is the case among the Wana of Sulawesi for whom "ritual operates as a primary means of political organization and integration" (Atkinson 1989: 8), it is above all in rituals that the Luangan communities historically have, and in many cases still, come together.[6] Even though Luangan rituals cannot be described as political arenas in the sense that ritual officiants or families compete for political authority, they are, as Weinstock (1983: 64) has expressed it, "the primary source of social cohesion for the community." Community and family rituals are sometimes even explicitly arranged, as a man once expressed it, because "relatives have become distant from each other," and thus should be brought close again.

Ritual Repertoire

It is the last day of a gombok *death ritual, in a neighboring village of Sembulan's, for a man who tragically died on his way to Samarinda, the provincial capital, in June 1996. Together with a group of other villagers he was on his way to pursue a lawsuit against the logging company operating on their land. During the journey downstream along the Mahakam River he fell from the river ferry into the water, hit his head and drowned. As everyone is gathered in the house of the* gombok, *the sound of a gong suddenly tells us that another death has occurred in the village. Later, as everyone present at the* gombok, *sits down to eat the meat of a water buffalo that has been sacrificed earlier during the day, the* kepala adat *of the village enters the house (as a Christian he has chosen not to participate in the ritual proceedings before). He gives a speech before the meal, as is customary, and puts forward a request. He asks that the death ritual for the woman who just died should be postponed until the following month, so that there would not be two death rituals performed during the same month. People should get on with the work of slashing their fields now, he recommends. He also points out that the authorities would probably not be willing to issue a permit to stage another large ritual immediately after this one is finished. Furthermore, he asks the family of the deceased woman to consider not including the sacrifice of a water buffalo in the upcoming ritual. This would demand authorization from the police, which has proved a hassle during the now ongoing ritual as the buffalo intended to be sacrificed could not be caught, which prolonged the whole ritual and complicated the* kepala adat's *dealings with the authorities. People*

45

look uneasy as he speaks and finally one of the death shamans speaks up, pointing out that it is not up to the kepala adat *to say when and what kind of ritual should be arranged, but that this instead is a matter for the family of the deceased to decide, together with the death ritual specialists. Death, and the souls of the dead, do not see to timetables or permits from the government, he declares.*

There is a lot of local variation in style, details, as well as designations for rituals practiced by the Luangans. However, as reported for the Toraja of Sulawesi (Buijs 2006; Volkman 1985), a general division and separation between life rituals and death rituals can be seen (Weinstock 1983: 36). Whereas life rituals are conducted by *belian* (called *pemeliatn* among the Benuaq), death rituals are performed by *wara* (*pengewara* in Benuaq). Life rituals are generally performed for an even number of days (if they exceed three days) while death rituals are conducted for an uneven number of days, although this is, as Luangans often say, how it is "written" (*tenulis*), not how rituals often turn out in practice, because of different sort of delays. Different persons are generally specialized in either life or death rituals, but the same person may also be knowledgeable in both. Both death and life shamans go through a several year-long period of apprenticeship during which they are guided by and perform rituals together with already established specialists. During this period they learn the chants and origin myths of their respective specialization, before being formally initiated as *wara* or *belian*.

Like many other Borneo peoples, the Luangans practice secondary mortuary rituals (*gombok,* called *kenyau* and *kwangkai* among the Benuaq) which are carried out after the funeral of the deceased. Unlike the funeral, which is a brief one-day affair, the *gombok* is a major ritual and festive event which involves considerable expenditure, including food served to a large number of guests for the duration of the ritual, and sacrifices of chickens, pigs and, frequently, one or several water buffalos. The length of the ritual varies considerably between different Luangan subgroups and depending on the social status of the deceased, but the ritual lasts at least three days and sometimes up to several weeks or even months.[7] A *gombok* may sometimes be performed up to several years after death, but is nowadays usually performed within a year after the funeral, and, at least among the central Luangans, often immediately after it.

Upon death the *juus*, that is the "soul" or "life-force" of a person, ceases to exist while two different "souls" or "spirits" of the dead come into being: *liau* and *kelelungan*, which Weinstock (1983: 50) refers to as the "coarse" and the "refined" soul, respectively, the former associated with the body and the body bones, and the latter with the skull and mind. These spirit-like agencies are respectively conceived of as "bad" (*daat*) and "good" (*bue*), reflecting the idea that *kelelungan*, unlike *liau*, can become purified (*lio*) and act as a protecting spirit (*pengiring*), whereas *liau* is predominantly malevolent and essentially useless. During the *gombok*, *liau* and *kelelungan* are guided by two different groups of *wara* to their respective realms in the afterworld: *liau* to Mount Lumut and *kelelungan* to Tenangkai, its abode in heaven. This is done through chants in which the route taken is rendered in detail, with mention of all the rivers and streams passed, the mountains climbed, and so on. Sometimes a group of *wara* sit inside a decorated wooden canoe (*selewolo*) suspended from the ceiling while escorting *kelelungan*, while *liau* travels in a rattan basket (*ringka jawa*) tied to its stern. Along the way stops are made at fixed locations where they are given provisions for their stay in the afterworld, and where there is entertainment for *liau* in the form of special games (*gege liau*) in which the participants take part with much joking and merriment. The *liau* and *kelelungan* of previously deceased relatives are invited to the ritual and a special dance (*ngerangkau*) is performed for their entertainment, in which the *wara*, together with other ritual participants and the dead, dance together. Before reaching their final destinations the *wara* leave the spirits of the dead in the hands of those already passed away and return to the realm of the living.

In the death realms the souls of the dead are said to live in much the same way as living people, occupying houses and keeping livestock. Before the *gombok* has been carried out both *liau* and *kelelungan* are said to often hover about the place where the deceased lived and frequently disturb the living. They may also continue to visit their relatives (e.g., in dreams) after they have been escorted to the death realms, asking for food and making requests or giving advice, and quite frequently, stealing their souls. Soul searches to their realms are routinely performed by *belian* and both *liau* and *kelelungan* are often presented with offerings as a preventive measure during life rituals. *Gombok* rituals may also include secondary burial of the dead (*gombok empe selimat*, corresponding to what the Benuaq call *kwangkai*), in which case they are typically carried out twice and usually for several deceased at the same time. In such cases the bones of the dead are removed from the grave, washed, and placed in a wooden bone ossuary raised on posts (*temla, keriring*). Subsequently, the skull is sometimes brought to the house and installed as an ancestor skull stored above the *longan*, whereupon *kelelungan* is transformed into a house or community protecting spirit.

Belian are life-enhancing rituals in which one or several shamans negotiate with spirits so as to cure illness, keep away bad dreams and omens (*upi daat, baya sala*), and assure bountiful harvests. Illness, understood in a broad sense, including physical as well as mental symptoms, is typically seen as a result of soul-loss and spirit invasion, and its cure consists of soul retrieval and spirit abstraction. Through chants the *belian* summons spirit familiars (*mulung*) and negotiates with various malevolent spirits (*blis*) which are thought to have caused an illness. Like the Iban *manang*, the *belian* can be described as a shaman in the classical sense of a "ritual intercessor" (Sather 2001: 11), who is capable at will of passing "from one cosmic region to another" (Eliade 1964: 259). Like his or her Iban counterpart, a *belian* is "believed to dispatch his soul into invisible regions of the cosmos" and is thought to have "the power to direct [his soul's] movements and to perform deeds within these unseen regions with the help of personal spirit guides" (Sather 2001: 11). In contrast to Iban shamans, spirit possession is not unheard of among *belian*, but occurs occasionally, either spontaneously or as a result of the use of special techniques, such as fast spinning around during rapid drumming. Some *belian* claim to have learned *belian*-ship through possession by spirits, but like other *belian* these *belian* have usually gone through a period of apprenticeship with already established shamans at some stage as well. Again, as for Iban shamanism (Sather 2001: 185), trance is not a necessary or "defining feature" of *belian*, even if some sort of altered state of consciousness occasionally occurs.

Belian rituals may be conducted in different styles or genres, among which three—*luangan, bawo*, and *sentiu*—are the most common in the central Luangan area (with the exception of *belian sentiu* which is not commonly practiced in Central Kalimantan). These genres differ from each other in that they employ different styles of dance and music in negotiating with spirits, and in that partly different sorts of spirits are contacted in the negotiation.[8]

Belian luangan, or *belian bene,* "true" or "real" *belian,* as it is also sometimes called, is considered the oldest form of *belian* curing, said to have originated among the Luangans in the upper Teweh River area, the area which forms the Luangan mythological landscape. In addition to ordinary curing rituals, *buntang* family and *nalin taun* community rituals are also performed in this style among central Luangans. Drums are the only musical instruments used in the *luangan* style and the shaman does not dance. He is dressed in his ordinary clothes, except for wearing a head cloth (*laung*), and the chants are performed in the local language. The ritual paraphernalia (*ruye*), which includes offerings, spirit images, and houses for the spirits, is of central importance and together with the words of the shaman's chants "constitute" much of the action.

Belian bawo rituals resemble *belian luangan* rituals in their use of words and ritual paraphernalia, but include episodes of dancing by the shaman. The *bawo* shaman is dressed up in a specially decorated, colorful skirt (*sempet*) with a pattern of flowers or spirit figures, together with a belt embroidered with pearls and a wrapped head cloth. He also wears heavy brass wrist bracelets (*ketang*), two or three on each wrist, which he shakes so that they strike against each other while he dances, producing a rattling sound. His chants are in the local language with some elements of Bawo Pasir, the language of the region whence this style of curing is said to originate. The audience is involved as drummers, hitting long drums suspended by rattan strings, leaning at an angle, hard and fast with two rattan or split bamboo sticks, in contrast to *belian luangan* rituals in which the same and smaller drums, kept on the floor, are usually played at a much slower or more moderate pace.[9] The *bawo* shaman characteristically spins around at a very fast pace while the drums are hit violently (e.g., when looking for the cause of the patient's illness) and he sometimes goes into a trance-like state. As in the other styles of *belian,* the ritual may last for one evening only, but more commonly extends over several nights.

Belian sentiu is a much newer style of curing, introduced to the central Luangan area in the 1970s. Unlike *belian luangan* and *bawo* it is usually performed partly in Kutai Malay or Indonesian, and partly in the local language, as the spirits contacted consist

49

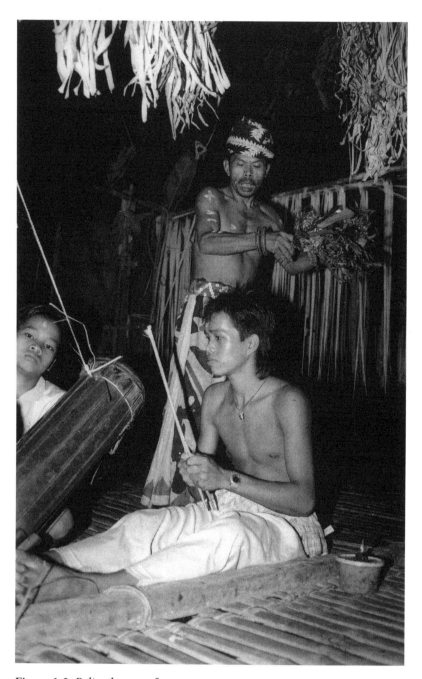

Figure 1.3. *Belian bawo* performance

of foreign, downriver spirits as well as local spirits. As in *belian bawo* the similarly dressed-up shaman dances during the ritual, but wears ankle bracelets with jingling bells, *junung*, instead of *ketang* wrist bracelets. The music played on drums and the *kelentangen*, a xylophone-like percussion instrument consisting of small gongs, is also more melodious, the dancing more delicate, but the chants often less elaborate than in *bawo* or *luangan* rituals. The sacrifice of pigs is often banned from *sentiu* rituals as many of the spirit familiars and spirits contacted are considered to be Muslims. *Gaharu* incense wood (*Aquilaria* sp.) is burnt during *sentiu* rituals, whereas *bemueng* (*Agathis* sp.) is usually used in *luangan* and *bawo* curing.[10] Whereas almost all *belian* performing in the *bawo* and *luangan* styles in the central Luangan area today are men, there are some women practicing *belian sentiu*.

Any single *belian* ritual may be performed in one of these main styles, or in a mix of styles, so that a ritual which starts out as a *luangan*, for example, may continue as a *bawo* or *sentiu* after three days (cf. Gönner 2002: 69). Or, it can be predominantly conducted in one style, but incorporate sequences of another style, performed by the same or another shaman, a *belian luangan* containing phases of *sentiu* curing, for instance. Each style further contains a variation of sub-styles, with their own specific musical conventions, associations with particular spirits, and special ritual objects used. Individual shamans also have their own stylistical techniques, based both on their education and on inspiration received during rituals. A fair amount of improvisation is allowed in *belian* (cf. Weinstock 1983: 63). As Jane Atkinson (1989: 15) reports for the *mabolong* ritual performed by the Wana of Sulawesi, a *belian* "cannot be described or analyzed as a preordained progression of delineated steps to which ritual practitioners and congregants collectively conform. It is rather a repertoire of ritual actions available to performers acting independently in the ritual arena." *Belian* rituals are open-ended rather than self-contained, and display a reiterative rather than a linear structure. Program activities do not conform to a straightforward, linear logic according to which one moves from point A to point B, and from B to C, etc. Rather they involve doing the same or similar things over and over again during the same evening, and over several subsequent evenings, and in the process they adjust to changing circumstances arising from both inside and outside the ritual.

51

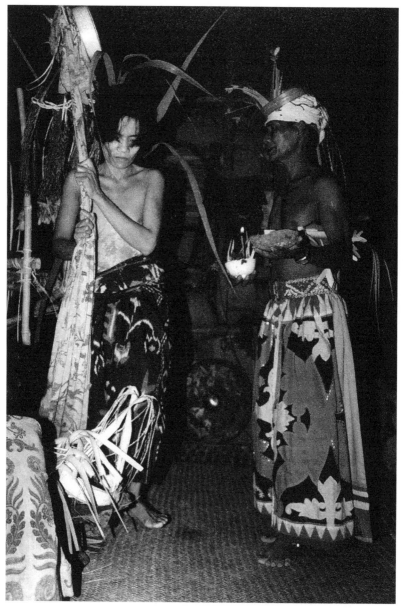

Figure 1.4. *Belian sentiu* performance

There are, however, a number of elements in the *belian* reper-toire without which a performance, especially a longer one, would not be considered complete and which pretty much are standard procedures in *belian* rituals. Central among these are "the calling of spirit familiars" (*mangir mulung*), "the presentation of offerings and respect" (*besemah*), "the purchase of the soul" (*sentous*), "soul searching" (*berejuus*), "the treatment of patients" (*bekawat, nyelolo, naper*), and "the presenting of rewards" (*nyerah upah*) to the spirit familiars.

During "soul search," *berejuus*, the shaman, together with his spirit familiars, verbally travels to search for the lost soul (*juus*) of the patient(s), normally visiting a variety of different places and spirits. The soul or life force (*juus*) of human beings may occasion-ally wander off during dreams, it is believed, and may be caught by malevolent spirits, causing illness and eventually death. For a variety of reasons, including breach of taboos, illness, or just young age, the soul may also be or become weak (*lome*), a condition which makes it susceptible to theft or fright. Based on the symptoms, the patient's life-history and recent experiences, and the outcome of a range of divination techniques (*pereau*), the *belian*, with the help of his spirit guides, selects some potentially guilty, offended, or otherwise rele-vant spirits, in order to direct his effort to buy back (*sentous*) and return (*pekuli*) the soul of the patient, and, as a safety measure, the souls of the patient's family and other ritual participants as well. These journeys and the actions performed at their destinations are described in detail during *belian* rituals, both verbally and materially. The shaman sometimes sits in a swing (*tuyang, bantan*) or swings a miniature ship (*sampan benawa*) as he travels, usually accompanied by drumming by members of the audience. As he reaches the desti-nation, he grabs the soul with his hand (an activity called *nakep juus*, or *kerek keker* with metaphoric reference to the sound made when calling chickens), and then puts it into a small brass tin or plastic jar before subsequently returning it through a hole (*kerepuru*) at the back of the patient's/participants' heads. He does so again and again during the course of a ritual, the soul being constituted of, as Luangans metaphorically say, a hundred parts and eight essences (*juus jatus, ruo walo*).

In treating (*ngawat*) the patient, something which is also done repeatedly during *belian* rituals, the shaman usually brushes off the illness (*roten*) thought to have entered the patient's body with a shredded banana leaf whisk (*daon selolo*). Sometimes he sucks it out with his mouth, washes it off with water, and fans it away with some leaves. Fundamental in these activities, and in *belian* curing generally, is what the Luangans call *pejiak pejiau*, the process of "undoing and redoing" whereby bad luck and adversity is turned into good luck and prosperity. This is done by enacting and verbally presenting something in the wrong way first, evoking death and adversity, after which the same operation is then redone in the right way, evoking continued life and prosperity. Thus, for example, flawed, incompetent spirit familiars are first called, rotten rice seeds are scattered to call the spirits, water is poured over patients in the direction of the setting sun. A transformation is then concretely executed as the *belian* "turns things around" (*malik*), and remakes them in the right way, calling competent spirit familiars, scattering unspoiled rice seeds, pouring water in the direction of the rising sun.

The spirit familiars summoned by the *belian* are mostly *belian* of the past, both mythological *belian* and more recent predecessors, but may also include other spirit beings of the local landscape and, especially in *belian sentiu*, beyond it.[11] The spirits that are thought to be the cause of an illness and who are the recipients of the principal offerings and requests for withdrawal are manifold, including a variety of loosely defined categories of spirits such as *naiyu*, *timang*, *wok*, *bongai*, *tentuwaja*, *juata*, to mention only some of the most frequently addressed, besides the spirits of the dead. They come both from the local milieu and from more far-away places (such as downriver regions and various heavenly locations), and even though there is sometimes only one or a few particular suspects to whom a journey of soul search is conducted, the typical pattern is to conduct such journeys to or negotiate for such purposes with invited representatives of an abundance of spirits. As among the Wana (Atkinson 1989: 120), spirit guides are not summoned just once during a *belian* ritual, but repeatedly, and new spirits keep arriving during the course of events.

Even though the word *blis* is used as a generic designation for spirits in a malevolent capacity, there is no clear line between malevolent and benevolent spirits, most being able to take on both capacities (see also te Wechel 1915: 15). Thus, the "refined head souls" of the deceased (*kelelungan*), that are often described in contrast to the dead's coarse "body souls" as good (*bue*) or purified (*lio*), may protect human beings as well as hurting them. Spirits are not always contained in neatly bounded categories either but can change form; *kelelungan* may become *naiyu* for instance—most spirits indeed have a more or less recent human origin—or spirits may appear as animals. Spirits of a certain category often take on a variety of manifestations and occupy a variety of locations. *Juata*, the water spirit, to give one example, comes in the shape of a water dragon, snake, crocodile, turtle, leech, and crab, among others, and inhabits river environments both on the earth and in heaven. Luangan spirits share the environment with the Luangans and they are generally said to lead roughly similar lives as people, although mostly remaining invisible (*gaib*). According to the origin myth of human beings (*Tempuun Senaring*), they are the older siblings of human beings, and their common origin with man is often emphasized in communication with them (for more on this myth, see chapter 6).

All *belian* rituals require the construction of a variety of ritual objects or paraphernalia (*ruye*), which the *belian* present (*nyemah*) to the spirits as rewards for help and as gifts in exchange for people's souls and general well-being. The larger the ritual, the more *ruye* are called for. At the very least, some bowls filled with uncooked rice (both ordinary rice and sticky rice), some flowers (*bungen dusun, bentas*, etc.) and plaited coconut leaf decorations (*ringit*), an egg, and a burning candle are required, together with some rice paste figurines and a plate of burning incense (*jemu*). During larger rituals considerable time is put into the preparation of ritual paraphernalia, including images of human beings and spirits made of wood, rice paste, sugar palm fiber, banana plant wood, and other materials; various small houses (*blai*) and offering trays (*ansak*) specific to different spirits, made of a wide range of wild-growing or cultivated plants; and *balei*, large shrine-like worship structures constructed inside or outside the house, in which offerings to several different categories of spirits are usually made. The ritual paraphernalia is considered essential to rituals and their efficacy. Even if a ritual can start out with only a minimum of *ruye*, its completion usually requires the construction of a diversity of paraphernalia, the correct preparation of which is regarded as essential (the *belian* normally gives orders about the objects that should be made, and in what materials they should be, at an early stage of the ritual and then complements them during the course of the event). In his chants, the *belian* then presents the paraphernalia to the spirits, elaborately describing the objects in poetic language, evoking them for the spirits.

Besides these material offerings, the sacrifice of at least a chicken should be included in a *belian*. During larger rituals a dozen of more chickens may be sacrificed, together with several or sometimes as many as ten pigs, and in addition, one or two water buffalos. Since domestic animals are not killed outside ritual, the killing of pigs and water buffalos, and the serving of their meat with rice to the people congregated, usually draws a large audience. Plants, such as banana or areca palms which are felled for the purpose of the ritual, may be counted among the offerings as well. Barbecued chicken, sticky rice parcels, and cakes made of rice flour, sugar, and coconut milk make up standard food offerings to the spirits (*okan penyewaka*), which during most *belian* rituals are then served late at night to the people still present at the end of the day's program.

The language of *belian* chants is composed of a mixture of "stock formulae and improvisation" (Atkinson 1989: 16), and marked, like ritual language in Eastern Indonesia (Fox 1974) and elsewhere in the archipelago, by frequent use of parallelism, words and lines being repeated by paired, roughly or strictly synonymous words and lines, which sometimes have no referential meaning of their own (what Metcalf 1989: 41 calls blind dyads). As among the Berawan (Metcalf 1989: 39), the parallelism of Luangan chanting is "less structured" and "less formal" than the parallelism of Eastern Indonesia: "There are words that are frequently heard together, but one of them may occur in a novel pairing without exciting comment." Rhyme, alliteration, assonance and consonance are common elements of these parallel expressions and a characteristic of *belian* language in general. Again, as among the Berawan (ibid.: 44), rhyming is "generally within lines, rather than between lines." Even though chants are mostly in the vernacular language (with the addition of Malay in *sentiu* curing, and Pasir Luangan as in *bawo*) they characteristically include numerous archaic words and loan words from other languages as well as special ritual words which are not used in any other contexts than *belian* or cannot be understood separately from words that they replicate.

The potency of *belian* curing is considered to lie as much in the beauty of its language—constituted by conventional couplets, rhyming, and a number of more or less standardized metaphors regularly used in the chants—as in the meaning of words, the words (*bukun*) forming offerings in their own right. Lists of names of spirits and places make up a considerable part of many chants, the pronunciation of these names functioning to call and thus bring forth the spirits (cf. Morris 1993: 110). Since the chants are primarily addressed to spirits, they are often sung too quietly or inarticulately—the *belian* mumbling or rushing through the words, often with their mouths full of betel—to be fully audible to the audience, but the latter are familiar with stock expressions and many of the metaphors and special ritual words used, and often find pleasure in these. The extent of improvisation varies between individual shamans, some improvising more than others, as well as between styles of *belian*: *belian sentiu* usually contains more improvisation than the other styles, as do curing rituals in general, in comparison with harvest and community rituals (or death rituals, for that matter).

Belian rituals include moments of high intensity—people gathering together to prepare food, kill and slaughter an animal—but they also include long stretches of inactivity, with participants sleeping through much of the event, and a *belian* chanting alone in a house during the daytime while everyone else is out working on their fields. Ultimately, the course of a *belian* ritual is unpredictable; a small ritual may turn into a several-week-long performance because a patient gets worse, or because this is demanded by the spirits, and a planned ritual may be delayed or postponed because sufficient rice to feed participants is lacking, or a shaman intended to conduct it is busy. There is no prescribed regularity to *belian* rituals; weeks may pass in a village without a ritual, and then again rituals may follow on each other, the sound of drums penetrating the darkness of village and forest from several directions at once. Except for harvest rituals (*kerewaiyu*), *belian* rituals are not calendrical but performed when the need arises or when resources allow. Whereas family, community and mortuary rituals are mainly performed in village longhouses (*lou solai*) and extended family houses (*lou*), *belian* curing rituals are regularly performed in single-family village houses or swidden houses as well.

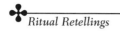

A History of Marginalization

> Ask him [God] for oil from the realm of the dead, so that we can become invisible ... So that we won't be hit by the orders and commandments of the Dutch. Because those orders and commandments do not make sense, they do not seem reasonable.
>
> —Excerpt from an unpublished manuscript on Luangan myth and history written by Lemanius (1996, my translation). The excerpt is from a story of how some Luangans searched for invisibility as a means to escape the unreasonable orders of the Dutch, who requested them to make ropes of sand and canoes of ironwood (which does not float).

When the Norwegian natural scientist and explorer Carl Bock (1881: 143), commissioned by the Sultan of Kutai, traveled through the central Luangan area in 1879 he noted that Dilang Puti (the present-day district capital of Bentian Besar) was the "furthest extremity" of the dominions of the Sultan. Beyond that the Dayaks were noted for their "ferocity" (Bock 1881: 146; see also Dalton 1831: E4–E5). Although this reputation may have expressed fear of the unknown—Bock was reaching into territory outside the control of the sultanate—more than any real state of affairs (the central Luangans seem to have participated only marginally in headhunting and were more often the prey than the predator in the context of this activity), it is indicative of how the Luangans, like many other Dayaks, have generally been viewed by both colonial and post-colonial authorities. As they did not generally, or at least not actively, pay tribute (*suaka*) to the coastal sultanates (Bock 1881: 147; Knappert 1905: 626), the central Luangans were considered dangerous and unpredictable. Even though they traded with Bekumpai Malays resident on the Teweh River (Schwaner 1853: 120), and with traveling Kutai Malay and Buginese traders on the tributaries of the Mahakam River and in interior Pasir, at least from the early nineteenth century, the relative remoteness of their area and the lack of navigable rivers meant that travel to and through the area was difficult and sporadic. As a consequence, they maintained for most practical purposes an effective political autonomy much longer, and settled in permanent, nucleated villages much later than most of their downstream neighbors, in some cases only in the 1920s. However, since the late nineteenth and early twentieth centuries, as the Dutch established effective control over the interior of Southeast Borneo, introducing a "head tax" (*uang kepala*) and prohibiting headhunting and slavery, the Luangans became increasingly drawn into the orbit of an administrative order and a political rhetoric which has shaped the basic contours of their self-understanding and relationships with other peoples and government authorities ever since.

As Luangans conceptualized it during my fieldwork, however, it was to the period of Indonesian independence that they assigned the most significant changes in their ways of life. In discourse, the time of Indonesian independence had gained a reified symbolic status, marking the end of an era and various practices associated with it, which in many cases were, in fact, either abandoned long before independence—such as headhunting, slavery, and human sacrifice (in the late nineteenth century)—or a few decades after it—such as the use of loincloth, tattoos, and long hair by men, or tree plugs inserted in the ear lobes by women—or even still persist—such as dispersed settlement and polygamy. As they expressed it, before independence they were still "wild" (*liar*), while after it, in "the age of development" (*jaman pembangunan*), they became ordered (*diatur*). During my fieldwork, local history—especially to the extent that it invoked dispersed settlement, residential mobility, swidden cultivation, slavery, headhunting, and polygamy—was usually only recounted reluctantly and with great caution. Even personal history, in the form of personal swidden or kinship histories, was frequently recounted only with much suspicion. This was not so much, or at least not unambiguously, because the past was considered shameful as such—in discourse, the ancestors (*ulun tuha one*) and tradition (*adat*) were, on the contrary, repeatedly invoked as paragons of exemplary behavior and moral ideals—as because of a fear of how history might discredit them in the eyes of others, or even make them susceptible to government intervention in the form of development programs (*bina desa*), for instance. Silence here functioned somewhat like invisibility, allowing certain aspects of tradition to remain out of gaze, and thus in some sense served to protect, and even maintain, them. As James Scott (2009: 237), investigating similar strategies of "state-evasion" by the hill peoples of mainland Southeast Asia, observes: "how much history a people have ... is always an active choice, one that positions them vis-à-vis their powerful ...

neighbors." In order to better understand the predicament of the Luangans in the Indonesian nation-state after independence, and especially during the New Order era which still held sway during my principal fieldwork in the 1990s, I will here briefly present some aspects of the rhetorics of Indonesian state rule at the time, as well as its politics of religion.

The Indonesian center of state rule being located on Java, Javanese notions of order and power, mediated by colonial influence (see Day 2002: 64), pervaded the national ideology of the New Order. In Javanese political thinking, power is, according to Benedict Anderson's famous characterization, conceived of as something concrete, which exists independently of its users (1990: 22–23). It is "that intangible, mysterious, and divine energy which animates the universe" (1990: 22). The quantum of power is constant; its concentration in one place entails diminution of it in another place. Rulers hold power to the extent that they are able to concentrate it and maintain order. Lack of order is not a sign of someone losing power, but of power already lost. Power, according to this notion, is typically concentrated at exemplary centers, the influence of which diminishes the farther away from the center one goes (Anderson 1990; Errington 1989; Geertz 1980). Stability is a vital requirement for the concentration of power, and in the New Order era national unity was seen as a necessity for keeping up the Indonesian nation state. Plurality was accepted only as long as it did not threaten national unity and order.

During the New Order, the inhabitants of the periphery, especially so-called "primitive peoples," were seen as living on the fringes of order and power (see Tsing 1993: 28). They trespassed, in a double sense, the limit of the known and controlled. They did so in actuality, in that their geopolitical marginality made them hard to administer, but equally importantly, they did so because it made them appear to do so in the eyes of their observers.

In this master narrative of order and disorder the swidden cultivating Dayaks represented wildness per se (and in many ways continue to do so; see Chalmers 2006: 19). As Scott (2009: 77) points out: "swiddening has been the anathema to all state-makers, traditional or modern." The mobility entailed in swidden cultivation made the Dayaks hard to locate and control. In order to subordinate them and other so-called "isolated" or "estranged" peoples (*suku terasing*) to the national order, they were resettled in less distant locations through state-run resettlement programs (see, e.g., King 1993: 287–288; Tsing 1993: 92–93). Several studies and reports of Luangan subgroups or villages were conducted with this aim in the 1970s (see, e.g., Team Survey Suku Bawo 1972; Badan Koordinasi Penelitian Daerah 1975). In parts of Borneo, wet rice cultivation was introduced even if swidden cultivation is better suited for the ecological conditions of most of Kalimantan (see Avé and King 1986: 29–32; Dove 1993: 174). As Stephanie Fried (2003: 148–149) has aptly noted, for outsiders visiting a swidden rice field, with its diversity of vegetables and fruit trees growing seemingly at random in the midst of the rice, rattan shoots rising here and there among the charred remnants of tree trunks, it often seems disorderly in comparison to the neat rows of vegetables grown by immigrant farmers practicing sedentary or intensive cultivation. The fact that the swidden fields, which in a majority of cases are cultivated on regrowth of forest which has been used for farming for generations, will revert into forest in a few years, while still producing rattan and fruit for their users for many years after, escapes their attention (ibid.). Instead, these practitioners of "disorderly farming," *pertanian yang tidak teratur* (Tsing 1993: 156), are blamed for their irrationality, and even for the ecological damage produced by immigrant sedentary farmers.

A central concept in the New Order state ideology was *pembangunan*, "development" (Heryanto 1988).[12] The Suharto regime, appositely labeled *Orde Baru*, "the New Order," saw the promotion of development and "progress" (*kemajuan*) as one of its main tasks. What primarily seems to have been meant by "development" and "progress," however, at least with regards to "backward" tribal populations, was not so much the promotion of human welfare as the eradication of primitiveness and the establishment of order and stability. Rather than trying to improve the living conditions of the inhabitants of the periphery, the authorities tried to impose order and power on them—and ultimately to confirm their own order and power (cf. Tsing 1993: 91–93).

The building served as a powerful symbol of this development ideology (Bowen 1991: 125; Tsing 1993: 91).[13] It was not just the banking complexes of Jakarta that stood as monuments of development; the organization of private housing also functioned as a measure of development. The longhouse habitation of the Dayaks was considered primitive and unorganized. Especially during the 1970s, but also after that, campaigns were held to encourage the Dayaks to build small, numbered, single-family houses. These "development houses," built in a neat, straight row on both sides of a single street, were evidence of the capability of those in power to control wildness and disorder. The place of the longhouse was at the outdoor museum of ethnic exhibits at the *Taman Mini Indonesia Indah* (Beautiful Indonesia Miniature Park) in Jakarta. There it stood, together with other traditional houses of the archipelago, as an icon of national plurality, valued as long as it remained on the level of, what Greg Acciaioli has termed, "display, not belief, performance, not enactment" (1985: 161; see also Bowen 1991: 126; Pemberton 1994: 152–161). With increasing tourism in the 1980s, a few longhouses along the major rivers of Kalimantan were refurbished to provide accommodation for tourists, and serve as centers for well-scripted cultural performances.

What in many cases denoted the wildness of the wild man in this Indonesian master narrative of order and disorder was his lack of affiliation with a religion, *agama*. Indonesians have freedom of religion, as long as they confess to one of the six officially recognized world religions—Islam, Hinduism, Buddhism, Catholicism, Protestantism, and Confucianism—the primary criterion of which, inscribed in the first principle of *Pancasila*, the national ideology, is belief in the almighty God (*Tuhan yang Maha Esa*). Indonesia's various local religions are not viewed as true "religions" (*agama*), but as constituting merely "beliefs" (*kepercayaan*), and those who follow them are seen as primitive animists, lacking national consciousness. In an often used phrase, they are referred to as *orang yang belum beragama*, "people who do not yet possess a religion," the "not yet" formulation here connoting anticipated future conversion (Atkinson 1987a: 174–178). While members of world religions are granted protection from proselytization by members of other world religions, the government encourages missionary work among those still not possessing one (Kipp 1993: 91; Ramstedt 2004a: 9).[14]

It is in his pact with the magical, the unpredictable, with chaos raised to order, that the wild man emerges in all his primitiveness. As he turns his back on the almighty God he turns his back on ultimate control. In the wake of the communist killings after President

Sukarno's fall from power in 1965, many Dayaks converted to Christianity or Islam as a safety measure, afraid of being accused of communism (Whittier 1973: 146), which lack of world religion affiliation was sometimes taken to imply. Lack of religion still entails many practical complications in the lives of those who, like many Luangans, do "not yet" belong to an *agama*. In order to apply for official identity cards, needed for voting and for traveling, among other things, they must state religious affiliation, usually forcing them to adopt Christianity at least nominally (thus becoming what is called *Kristen kartu penduduk*, "identity card Christians"). Children are also required to take lessons in *agama* in school, even if they do not belong to an official religion (cf. Kipp 1993: 91; Ramstedt 2004b: 213). Similarly, village heads have often felt compelled to classify villagers as Christians in village-level statistics, which until 2000 recognized religious, but not ethnic, affiliation. In one case which I encountered during my fieldwork, a Luangan village head refused to do this, but the papers still came back with Christianity marked on them.

A few of Indonesia's local religions have, however, succeeded in obtaining status as *agama*, by stressing their similarities with Hinduism. One of these is Kaharingan, which received official recognition as a Hindu sect in 1980, and came to be called Hindu Kaharingan (other examples are Aluk To Dolo and Ada' Mappurondo in Sulawesi and Pemena in Sumatra). Kaharingan, or Hindu Kaharingan, is the designation used today for the local religion of the Ngaju in particular, but also of other Central Kalimantan Dayak groups, including Luangans living in the province.

The recognition of Hindu Kaharingan as an *agama* was the result of a long struggle carried out mainly by the Ngaju in Central Kalimantan. This process had already started in the colonial period, with the foundation of the Sarikat Dayak political party in 1919, which was established to promote Dayak interests and identity in the face of the increasing political and economic presence of Banjar Muslims in the area (Miles 1976: 108–110). Upon Indonesian independence in 1945, Kalimantan was divided into three provinces: West, East, and South Kalimantan. Among the Ngaju, and especially the educated elite of the group, discontentment with belonging to the same province as the more numerous Banjar Malays was widespread and resulted in attacks against government installations and clashes with Muslims. Dayak rebels threatened to continue these attacks if the national government did not announce Central Kalimantan as an autonomous province. At the same time, claims were raised that the local religion, Kaharingan, should become officially recognized. In order to resolve the conflict, President Sukarno founded Central Kalimantan in 1957, and Tjilik Riwut, a Ngaju military commander, national hero, and adherent of Kaharingan, was appointed as its first governor. Even though the majority of the population in the new province, contrary to Ngaju expectations, was still Muslim, all the higher posts in the province were given to Dayaks (Miles 1976: 120–123). Official recognition of Kaharingan was only achieved more than twenty years later, however.

What finally enabled Kaharingan to become an *agama* in 1980 was its alleged similarity with Hinduism, which allowed it to become classified as a variety of Hinduism. Among other things, similarities between the names of the Kaharingan Sangiang deities (*seniang* among the Luangans) and the high God Sang Hyang Widhi of Balinese Hinduism was emphasized, as was the use of a specialized ritual language (*bahasa Sangiang*) seen as characteristic of religions (Schiller 1987: 23). Archeological findings suggesting an early Hindu presence found in various locations on Borneo were also advanced as evidence of Kaharingan's Hindu connections and origins. By committing themselves to the doctrines and books of Hinduism, Ngaju representatives thus finally succeeded in receiving official recognition of Hindu Kaharingan (Schiller 1997: 119).

In order to bring Hindu Kaharingan closer to other world religions, it has since its recognition undergone an extensive process of rationalization (see Baier 2007; Mahin 2009; Schiller 1997: 109–131).[15] A Supreme Council of the religion (*Majelis Besar Agama Hindu Kaharingan*) has been established largely for these purposes. In addition to formalizing and standardizing rituals, the council has compiled a holy book (*Panaturan*), and constructed prayer halls for worship of the almighty creator God, Ranying Hatalla Langit, who has achieved an increasingly prominent role, thus fulfilling the demands for monotheism in the national ideology. Local variation in beliefs and rituals are condemned and dismissed as results of villagers' inability to maintain traditions over time and as consequences of difficulties of communication (Schiller 1997: 24). As Anne Schiller (1997: 24) notes, it would only "be fair to describe the Supreme

Council as intolerant of variation within the faith." Today the council has branches on both district and sub-district levels in Central Kalimantan, and its authorization is needed for the arrangement of major rituals. Its influence is perhaps most clearly manifested in the weekly services (*basarah*), during which, in addition to worship, administrative meetings of the village-level organization of the council are held.

Hindu Kaharingan was originally, and still is to a large extent, a Central Kalimantan project. As such, it has influenced Luangans in different areas differently. For Central Kalimantan Luangans, as for other Dayaks in the province, Hindu Kaharingan is today a legitimate alternative for official religious affiliation. On the upper Teweh River in Central Kalimantan, Hindu Kaharingan meetings and services were occasionally held during my fieldwork and a prayer hall was built in one village (in the large village of Benangin on the middle reaches of the Teweh River there was already a prayer hall as well as regular weekly services, which were mainly attended by school children). A few young locals also studied in Palangkaraya to become Hindu Kaharingan teachers.

In the Muslim-dominated province of East Kalimantan, however, Hindu Kaharingan had not been recognized as a religion by the local authorities. Here it remained a much idealized utopia for the province's Luangan population (see chapter 2 for more on some of the implications of this). Attempts by East Kalimantan Luangans to state Hindu Kaharingan as their religion when applying for identity cards were met with refusal by subdistrict leaders.

The apparent benefits of the official recognition of Kaharingan notwithstanding, Hindu Kaharingan and the policies of the Hindu Kaharingan Council have not been accepted unconditionally. There have been worries among Ngajus as well as among members of other Dayak groups that their traditional practices have become "etiolated" as a result of the standardization process (Schiller 1997: 10). Dayaks from other ethnic groups than the Ngaju also complain that they do not understand the language of the holy book, which is in the Ngaju ritual language; this is why the Luangan author Lemanius, quoted above, set out to write the Luangans' own version of a holy book. The Hindu Kaharingan Council's emphasis on eschatology and mortuary rituals (*tiwah*), at the expense of curing rituals, does not make much sense for Luangans either, who regard their life rituals as at least as important as their death rituals. Thus, while providing the Luangans of Central Kalimantan with a viable course to fuller citizenship in the Indonesian nation state, Hindu Kaharingan has simultaneously served to marginalize them in some new ways in relation to powerful others, this time the more numerous and politically influential Ngaju Dayaks. The Hindu Kaharingan Council's notions of what should be, and not be, part of the domain of religion have induced some Luangans to claim that while they officially belong to Hindu Kaharingan, they still also practice Kaharingan, or "the old Kaharingan," as they sometimes call it.[16]

When the Luangans made themselves invisible in the story of Lemanius, referred to in the beginning of this section, with the aim of evading the unreasonable requests of the Dutch, they did so through recourse to a strategy of avoidance rather than confrontation. Instead of overt resistance the Luangans, like other Borneo peoples, have often chosen evasion, dispersion, or flight as strategies of adaptation. There are numerous historical examples of this, including of groups that fled further upriver to escape aggression from other groups, colonial exploitation, resettlement or other policies, and Muslim influence (Knapen 2001: 88; cf. Li 1999: 6; Scott 2009). In this sense these groups, to quote Scott, "are where they are and do what they do intentionally" (2009: 186).

The central Luangans often remain "invisible" also in the sense of being unnoticed on the larger cultural map of Borneo today, even within the two provinces of Central and East Kalimantan that they inhabit, where other Dayaks are more prominent. Living in a remote area, with few distinctive or ostentatious cultural attributes to distinguish them from other peoples (such as the headhunting practices, grand longhouses and elongated ears of northern Dayak groups, or the months-long *tiwah* mortuary ceremonies of the Ngaju or the *kwangkai* of the Benuaq), they have not been spectacular enough to attract much tourist or ethnographic interest, while remaining too remote to enjoy the full benefits of "development." Like other upland populations, central Luangans do not resist development as such: "complaints ... relate not to the concept of 'development' as articulated by 'the state,' but to particular, localized experiences with a development which removes sources of livelihood without providing viable alternatives, fails to bring promised benefits or distributes benefits unevenly" (Li 1999: 22; cf. Peluso 1992). Still, their relative "invisibility" is perhaps what has kept central Luangan religious "tradition" not only alive, but in many respects more vital than that of most Dayaks. Today there are, in fact, in relative terms proportionate to population size, more Kaharingan Luangans than there are Kaharingan Ngajus. Indeed, the central Luangans are among the least christianized of all Dayaks, not only in Central Kalimantan, but also in East Kalimantan.[17]

While in some senses highly marginal, the central Luangan area remains a cultural center in some other respects, including that of representing a center of magical knowledge in Malay perceptions (somewhat like the Tengger Highlands in Java, where the residents used to be both feared and admired by lowlanders; see Hefner 1990), and that of representing a center and place of origin of an indigenous religious tradition of the Dayaks of Southeast Borneo, distinct from (the Kahayan River) Ngaju tradition which holds a dominant position in Central Kalimantan. This status is apparently quite ancient. Its importance as a religious center was illustrated by several millenarian messianic movements in the early twentieth century (see Mallinckrodt 1974; Feuilletau de Bruyn 1934; Weinstock 1983: 118–126). Motivated by discontent with Dutch politics, the people following these movements wanted to bring back an original mythological state of immortality and reunion with the ancestors. Then, as now, the characteristic Luangan method of confronting the unpredictability of outside sources of power of various kinds was largely through the authority of spiritual and ritual knowledge and through ritual mediation.

Today the Luangans have become increasingly engaged in overt confrontation when it comes to land right issues and some of them have engaged in lawsuits and road blocks against logging and, in recent years, palm oil companies, invoking a discourse of indigenous rights influenced by visiting NGOs (see Fried 2003). Still, during the time of my fieldwork, many Luangans felt highly ambivalent about these efforts, as they were wary of the politicking and self-interest (designated by the negatively loaded Indonesian term *politik*) of protagonists on each side of the negotiation table. As among the Meratus, who like the Luangans are often "defined by externally imposed categories of cultural difference," Luangans simultaneously "resent and embrace those categories" (Tsing 1994: 280), wishing to be seen as lawful citizens of the nation-state, while not fully accepting the terms of its definitions. Turning to ritual and spiritual negotiation rather than overt confrontation is not just a way to return to past tradition, but also to claim real indigenous potency. Government representatives visiting central Luangan villages might as often be met by a welcoming ceremony, complete with speeches molded in an official-sounding rhetoric, as by a near-empty village, or, as in one case that I witnessed, by the locked up house of a *kepala desa*, who due to illness in the family and taboos set by a *belian* had moved to another house and was too busy with ritual "work" to meet them. Avoidance in such a case might not primarily be intended as an act of resistance (even if it sometimes works out as such and at other times quite consciously is used as such), but should be seen as an expression of the proportion of "obstruction" (*aur*) that illness and rituals may constitute. The fact that the cause for this illness, and the means employed to resist it, seems to derive from outside the Luangan area ever so often these days shows both the constraints of power and knowledge and the creative possibilities of Luangan agency (cf. Tsing 1993: 18), something which is reflected in the politics of their aesthetics.

Notes

1. The pronunciation "Lawangan," or "Lowangan" is more common among the more southerly Luangan subgroups in Central Kalimantan, whereas "Luangan" prevails in the north, on the Teweh River and in East Kalimantan. "Lawangan" also designates a specific Luangan subgroup who live on the Ayuh and Paku-Karau tributaries of the Barito in Central Kalimantan, which is the one Jacob Mallinckrodt (1928) took as the model for the tribal group. As a designation for the entire "tribal group," or a larger number of subgroups as opposed to just one, the term is best known among the people that I call the central Luangans.

2. Among the Bentian subgroup of the Luangans, a stronger ethnic identification as "Bentians" emerged in the late twentieth century, in part as a result of contacts with NGOs, and especially among younger people living in cities outside the subdistrict of Bentian Besar itself (as can be seen in groups on Facebook, for example).

3. The term "religion" is used with some reservations here. Kaharingan is recognized as an Indonesian "religion" (*agama*) for only part of the Luangans. Furthermore, as Weinstock (1983: 14) acknowledges, there are also Christians who consider themselves as Luangans, on the basis of their Luangan origin.

4. The isolect of Luangan spoken on the upper Teweh is, for example, used in rituals by Luangans living in other areas and by the Ma'anyan of the lower

Barito (Weinstock 1983: 41). The Ma'anyan also share some mythological elements with the Luangans (Mallinckrodt 1974: 14).

5. The Malay words *suku* and *bangsa* mean "ethnic group," or "tribe," and "nation" or "people," respectively. I could not elicit a meaning for the words *jumben* and *barung*, but the expression, which was also known by some other informants, obviously fuses the ethnonyms Lewangan (Luangan) and Tewoyan (Taboyan) to designate a composite unity.

6. Other occasions are *perkara*, lawsuits, and *beru*, collective work parties, which are arranged to sow rice, for instance.

7. The recognized standard length for a *gombok* is three, five, seven, nine, two times seven, and three times seven days. There are particular formats associated with *gomboks* of different lengths, and longer rituals involve more ritual activities and animal sacrifices (e.g., a seven-day *gombok*, which is perhaps the most common format, requires the sacrifice of a water buffalo).

8. These styles may be known by different names among different Luangan subgroups. *Belian luangan*, for example, seems to be what some Benuaq call *belian turaatn* (whereas it seems to be a different style among others, see Gönner 2002: 69; Massing 1982: 60). There are also a number of other styles of *belian* practiced by central Luangans, probably mostly East Kalimantan Luangans, such as *belian bawe, belian kenyong*, and *belian dewa-dewa*. The first is said to originate among the Benuaq, while the two latter are associated with the Kutai Malays and are quite similar to *belian sentiu* in stylistical conventions. None of the three are nearly as common as *belian sentiu, bawo*, or *luangan*. In Central Kalimantan Luangan villages there exists a style of curing called *belian dewa*, which resembles *belian sentiu* in that it incorporates Malay elements, but in this case Banjar Malay as opposed to Kutai Malay.

9. Anyone in the audience may play drums in rituals, including children. Some forms of drumbeat are complex, however, and require a more experienced drummer as well as attention to the shaman's chant. Both men and women strike or play melodies on the large gongs (*gendring*), which are used principally in *buntang* and *nalin taun* family and community rituals, and *gombok* mortuary rituals. In these rituals, and sometimes in *belian luangan* and *sentiu*, the shamans themselves play small hand-held drums that they hit softly with the palms of their hands, but they do not usually play any of the other instruments.

10. *Gaharu* is an incense resin collected mainly for export to the Middle East, Saudi Arabia and Hongkong (see Momberg et al. 2000: 271) and hence associated with foreign tastes.

11. Similarly, the spirit familiars of death shamans are mostly *wara* of the past, but also include spirit animals of various kinds.

12. As Ariel Heryanto (1988: 11) has shown, *pembangunan* came to be a key concept in the politics of President Suharto. The president was called *Bapak Pembangunan* ("the father of development") and his cabinet *Kabinet Pembangunan* (cf. Dove 1988: 33).

13. The literal meaning of the word *pembangunan* is "construction" or "build-ing." Bowen (1991: 125) and Tsing (1993: 91) have both emphasized how the Indonesian development policy was largely about promoting building projects. According to Tsing, these projects functioned like state rituals through which the state demonstrated its own power.

14. During the pro-Islamic campaigns launched by Suharto in the beginning of the 1990s, the Indonesian Council for Islamic Predication was, however, permitted to operate among Christian and Hindu Javanese in the country-side of Central and East Java (Ramstedt 2004a: 17).

15. For a similar process in Bali and highland Java, see Geertz (1973a), Hefner (1985) and Picard (2004).

16. An example of this was provided when I visited a village where a Hindu Kaharingan meeting was held in one house while there was a *belian* ritual going on in another house, and the people in the latter house remarked that Hindu Kaharingan was practiced in the former, while Kaharingan was practiced in theirs. Schiller (1986: 233) similarly provides an example of a Ngaju ritual specialist preferring to call his beliefs the "old religion," as he perceived much of what was called Hindu Kaharingan to be spurious. Since the beginning of decentralization after President Suharto's fall from power in 1998, a split within the Hindu Kaharingan organization has occurred, with some of its members advocating leaving the Hindu associa-tion (Mahin 2009).

17. Statistics on ethnicity and religious affiliation in Central Kalimantan pro-vided by Ian Chalmers (2006: 17) do not include specific data on Luangans or Luangan sub-groups, but they are presumably included in the Dusun group which had a 63 percent Hindu adherence in 2000, the highest in the province. According to government statistics for the subdistrict of Gunung Purei on the upper Teweh from 2007, 52.4 percent of the district's non-Muslim inhabitants are registered as Hindu, while 47.6 percent are Christians (see *Barito Utara Dalam Angka* 2007).

♣ Chapter Two
Representing Unpredictability

Everyone is aware that life is parodic and that it lacks an interpretation.

—Georges Bataille (1985: 5)

Dancing with Spirits

Tak Dinas is dancing, moving her hands up and down along the sarong cloth (*penyelenteng*), which hangs down like a rope from the ceiling, connecting spirits and human beings. This is a dance of gracefulness, of vivid color, of sweet scent. Black oily hair, white powdered skin, shining, glittering clothes in gold and silver, ankle bells jingling with the steps. These are women dancing, first just Tak Dinas, then Tak Lodot, Tak Tiku, Nen Bujok, Nen Bola, Nen Neti, joining in, one after another. Women dressed up, perfumed, made-up. Then suddenly Nen Pare gets up, moving slowly at first, her feet gaining confidence, but in the next moment already dancing, on stumbling, shivering legs, swinging her hands gracefully, her palms moving outwards, her body opening up like a flower. "In four days time you will be able to walk," Tak Dinas told, exhorted, Nen Pare yesterday. And here she is now, dancing, following the others, circling, swaying. There is an uncanny feeling—surprise, confusion, hope—spectators not knowing whether to cry or laugh, what to make of this, whether to believe it or not. Nen Pare has not been up walking for months, she is hardly considered alive, having been lying invisible beneath her blue cotton mosquito net for such a long time. Tak Dinas' dance is getting wilder, faster along with the beat of the drums, the frenzied clangs of the *kelentangen* speeding up. Then suddenly she stops, the music ceases. There is complete silence for a couple of minutes.

71

"This is what we have to offer you tonight, I don't know what other people are giving you but this is what we have." Tak Dinas is holding a tray with colorful cakes made of sticky rice; blue, red, green, and yellow cakes. She is addressing the spirits in Indonesian, the national language. She has been called to perform a *belian* curing ritual for Nen Pare, who in May 1996, when this ritual was performed, had been sick for over a year. At first Tak Dinas refused when asked to perform a *belian* for Nen Pare, for whom some fifteen rituals had already been arranged during the past year, and who had just returned from a trip to seek medical help in the regional capital of Tenggarong, several hundred kilometers downstream. Then she changed her mind, partly encouraged by the news that Nen Pare was feeling a little bit better, that she was eating again.

The ritual performed by Tak Dinas here is a *belian sentiu*, or *belian dewa-dewa* as she herself sometimes preferred to call her version of this curing ritual. What separates *belian sentiu* from other styles of *belian* curing is, as we have seen, the particular set of spirits contacted in the ritual, the way in which these are contacted, and the language used in contacting them. In contrast to the other styles of *belian*, the chants of *belian sentiu* are not just in the local language, but partly in Indonesian or Kutai Malay, and partly in Luangan. The same chants are sung in both Luangan and Malay/Indonesian, with different sets of spirits being addressed in different languages: those of the local world and forest environment in Luangan, those of the foreign and downriver worlds in Malay/Indonesian.

Tak Dinas received her version of *belian sentiu* in a dream when she was fourteen. She became possessed and then started to practice *belian*—in discussions she stressed that she got her knowledge of *belian* curing through possession (*keturunan*), not by studying under other shamans as is the common practice. Except for her own apprentices, Tak Dinas was the only female shaman in the area during my fieldwork (she was also a renowned midwife). Her grandmother was also a *belian*, although an exceptional and "crazy" *belian* "running around in the woods" (female *belian* are said to have been much more common in former times, as were female leaders, *manti*). Having learnt *belian* through possession Tak Dinas relied more on visual effects, "charisma," and performance than "ordinary" (mostly male) *belian* usually did (these *belian* were generally more concerned with correct chanting, and "the power of words,"

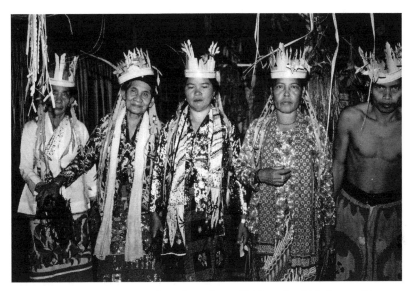

Figure 2.1. "Dressed up, perfumed, made-up." Tak Lodot, Tak Dinas, Nen Bujok, Nen Bola, and Mancan

although this, of course, was a matter of degree). Her hesitance to perform a *belian* for Nen Pare probably had much to do with a wish to maintain her reputation as a successful *belian*. She did not want to take the risk of Nen Pare dying during the ritual (*belian* curers seldom refuse to cure someone when asked; their own illnesses or previous engagements are among the only acceptable excuses).

Nen Bujok, Nen Pare's sister, bursts into tears. These have been hard times for her. She and her husband have moved in with her sister (and her two husbands) to help take care of her, and assist with the work in the swidden field. There has been a feeling of hopelessness, especially after the unsuccessful trip to Tenggarong. The doctor whom they consulted there told Nen Pare that she had a tumor and that an operation was her only option, but Nen Pare refused to be operated on; she said she did not want to die away in town, and ordered her husbands to take her home. There have been accusations: Nen Pare's husbands interpreted the doctor's words to mean that the illness was "man-made," afflicted on her on purpose by some fellow-villager. They sued a young man, generally believed to be innocent; he, in his turn, accused Nen Pare of polygamy and told her that her illness was related to her living with two men. The

73

whole affair resulted in hurt feelings and resentment. The fact that one of her husbands stole and sold a carved *blontang* pole from the village graveyard in order to get money for the trip to Tenggarong did not improve relations between her family and fellow-villagers.[1] And here now, Nen Pare is dancing, twirling and whirling even after the others have stopped—dancing against death.

Tak Dinas comforts Nen Bujok, talking in a play-like voice, a voice of spirits. "Let's wash ourselves—*ayo mandi*," she suggests. "*Yaaa…*," there is laughing and shouting, joking—"let's bath, *mandi selalu!*" Water is brought in, people undress themselves, the music starts again. Dancing, Tak Dinas with the help of Mancan, her apprentice and the only male shaman taking part in this ritual, pours water over the participants who are sitting in a row on the floor, wrapped in sarongs. She splashes scented water on the heads of those of us not joining in. People get possessed; Mancan jumps up and down, stamping his feet on the floor, dancing standing on a gong, dripping with water, having himself been bathed by Tak Dinas; Nen Bujok soaking wet, giggling, stammering, pronouncing unintelligible words; and Tak Dinas, talking with that spirit voice, making you wonder: is this for real, or is it some kind of play?

"Assalamu' alaikum," Ma Sarakang, one of Nen Pare's husbands, walks in, speaking out into the air, probably addressing Tak Dinas, with a loud and official sounding voice, dressed up in a checked cotton sarong, a white well-ironed, long-sleeved shirt and wearing a *kopiah* (the black cap worn all over Indonesia mostly by Muslim men, often as a symbol of national identity). I have to clench my teeth not to laugh, his entrance is so unexpected, and seems so out of place—Ma Sarakang mimetically embodying Muslimness. He offers Tak Dinas a lit cigarette, referring to it in Indonesian as the "signature" (*tanda tangan*) of his sister, who lives in another village and is unable to attend the ritual. Then he sits down and puts his hands together to pray, whispering prayers, concentrating with his eyes shut, his head bent. Some girls are giggling, a group of young men who are playing cards look amused, but most other spectators do not pay much attention to him.

The dance goes on, the dancers dancing around the ritual construction, the *balei*, which occupies the center of the room. The *balei* is an altar-like construction made of yellow bamboo, with walls of colorful clothing and a roof of yellow cloth with a hornbill effigy on the top. It is decorated with figures made of plaited coconut leaves (*ringit*), bright red flowers (*bungen dusun*), and young leaves of various forest plants. In front of the construction, on each side of its entrance, are two heavy Chinese jars filled with uncooked rice. In between there is a ladder with its base on a gong on the floor, leading up to a shelf on which the dancers are putting trays of rice, beeswax candles, eggs, incense, flowers, cakes, cigarettes, 5000 rupiah bills, and small rice flour images representing human beings (*sedediri*), after first having danced around the construction with the trays in their hands. Tak Dinas is singing while she and the others dance, naming the objects placed on the altar, presenting them for the spirits. As the ritual is proceeding, more and more decorations and offerings are added to the *balei*; on the second to the last day the coconut leaf decorations are dyed in red and yellow, and a human skull wrapped in *kajeng* leaves is hung under the shelf. The beauty of the *balei* and the abundance of its offerings are attracting *mulung*, spirit familiars, from their places in heaven, and from Tanjung Ruang, the ancestral village. Then, suddenly, there are spirits from Palangkaraya, the capital of Central Kalimantan, announcing their presence, "ancestor spirits" Tak Dinas calls them, "friends of the ancestor spirits from Tanjung Ruang," she explains. This multitude of spirit beings, drawn to the ritual and the *balei* at its center, bring Tak Dinas the power she needs to fight whoever, whatever is hurting Nen Pare and her family.

Someone puts on the radio. It is Thursday night, the night of *kesenian daerah*, "regional arts," broadcast from Palangkaraya, the capital of Central Kalimantan and the center of Hindu Kaharingan. Palangkaraya and Hindu Kaharingan have been on people's minds ever since the ritual started. Langkong, back from a visit to Central Kalimantan, to Benangin where his daughters live, has witnessed *basarah*, the weekly Hindu Kaharingan service arranged for Ranying Hatalla Langit, the almighty God (*Tuhan Yang Maha Esa*). He describes the newly built "prayer-hall," the crowd of people attending, the decorations used, the unison hymns and the preaching, the holy book—how good all this was, to have a religion. Mancan takes a break, asks us if it is true that we have shown pictures of him performing *belian sentiu* while we were in Palangkaraya recently. I do not know where he has got the idea from, but he clearly seems to wish we had. Ma Putup, Nen Bujok's husband, a *belian sentiu* who received his calling directly from the spirits, just like Tak Dinas, asks if he can come along if we are going there again, to meet the Great Council of the Hindu Kaharingan religion, to visit the radio station. Some people in the village listen to the broadcasts from Palangkaraya every Tuesday and Thursday, the sound of *dongkoi* ("traditional" love songs) permeating the darkness of the village, entering every house.

"Darma, your new name shall be Darma," Tak Dinas announces, addressing Nen Pare. "What? Darma?" This is the last day of the ritual, a pig and some chicken have just been sacrificed—and now Tak Dinas is giving Nen Pare a new name, a new name to enter a new, cool life. Darma. Ma Putup writes it down with his finger in the dust on the floor. "Derma," Ma Lombang suggests, proposing a pronunciation more consonant with the local language. "No, Darma," Tak Dinas insists. "Dar-ma." The name sounds unfamiliar, foreign. Most people present do not know what to associate it with, except that it is foreign. Afterwards, I ask Mancan what he thought about the name. Tak Dinas got it from the Kayangan spirits he explains, and then he mentions the Indonesian concept of "Darma Wanita."[2] My association of the word *darma* with the Hindu concept is received enthusiastically: "of course," he says, "the Kayangan knew what they were talking about." Later Tak Dinas asks me if it is true that I think the name was a good one, and she assures me that she had never heard it before, it just came to her as she spoke, appeared automatically.

A Politics of Spirits

For Nen Pare, for her husbands Ma Buo and Ma Sarakang, her sister Nen Bujok and her brother Ma Geneng, the dancing, the chanting, the embodiment of spirits during the eight-day ritual has been an uneasy balancing between hope and despair, between life and death. Lying on her mattress under her mosquito net—for that is where Nen Pare, in accordance with general Luangan practice, still spends most of her time during the ritual—she does not care much about the politics involved in curing, in contacting spirits. For her it is enough that spirits are contacted, that someone knows what should be done; the music and other "denotatively implicit forms" (Briggs 1996: 208), such as intonation, speech style etc., telling her what was going on, even when she is not watching or paying attention. For

Tak Dinas, on the other hand, it is crucial to give the impression that she does know what to do; she must, to put it in Tsing's (1990: 122) words, "convene an audience," and this is a matter of spirit politics as well as social politics.

The spirits that Tak Dinas contacts in the ritual are either *mulung*, spirit familiars, or *blis*, various kinds of malevolent spirits, which cause Nen Pare and her family suffering. Some of these spirits, in both categories, are part of the local world, and some come from foreign, downriver or celestial worlds. The spirit guides consist of both ancestors, great shamans from the mythical village Tanjung Ruang, and Kayangan, gods (*dewa*) who reside in heaven, and who are vaguely associated with Islam, and the court of the Sultanate of Kutai (which was Hindu-Buddhist until sometime between 1500 and 1700, then Muslim, but with persisting Hindu and earlier "animist" influences). Through these spirit guides she negotiates with local *blis* as well as *blis* coming from downriver locations. She is, according to Langkong, calling on two different religious centers here, that of Tanjung Ruang, which represents Kaharingan, the local religion, and that of Pahu, which represents Islam.[3] The dualism which Langkong intends to invoke here is not really as clear as it might seem though, as Tak Dinas is working in a world where influences keeps flowing in, where other centers are announcing themselves, where borders are formed in fluidity.

It has been suggested that the *sentiu* style of *belian* curing first appeared when Dayaks on the Pahu River converted to Islam in the beginning of the twentieth century (Weinstock 1983: 41–43). Many locals, however, claim that *belian sentiu* actually originated on the river Ohong, among non-Muslim Benuaq Dayaks.[4] What is generally agreed on is that *belian sentiu* is a relatively new form of curing. Similarities between *belian sentiu* and curing rituals practiced by Kutai Malays, including those held at the court of the former Sultan of Kutai, are apparent and recognized by the Dayaks. These rituals use the same kind of ritual paraphernalia and ritual techniques as *belian sentiu*, including ankle bracelets with jingling bells (or calf bracelets in the case of the Malays and some Benuaq Dayaks), an emphasis on the color yellow (symbolizing magical power and royalty), summoning of the Kayangan (a category of spirits widely known in the archipelago), the use of identical ritual paraphernalia, etc. *Belian sentiu* was introduced to the central parts of the Luangan

77

region, the area where the ritual led by Tak Dinas took place, in the 1970s. In Tak Dinas' understanding, however, the fact that *belian sentiu* was developed quite recently does not mean that it cannot be, at the same time, a quite ancient form of curing. According to her, Kakah Make, a Benuaq Dayak living along the Jeleu River, was the founder of *belian sentiu*. He once dreamt about *belian sentiu* and in his dream went to Tanjung Ruang to study it from his mythical ancestors. Waking up and recovering from the eight-day possession following the dream, he started to practice *belian sentiu* and to teach it to his neighbors. What could be seen as something new then, was in fact there all the time, known by Luangan mythical ancestors, but concealed from their descendants until Kakah Make gained access to it through his dream.

Tak Dinas' performance bears out her conviction that *belian sentiu* is a form of curing with a local origin. In the ritual performed for Nen Pare (which she referred to as a *belian dewa-dewa*, with reference to the spirit familiars assisting her in the ritual bathing), she mixes elements of what she calls *belian bene* ("true" *belian*, that is, *belian luangan*, the curing style considered to be the original form of *belian*) with the *sentiu* style. While this was also true of most other *belian sentiu* curers in the area, Tak Dinas does so much more explicitly and self-consciously. When other *belian* often asserted that pure *belian sentiu* should actually be conducted exclusively in Malay, and that pigs should not be sacrificed in the ritual (as downriver spirits do not eat pork), Tak Dinas seems to consider the hybridity to be original, not a consequence of deficient knowledge or an adjustment to local conditions. *Belian sentiu* (or *belian dewa-dewa*) as practiced by Tak Dinas here is a form of curing which "borrows" the power of foreignness (Tsing 1993: 128), just to claim that it is, in fact, originally local.

In this interplay between the autochthonous and the foreign, Tak Dinas accentuates both locality and foreignness, both similarity and difference, at times with much more elaboration than most *sentiu* shamans. Tanjung Ruang is invoked in her chanting again and again, almost over-explicitly, as if only the repeated enunciation grants it an existence. The diversity of Luangan origins is simultaneously played down, the multitude of ancestral villages summoned in *belian luangan* reduced to Tanjung Ruang. Tanjung Ruang stands out as a background, representing a clearly marked ancestrality, contrasting with the overwhelming richness of foreign influences flowing in. Tak Dinas' dance, in its gracefulness and femininity, in the smoothness and delicacy of her movements, in the splendor of her appearance—the other women mirroring her, following her steps—stresses the performativity, the artfulness, promoted in dances at cultural festivals (cf. Tsing 1993: 235), evoking the kind of entertainment promoted on national television. The plenitude and colorfulness of the cakes served during the ritual are reminiscent of cakes served in *warung* in market towns and cities on the coast, giving an impression of prosperity, even overabundance. The *balei*, with all its decorations—the burning incense, surrounding it with the heavy odor of *gaharu*, the offerings of rice, coconuts, and flowers—has the appearance of a temple (in some chants it is referred to as a *keraton* or palace) with dancers expressing their devotion, while calling on spirits from distant places, speaking foreign languages.[5] But then again, hung under the *balei*, wrapped in dried leaves, there is also the ancestral skull, symbolizing ancestral tradition, or maybe just the power of ancestors, causing thunderstorms and calamity if left out. Tak Dinas is playing with distinctions, emphasizing them, bringing them into contact by juxtaposing them. It is through a "poetics of shock" (Rutherford 1996) that she creates her authority, drawing on both local and foreign powers, creating unexpected encounters between them, and claiming the mastery of both.

When the spirits from Palangkaraya announce their presence in the ritual, they are simultaneously unexpected and well prepared for. Palangkaraya and what it stands for was present in the villagers' discussion and imagination from the beginning of the ritual, invoked by Langkong's recent visit to Benangin, Mancan's and other participants' frequent listening to the radio broadcasts from Palangkaraya, and the anthropologists' stories of Hindu Kaharingan. Yet, they are unexpected; ancestors from Palangkaraya have not been heard of before, and have certainly not been called on in *belian* curing. There is something unsettling in this, in the relationship between ancestors, in the coupling of past and present, and in the blurring of origins. Palangkaraya is, in fact, a relatively new town. It was created in 1957 as the capital of what was meant to become the new Dayak province of Central Kalimantan (Miles 1967: 114–117). How the spirits from Palangkaraya have come to be ancestors of the Luangans, friends of the "real" ancestors from Tanjung Ruang, is something of a mystery then, although a mystery more thrilling than confusing, it seems. Their emergence, at least to some extent, appears to have been brought forth by their pertinence, and their pertinence could perhaps also explain why their unexpected appearance succeeds so well in attracting the attention of the participants, drawing them into participation, with more and more people taking part in the dancing as the ritual progresses, and people arriving from neighboring villages. The emergence of these spirits is exactly what constitutes Tak Dinas' ritual authority during this ritual: they are the very stuff that makes up her ability to create relevancy, to convene an audience.

By joining the ritual, the spirits from Palangkaraya situate *belian sentiu* within the same framework as Hindu Kaharingan, in an analogous relation to the national politics of religion. Whereas Hindu Kaharingan is not practiced outside Central Kalimantan, *belian sentiu* is almost exclusively practiced in East Kalimantan (with the exception of a few border villages in Central Kalimantan). The recognition of Hindu Kaharingan as a state-approved religion, *agama*, was the result of a long history of resistance (mainly carried out by Ngaju Dayaks) against the suppression of Dayak identity and religion by Muslims and state officials (see Miles 1976: 102–124; see also chapter 1 of this book). The recognition of Hindu Kaharingan has helped the Dayaks to maintain their Dayak identity, at the same time as it has also involved an extensive process of religious rationalization, adapting Hindu Kaharingan to the criteria defining world religions in the national ideology. Whereas the details of the process of recognition, as well as the exact contents of the newly rationalized religion, were largely unknown to East Kalimantan Luangans at the time of my fieldwork, the idea of belonging to a distinct Dayak religion was extremely appealing to most of them.[6]

At least at the time when this ritual was performed, however, there seemed to be no real prospects of an inclusion of Kaharingan in East Kalimantan into Hindu Kaharingan. While the Central Kalimantan government, which to a significant part consisted of Dayaks, had been generally sympathetic to Dayak interests, the Muslim dominated East Kalimantan government had so far been unwilling to even consider the question. Seen against this background, it is not surprising that *belian sentiu* had taken on a special significance for some Luangans living in East Kalimantan. Tak Dinas' introduction of the spirits from Palangkaraya, together with the persistent talk about Hindu Kaharingan during the ritual, points to this significance.

In certain respects, *belian sentiu* can be said to represent a local alternative to Hindu Kaharingan, or maybe more to the point, the attraction of both lies in how they represent ways to maintain and modernize local tradition in the face of national integration. In the relatively short time that it has been practiced, *belian sentiu*—and related curing forms such as Tak Dinas' *dewa-dewa*—has rapidly gained great popularity. In many villages downstream from the village where Tak Dinas' ritual was held, few of the younger *belian* are learning the older forms of curing these days, most just study *belian sentiu* (Massing 1982: 73). Part of the explanation for this undoubtedly lies in the fact that *belian sentiu* is easier to learn than the older *belian* forms (which use many more words, and so demand much more time and practice to master). Another, and perhaps more interesting reason for this, is the use of foreign languages in *belian sentiu*, and what could be called a "downriver aesthetics," with a greater stress on artistic performance and refined (*halus*) conduct, which many younger people find attractive.[7]

That *belian sentiu* was recognized as akin to Hindu Kaharingan in discussions among the ritual participants, as well as through the presence of the Hindu Kaharingan spirits visiting the *sentiu* ritual, is no wonder then. *Belian sentiu* and Hindu Kaharingan are alike in that they both reformulate local tradition. They are, of course, also similar in that they use foreignness to achieve this; foreign elements are not only borrowed but encapsulated in the local world, and thus made part of it. They are, to make an analogy with the Biak of former Irian Jaya (today West Papua), "resisting what is strange by making it [their] own" (Rutherford 1996: 600). In order to resist the power of others—so as to counter the accusations of primitiveness connected with "lack of religion," among other things—both similarities and differences have to be stressed. By making oneself similar to the other, one gains the power to be unlike. The issue here, clearly, is "not so much staying the same, but maintaining sameness through alterity" (Taussig 1993: 129). Tak Dinas, as well as many of the other ritual participants in this particular ritual, was engaging in a project in which *belian sentiu* was about much more than curing; for them, *belian sentiu* formed part of an attempt to sustain a distinct, local tradition.

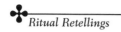

Truth as Experiment

Ma Sarakang, suddenly walking in during the ritual, looking as if he was performing a parody of Muslimness, unsettles any simple understandings about what it might mean to speak from the margins, much like Uma Adang does in Tsing's (1993) study of Meratus Dayak marginality (cf. also Rutherford 2000). Margins, as Tsing has conceptualized it, are the "zones of unpredictability at the edges of discursive stability, where contradictory discourses overlap, or where discrepant kinds of meaning-making converge" (1994: 279). Influenced by this conception, my intention here is to show how some people, participating in a particular ritual, who are occupying a space that is in many ways marginal, engage in a project not so much intended as overt resistance, but formed as an experiment in which the complexity of the surrounding world is invoked, and its power relations played with. This is an experiment rooted in sensuousness, infused by the unpredictability of life. As such, this experiment is both political and existential for the participants, and marginality, although clearly important, is not all that is at issue for them. My intention is to move beyond the political ground explored by Tsing (1993) in her inspiring study of Meratus Dayak marginality, aiming to add an existential dimension to the query at hand, and thus, to some degree, to de-emphasize the political rationality of peoples inhabiting such marginal spaces.

The foreignness introduced by Ma Sarakang at this point of the ritual is not in any easy way part of the engagement with foreignness otherwise sought for in the ritual. Ma Sarakang is not integrating his Muslimness with the *sentiu* style (although he could do that, as he was a fully learned *belian sentiu* himself), but keeps its foreignness intact, so to speak, turning it into prayer instead of dancing, for example. This does not mean that his intentions are to overthrow or lessen Tak Dinas' authority; instead, he is bringing in a power of his own, although in a somewhat "obtuse" (Barthes 1977) way, through a behavior which in another context would seem ordinary, but which here appears misplaced, strange.[8] He is acting in accordance with personal experience—having traveled widely in East Kalimantan, but not to Central Kalimantan as some other participants (e.g., Langkong)—bringing in his knowledge of Muslim behavior as still another possibility (we should not forget that Nen Pare was his wife, and that her well-being was thus of much more concern to him than to most other attendants, some of whom had not forgotten accusations in the recent past). His behavior reminds us of how uncontrollable life is, how ambiguous every attempt at coming to terms with its indeterminacy ultimately must be.

Interacting with spirits (and many times with people, for that part), one is confronted with what Mary Steedly has described as a "question of plausibility" (as opposed to certainty), that is, a question of "how one goes about making sense of something you can never get to the bottom of" (1993: 35). As Steedly argues for Karo spirit mediums, attitudes toward spirits are not characterized by "belief in the existential sense" (faith is really not very relevant here) (1993: 35). Spirits, whether Karo or Luangan, are not blindly believed in, but rather actively made sense of, frequently distrusted, and casually rather than devoutly accepted, because ultimately they are not known, and no one even pretends to know them completely. By stressing the bottomlessness and the uncertainty involved in spirit interaction, I want to draw attention to how ritual sense-making is formed in an emergent present (Schieffelin 1996), viable "in between the segments of ritual" (Taussig 1987: 442), but not necessarily applicable or even thought to be so outside. I thereby join Taussig in a critique of an anthropological tendency to explain ritual—and authorize interpretations—through "the imagery of order" (1987: 441). In particular, I want to raise a criticism against a somewhat instrumental or goal-oriented view of ritual, according to which its meaning can straightforwardly be equated to the anticipated outcomes outside it, which is implicit even in some analyses which are otherwise attentive to the emergent and responsive qualities of ritual. As in V. Turner's understanding of the dialectic between communitas and structure, which involves the view that people who go through *rites de passage* return to structure "revitalized by their experience of communitas" (1969: 129), ritual action in anthropological interpretations often seems to translate rather too easily into concrete effects in the realm outside ritual.

An interesting parallel to the Luangan case can be found in an interpretation by Marina Roseman (1996) of a healing ritual of the Temiar of peninsular Malaysia, which in many ways is strikingly similar to that led by Tak Dinas, in terms both of the types and wide range of concerns it addresses, and, it would seem, in terms of its evocative account, the manner whereby it does so (through address of spirits, and the media of chants and ritual paraphernalia). This ritual, set in a contemporary context of dramatic social transformation brought about by resettlement, logging, market integration and invasive interethnic encounters, expresses what Roseman calls a "cosmology gone wild," exemplified by a spirit medium treating illnesses with both "forest" and "foreign" etiologies, invoking spirits from both "upstream" and "downstream," which themselves form spatio-cultural categories with boundaries and meanings no longer as clear as they used to be. Like the ritual performed by Tak Dinas, it is focused on the healing of a particular patient—in this case an infant suffering from constipation—but it nevertheless emerges as a multidimensional reflexive project of collective self-deliberation. Through the performance of this ritual, as Roseman describes it, "community members join to choreograph and orchestrate their animated spirit world, bringing the presence of invasive outforesters temporarily under their control" (1996: 262). The author concludes the analysis by stating that:

> Temiars invent a poetics from the clash of competing societies. Through such creations, cultures carve their musics of survival, and gain the strength to carry on. Refreshed by the cool liquid of the spirits, "lightened" ... as if a load were removed—"empowered," to use a cosmopolitan metaphor—Temiars return to the realm of daily life. (Roseman 1996: 264)

Where this interpretation differs from mine is on the emphasis on a return to the realm of daily life and the suggested (but undemonstrated) transmittal to it of a catharsis-like state attained in the ritual amounting to "social healing."[9] From the perspective of my experience of the Luangans, the significance of what takes place in this ritual appears to articulate, a little too well, with the realm of daily life outside it. Social healing, in the Luangan case, or what would come closest to it, was nowhere near as concrete or straightforward. As for the Wana described by Atkinson (1987b: 344), who criticizes Claude Lévi-Strauss's (1963) analysis of the cathartic efficacy of a Cuna ritual, "abreaction is a potential neither systematically sought nor invariably realized in ritual performance." Missing in Roseman's interpretation, at least if it was to be adapted to the Luangan case, is an appreciation of the delicate sense of how rituals are formed in a play of unstable ritual representations emergent and uniquely viable in—and especially—between the segments of the ritual. Also missing in a sense is the unpredictability of events as they unfold in time (cf. Bourdieu 1977: 4–9), success never being fixed and conclusive, but measured and re-measured in "a continually changing present situation" (Steedly 1993: 11), and among the Luangans, seldom and only reluctantly evaluated after a ritual in the first place. Based on my Luangan experience, it would seem that the interpretation somewhat glosses over the vagueness and ambiguity of the relationship between the ritual and non-ritual realm, between representations and the represented. As I have tried to make clear, Luangan ritual representations, like those of Brechtian epic theater, are "never complete in [themselves], but ... openly and continually compared with the life represented" (Mitchell 1973: xiii, quoted in Taussig 1987: 445). This inescapable incompleteness of representations, we may note, is a problem which bears upon the above-mentioned one of ritual plausibility, which in the particular Luangan case presented here, is a question about how a technique aimed at curing, admittedly uncertain in its outcome, is made to seem credible and meaningful even when the curing fails. In this case, as apparently in the Temiar and many others too, this question essentially pertains to the open-ended relationship between spirits and human beings, which is created and re-created in the ritual, but not easily or lastingly transmitted beyond.

The participants in the ritual led by Tak Dinas did not return to daily life refreshed or empowered, at least not all of them, and none of them unambiguously, although the ritual certainly contained its moments of refreshment and empowerment.[10] As for Nen Pare, she did feel a little bit better for a couple of weeks after the ritual ended, but then got worse again, refusing to eat, and within two months literally starved to death. She never became Darma, at least not for most of the villagers, who continued to call her by either her personal name or by the teknonym Nen Pare.[11] Nen Bujok continued to care for her sister, feeling hopeful at times, but most of the time rather depressed. Many of the participants were in fact skeptical about the possibility of curing Nen Pare through a ritual in the first place. Kakah Ramat, an old *belian* specialized in the *luangan* and *bawo* styles of curing, and considered one of the most knowledgeable shamans in the region, made it very clear that he considered Nen Pare as not really standing a chance if she did not have the operation (Kakah Ramat himself had already performed several *belian* rituals for Nen Pare, and in fact even did so once more—although he was no less skeptical than before—the day before she died, when asked to by her family). Ma Geneng, Nen Pare's brother and one of the organizers of the ritual, remarked that Nen Pare was already rotten inside, and that it was therefore most unlikely that she would recover. Tak Dinas herself was hesitant to take up the case, and was persuaded to do so as much by kin obligations and expectations among her apprentices, as by assurances that Nen Pare was feeling better (Tak Dinas, resident in a downstream village some distance away, was first called to conduct another ritual in a neighboring village, then asked to perform the *belian* for Nen Pare by her family, who took the opportunity to do so when she was in the neighborhood).

The authority of Tak Dinas did not derive from her ability to control an uncontrollable world, but from her power to make sense of it in its arbitrariness. The ritual discussed in this chapter can be said to have formed itself like a montage; things happened, not always as planned, sentiments and moods shifted, spirits arrived, people entered the house, talked, danced, became possessed, slept. There were interruptions: dogs trying to get in that were thrown out (Tak Dinas did not allow dogs to enter the house during the ritual, in respect for her Muslim spirit guests), discussions so interesting that dancers had to pause, delays relating to the preparation of ritual paraphernalia and food, prolonging the ritual. Like Walter Benjamin's preoccupation with montage, and like the *yagé* nights in South America, the ritual technique used by Tak Dinas can be said to be "not bound to an image of truth as something deep and general hidden under layers of superficial and perhaps illusory particulars. Rather, what is at work here is an image of truth as experiment, laden with particularity, now in this guise, now as that one" (Taussig 1987: 445).

Tak Dinas' sense-making takes the form of an exploration, allowing the complexity of the Luangan world to enter the ritual, the negotiation between people and spirits. What she does is open up a space of possibilities, one in which recovering is made possible. For ritual participants, this space can accommodate quite different projects; in the ritual discussed here, the use of *belian sentiu* to create a "different" place (de Certeau 1986: 229; cf. Spyer 1996:

43) within the Indonesian nation-state came to be a leading one, just like the Temiar ritual described by Roseman (1996) served to resituate the Temiars at the center of an increasingly complex environment. Another issue, which emerged as a prospect in the ritual, was the empowerment of women. A woman herself, Tak Dinas inspired other women to participate, encouraging them to stand up, to dance, to become *belian*. As the ritual proceeded there were more and more women actively taking part, some of them just following Tak Dinas' dancing, others performing as fellow *belian* or apprentices, "answering her" (*nuing*), repeating her words and gestures. For these women, Tak Dinas' somewhat feminine aesthetics, her way of accentuating them through movement, attire, and appearance, formulated a different way to gain ritual power, one in which performance was emphasized as much as formalization through words.[12] This does not mean, however, that her aesthetics were not attractive to men as well; Mancan, her male apprentice, was one example; he was very excited about performing with her, and when he performed a similar ritual in her absence a few months later, he was dressed up as a woman for part of the time. Although Luangan women are in no way excluded from the opportunity of studying to become *belian*, very few chose to do so in the late 1990s, partly because they found it uncomfortable to study with male *belian*. Some had, however, seen their chance in Tak Dinas, who in her turn willingly took on apprentices, the sheer number of them adding to her ritual authority. For these women Tak Dinas' curing thus formed a female project, one in which Tak Dinas encouraged them into participation, a participation at the center of things, not on its periphery.[13]

Nen Pare's dance—so unlikely and so unforeseeable, yet such an evocative image of what ritual plausibility in this ritual was about—shows us how the negotiation between spirits and people, in its sensuousness and mimetic excess, was practically experienced as formulating a possibility, an opening. Nen Pare did not dance because she was recovering, but because she was made to believe that she might do so (she was probably also dancing for the same reason as the other women, driven by a sense of female power and togetherness). Contacting spirits and negotiating with them, Tak Dinas cannot be sure of the outcome, but what she can do is try to persuade both spirits and people of what it could be. Tak Dinas is not denying the unpredictability of life in doing this, nor the constraints

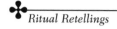

inherent in Luangan marginality, but with the help of her spirit familiars, in their "hybrid authenticity" (Clifford 1997: 187), she conjures open-endedness, and thus shows life to be changeable, illnesses curable.

The role of ancestor spirits in this process points to the importance of tradition, of making a connection between a future, ultimately unknown, and a past, already confronted and lived. Negotiating with spirits, Tak Dinas refers to both the continuity of tradition, and the unpredictability of life, and it is, it seems to me, from the tension between them that she evokes what I have referred to as a possibility.

Notes

1. A *blontang* is a carved hardwood pole (often anthropomorphic) used in secondary mortuary rituals for tying the water buffalo to be sacrificed.
2. *Darma wanita* is an association for the wives of civil servants, founded by the late Mrs. Suharto.
3. Pahu is the name of the nearest river area inhabited by a majority of Muslims. Like most Malays living close to or among the Luangans, these Muslims were originally Dayaks. Nevertheless, in the village where the ritual described in this chapter took place, present-day inhabitants use the word Pahu not only for the inhabitants of this river area but also as a generic designation for all Malays; even the national language (which is a standardized form of Malay) may sometimes be referred to as *bahasa Pahu*.
4. Regarding the question of the origin of *belian sentiu*, one has to consider that there are also some other forms of Malay curing such as *belian kenyong* and *belian dewa-dewa* (to be distinguished from Tak Dinas' *belian dewa-dewa*), which are used by some Luangans, and which are sometimes regarded as separate forms of curing, sometimes classified as variants of *belian sentiu*. Tak Dinas used to practise *belian kenyong*, in which she employed Muslim *blis* as spirit familiars, a dangerous enterprise which she abandoned on the request of her daughter, who feared for her mother's life. *Belian kenyong* is regarded as an older form of curing than *belian sentiu*, and Tak Dinas claimed that it was introduced to her home village when she was eight years old. It was not practiced in the village in which the curing ritual for Nen Pare took place.
5. Andreas Massing (1982: 73–74) implies that the *balei* is also seen as a mosque by some Benuaq Dayaks. Whereas Luangans make ritual constructions similar to the *balei* during all larger *belian* rituals (but outside the house, unlike this case), this one (which was called *balei mensigit lima*) was nevertheless made to appear special—more like a place of worship—by being unusually richly decorated and used throughout the ritual, as well as, more specifically, on account of the dance in front of it, with each dancer performing a solo dance standing on a gong, while holding an offering.

After Tak Dinas' ritual for Nen Pare had ended, members of the household which organized it lit a candle at the *balei* each night for a week, standing silently in front of it for a moment.

6. I am talking about Kaharingan Luangans here, not those Luangans who have converted to Christianity. Christianity, in the form of both Protestantism and Catholicism, was introduced to the central parts of the Luangan region in the 1930s. Today half of the Luangan population consider themselves as Christians, whereas the others regard themselves either as Hindu Kaharingans or as "still lacking a religion" (*belum beragama*). Some Luangans who "*belum beragama*" also consider themselves Kaharingans, as opposed to Hindu Kaharingans; the people in the village where the ritual lead by Tak Dinas took place all belong to this category.

7. Attraction to *belian sentiu* was especially evident in the case of Mancan, Tak Dinas' enthusiastic male apprentice and her co-*belian* in the ritual performed for Nen Pare. He, it is interesting to note, had an exceptional interest in development and modernization in comparison with other villagers.

8. His behavior would seem ordinary in Malay society, or in mixed Dayak-Malay villages, and some urban situations. Here, however, at a Kaharingan ritual in a village where all inhabitants were Kaharingans, it did seem a little odd, despite Ma Sarakang's interest in selective aspects of Islam, and the fact that he had chosen to categorize himself as Muslim on his identity card.

9. Also, there was in the Luangan case not really a sense of *control* of the patently unpredictable spirits and other external forces that were represented in the ritual. This admittedly seems to be the case among the Temiar as well, as suggested by Roseman in a later article (2002: 131): "The Temiar world is one in which the constituting of self and community is based on never-ending dialectical incorporation of that which is outside, be it spirits, other humans, neighboring forest peoples, non-foresters, or colonials. This process of dialectical incorporation, negotiated in sound and motion, destabilizes and decenters as much as it controls and contains."

10. After eight days and eight nights, involving not just participation through dancing and intense socializing, but also the work of bringing materials from the forest for the ritual paraphernalia and then manufacturing it, as well as drying, husking, and cooking rice for more and more attendants, most of the participants were, in fact, quite relieved when it was all over, feeling primarily tired, rather than refreshed. This highlights a difference between Luangan and Temiar curing rituals, as Temiar curing rituals do not require as much ritual work and care of guests by the hosts (Roseman, personal communication).

11. Luangans have both "personal" names, and names that can be regarded as teknonyms, that is, names that they get when they have children or grandchildren, or when they reach the age when they normally would do so. Female teknonyms take the form of Nen X or Tak X (i.e., mother of X, or grandmother of X) while male teknonyms, according to the same logic, read as Ma X or Kakah X. Central Luangan practice is perhaps unusual in

that many people get their teknonyms not from children or grandchildren but from other "things," such as habits or particular events associated with the person in question, or as the result of a wordplay connecting the teknonym with the personal name. Nen Pare, for example, means "mother of rice"; Darma was a substitute for her personal name. Personal names are normally used for persons on a lower generational level than the speaker, and sometimes also for people on the same generational level, and of the same approximate age as oneself; for older people, one is not allowed to pronounce personal names but must use teknonyms. For some reason, some people never get teknonyms which "stick to them." Both real names and teknonyms may be changed over time, personal names often after severe illness, teknonyms with changed status. A new personal name usually replaces the former one, whereas several teknonyms are commonly used at the same time.

12. Tak Dinas' way of stressing performative elements in the ritual was not just a way for her of establishing female shamanship (see Tsing 1993 on the creation of female shamanship among the Meratus Dayaks), but as much a result of her being a *belian* by "*keturunan*." Ma Putup, a male shaman who was also a *belian* by "*keturunan*," stressed performance as much as she did, although in a very different way. Being a *belian* by "*keturunan*" means that ritual authority is less attached to an office (cf. Bloch 1974) than it is for "ordinary" *belian*, and more dependent on "personal" innovations (which are normally received as gifts from the spirits).

13. During my fieldwork women participated in *belian* rituals as assistants (*penyempatung*), who helped the shaman to prepare offerings, and answered him (typically quietly, with backs turned to the audience) when he spoke with "spirit voices." Women also participated in rituals by playing the musical instruments (as did men and children) and by cooking the food for spirits and participants. Women very seldom performed as *belian*; when they did, it was as *belian sentiu*. There is also one *belian* style called *belian bawe* ("woman *belian*"), which in the past is said to have been practiced mostly by female shamans, but which today is practiced mostly by men. Exactly why female shamans have gradually become increasingly rare is unclear, but it may be related to "outside" influence (see Roseman 1991: 127 for similar issues among the Temiar).

Chapter Three

Making Tactile
Ganti Diri Figures and the Magic of Concreteness

Dewi Itak Silu Malik and Dewa Kakah Embung Mele were surprised to watch the work of God the Almighty. There was not one
of them [of the earthen figures that God had made] which had
turned into a real human being, destined to inhabit the earth that
had been prepared for them.

God then happened to overhear the talk of Dewi Itak Silu Malik
and Dewa Kakah Embung Mele. He told them so: my intention
was indeed to create human beings. But after I had turned around
those figures that I had made, they turned out to be the races of
wok and *bongai* instead [i.e., spirit beings].

Dewi Itak Silu Malik thus seated herself for a *belian* ritual, for a
turning around of the figures. She did so while holding a *biyowo*
leaf, an *olung* and a *jie* leaf. She started chanting, using a special
melody and special words. She whisked and waved, she fanned
and turned around those figures.

And thus they became human beings; human beings who could
move their feet, stir their hands, twinkle their eyes, turn their
bodies.

—Excerpts from the Luangan origin story as written down by
Lemanius (1996, my translation)[1]

In mythical times the goddess Itak Silu Malik turned around some
human-like figures, and by turning them she made them into real
human beings. While Allatallah, the almighty creator God, had
failed to make these figures into proper human beings, Itak Silu

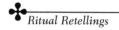

Malik succeeded. By turning them around, she transformed the copies into what they represented. Through her agency, they became real. This chapter is an exploration of the process by which Kakah Ramat and other *belian* curers call on Itak Silu Malik to help them turn around figures (*malik*, "to turn around," here means both to physically turn around, rotate, and to transform), assisting them in the making of representations that have magical power over what they represent. It is an exploration of the copies, the images creating what they are images of, and I will therefore start my analysis with a description of the images themselves, the objects—material objects as well as "objects" created through words—through which *belian* curers negotiate the relationship between human beings and spirits. I will thus attempt to describe the objects in their "objectness" (Taussig 1993: 2), trying to convey some of the concrete and sensuous qualities which I see as fundamental to how these images work.

Ritual Imagery

In order to apprehend this imagery, and the creation of it, we have to enter a *belian* ritual, the context in which the imagery is used. We are thus entering Kakah Ramat's house. It is a late evening in August 1996, and the sounds of drums are calling, telling us that a ritual has just started. Kakah Ramat's grandson's wife is feeling ill, she has suffered from sleeplessness and a general feeling of sickness for the last two weeks, and Kakah Ramat, a practicing shaman himself, has decided to hold a *belian* for her. This is not a big event, not a spectacular ritual, but a small curing session for a family member who is not very ill, but ill enough to cause concern.[2] Together with a few neighbors the family has gathered in the house, the necessary decorations have been made, and now Kakah Ramat starts the ritual by blowing on his bear tooth whistle. This is a *luangan* style ritual, a ritual focused on words and images, not on dancing and trancing which are characteristics of *bawo* and *sentiu* curing. Kakah Ramat, who at this time is an old man in his eighties, is an experienced shaman; he is considered by many of his neighbors as the most knowledgeable curer working in the *luangan* style. In his quiet and unobtrusive way he is a master of powerful words and images, words and images which here, once again, will take him, and us I hope, into the realm of ritual representations.

There is a *siur*, a large "fishing basket" (a rattan screen used to sieve for fish and river shrimp in flooded riverside grass) on the floor in the middle of the room, containing what might at first just seem to be pieces of wood, but which on closer inspection reveal themselves to be what you could call replicas. Some of them are wooden sticks, with eyes and mouths and traces of arms cut into them: rough representations of human beings. Others consist of small carved animal figurines: water buffaloes, pigs, chickens, goats. Still others represent musical instruments and heirloom objects: drums, gongs, Chinese jars, pearls. Then there are figurines resembling humans or animals, but not quite; some of them have a sharp, pointed head, others belong to anomalous categories of animals, such as tigers and water snakes—spirit figurines. All these different effigies are heaped together in the basket; some of them are old, shrouded with dust and cobwebs, others are new, smelling of fresh wood, still white in color. Next to the basket there is a row of miniature houses standing on the floor and hanging from the ceiling, all differently shaped, made of tree and plant parts, with roofs of various kinds of leaves. Inside each of these houses, which have open fronts and backs so that you can see through them, there are small white figurines made of rice paste, shaped like human beings with outstretched arms and legs, lying on pieces of banana

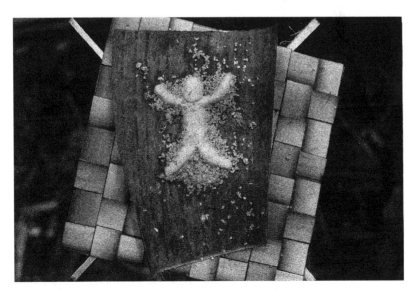

Figure 3.1. Rice paste figurine (*ganti diri*) depicting patient

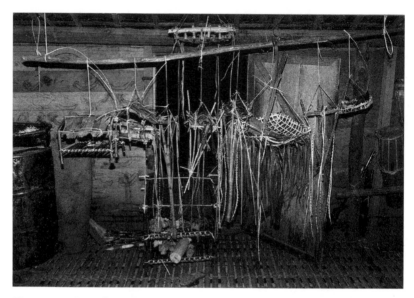

Figure 3.2. Spirit houses

leaf. Placed among these tiny figurines there are small portions of boiled rice, together with darkened clots of chicken blood.

Kakah Ramat is sitting cross-legged in the midst of these objects. He is chanting quietly, with his eyes closed—his gaze turned inward, his mouth full of betel. In his hand he holds a whisk of *biyowo* leaves as well as some *olung* and *jie* leaves, which he is moving slowly, back and forth.[3] On both his cheeks and on his bare chest he has yellow and white spots of turmeric and lime paste, decorations which make him visible and susceptible to the spirits. In front of him there is a plate with glowing-hot incense wood (*bemueng*), its smoke rising toward the ceiling along a sarong cloth twined as a rope (*penyelenteng*), which hangs down from the roof beams, connecting spirits and human beings. Next to the censer there is a white plate filled with uncooked rice, with a small porcelain bowl containing sticky rice placed on top of it, both decorated with red and yellow flowers, and the bowl has a burning candle in the center. Kakah Ramat is picking up a few seeds of rice, throwing them up into the air, letting them disperse at random. Tak Ramat, his wife and assistant who is sitting at his side, is squashing turmeric in a flat turtle-shaped ironwood mortar, making it into a bright yellow paste.

It is dark in the room; there is just a small oil lamp lighting up Kakah Ramat who is sitting close to it. The young woman for whom the ritual has been arranged is lying on the floor in a corner of the room, sleeping, together with her two small children. Mancan, her brother-in-law, is playing with a kitten, teaching it to chase mice. The attention of the few of us who are still awake is turned toward Mancan and the cat and toward the dead mouse he has fixed to a string as a toy for the indifferent kitten. Tired from the day's work of slashing undergrowth in their swidden fields, most of the people present have lain down on the floor, and they are soon falling asleep, lulled by Kakah Ramat's monotonous chanting.

It is, however, precisely in the chanting, in Kakah Ramat's mumbling words, that most of the action takes place at this moment. With his words Kakah Ramat has created a connection between spirits and human beings, he has opened up his body to the spirits, invited them to participate. It is at this point that we should pay close attention, because it is now that he turns his attention toward the effigies, toward the human-like figures, and the miniature houses. He does so with a hardly noticeable change of tune, starting a new song, initiating a process which is called *malik sepatung*, "turning the figures." He is whisking the *olung* and *jie* leaves back and forth over the figures in the basket, over the houses with their rice-paste inhabitants, the smell of dried leaves spreading in the room. Through his words he is turning the figures, first in the wrong way—seven turns— toward the setting sun and the waning moon, and then in the right way—eight times—toward the rising sun and the new moon, thus making them into substitutes for the patient, "the myna bird struck dumb," as she is here metaphorically called.[4]

Kakah Ramat's words make things happen as they are enunciated. They create and re-create objects and events—some visible, others invisible—through description and invitation. In order to perceive this process we have to open ourselves to Kakah Ramat's words, and step into the "empowered cognitive space" (Tsing 1993: 97) of his chanting, into the song of turning the figures. Kakah Ramat begins the song (which is presented below in full) by summoning some spirit familiars. With a hoarse voice he calls them.[5] Following the pattern of "undoing and redoing" (*pejiak pejiau*) he does everything incorrectly first. He thus calls flawed spirit familiars, lights charred incense wood (incense is thought to open the way of communication between a *belian* and the spirits), pours cloudy oil, smears rotten turmeric, rice paste turned sour (oil, turmeric, and rice paste are smeared on the chest and forehead of the *belian* as a sign that he opens himself for his spirit familiars). He then proceeds with the actual turning, here again doing it wrongly first, turning effigies made incorrectly in the wrong direction. Then, finally, he does it all over again, doing it in the right way this time. He sings hurriedly during this process, swallowing part of the words, just hinting at their constitution. Occasionally during the chant he pauses to clear his throat, or to spit out some betel nut juice. At points of transition he slows down and stretches vowels and syllables, including an "ooo-lololoooo" at regular intervals, assuring himself that the words will reach their destination.

MALIK SEPATUNG	TURNING THE FIGURES[6]
Nook Suit Ine Sao	Calling Suit, mother and wife
bero Bobok Uma Bao	with Bobok, father of Bao
bero Tiwak Ma Tawai	with Tiwak, father of Tawai
Silu Bisu Lintai Ngongo	Silu the Dumb One, Lintai the Idiot
Ayus Buok Intong Reboi	Ayus Buok, Intong Reboi
sulet Suit Ine Sao	come Suit, mother and wife
bero Bobok Uma Bao	with Bobok father of Bao
Silu Bisu Lintai Ngongo	Silu the Dumb One, Lintai the Idiot
Ayus Buok Intong Reboi	Ayus Buok, Intong Reboi[7]
nutung jemu areng	lighting the charred incense wood
nili olau burang	pouring the cloudy oil
matik jomit boto	smearing the rotten turmeric
burei benes	the rice paste turned sour
balik jurun sepatung	turning the wooden effigies
bera rentang kesali	together with the spirit houses
batek sepatung burei	complete with the rice paste figurines inside
butin Luing senenaring	the grains of Luing made human beings[8]
turu kali berebalik	seven times they're turned upside down
turu user berebele	seven turns they're turned around
turu jiak penejiau	seven falls they're felled down
dero balik sala belisei	this is the wrong turning
puput sala belisei	the defective manufacturing
sepatung sala kotek	the wooden effigy is wrongly carved
bayar bulau sala pulas	the gold which is paid is badly cut
sedediri sala urai	the rice paste figurine is badly formed
ganti beau jadi gilir	the exchange object is not received

timbang beau jadi gade	the substitute does not become a pledge
leban roten beau uli	the maladies are not returning
saan beau unur	the illness is not backing off
dongo beau golek	the sick one is not recovering
roten beau meme	the injuries are not healed
oreng jiak penejiau	this is the end of the turning and whisking
napang maten olo tonep	in the direction of the setting sun
nelama bulan punus	toward the waning moon
nuju Batu Rimbung Apui	head towards the Stone of Eternal Fire[9]
napang Goa Luang Olo	toward the Cave of Daylight
baling dining upak putang	penetrating the wall of *meranti* bark[10]
jaba sasak boa oleng	breaking through the trap at the river's mouth
balik tou elang pesan	turning the sugar-cane across the squeezer
bele empa elang wale	moving the betel quid to the other chin
balik napang olo sulet	turning around toward the breaking day
ngenawe bulan ure	facing the new moon emerging
sulet rengin meroe	there is refreshing coolness arriving
empet lampung melimei	renewed prosperity coming
balik kunen belisei	the turning becomes proper turning
puput kunen tengkieu	the manufacturing becomes correct
berejadi pemakar ganti	becomes an object of exchange
Ma Renga ganti diri	Ma Renga substituting for the self
gantin tiong pererongo	in return for the myna bird struck dumb
jadi rentang kesali	the spirit house becomes a dwelling place
lenuang lambang olang	a raft to lie down on
adi jakit bantan unan	a barque to row with[11]
oongok roten uli	a place for the illness to return to
pengantai saan unur	an abode for the sickness
uli tuhan ka lei	return together with your master[12]
la langit awe ulun	to the skies where there are no people
la tana awe ulun	to the lands where there are no people
balik tou elang pesan	turn the sugar-cane across the squeezer
bele empa elang wale	move the betel quid to the other chin
balik Itak Silu Malik	turn with Itak Silu Malik
Kakah Mung Mele	with Kakah Mung Mele
Biyayung Memalik	Biyayung the Turner
Bensiang Ma Muser	Bensiang the Converter
malik jurun sepatung	turn around the wooden effigy
balik napang olo sulet	turn toward the breaking day
ngelama bulan empet	face the new moon emerging
balik rengin meroe	turn into refreshing coolness
lampung melimei	renewed prosperity

berejadi ganti gilir	become an object of exchange
timbang gade gantin unuk	a pledge substituting
tiong pererongo	for the myna bird struck dumb
bagin muung poyut bulet	so that the *muung* bush becomes full of berries
bekakang poyut bisa	the *bekakang* shrub hangs heavy with yields
adi kukup nunuk nyang tempung	so that the strangler fig follows the tree falling
pernalau nyang topa	and the staghorn fern weighs down the branch[13]
liang sepatung iro	take this wooden effigy
bagin belibet beau empet	so that what leaves does not turn back
belayar beau uli	what sails away does not return
enko telahui molo	what walks away gets lost
uaa telahui watun	what ends ceases completely
liang sepatung iro	take that wooden effigy
bagin bongai bawen mulang	for *bongai* and the *mulang* woman
bagin blis buhan setan	for *blis*, the family of *setan*[14]
kayu entun simpung	for the trees in the forest groves
raba entun ruo	for the trees in the groves of spirits[15]
penulek ka salung uli	to tell you visitors to leave
penungkeng ka pasang munur	to make you all withdraw
penous bundrung juus	having you restore the soul
penuker ruo walo	change back the eight essences[16]
juus tiong pererongo	the soul of the myna bird struck dumb
pulun bulau tungke kesong	the poor one with the heavy breathing
adi dongen busek golek renak galak	so that the sick will recover soon
torik otau lio toto	quickly with a clean glance
ketakar kunen awat kunen anam	after being touched by the cure
ngankar asi kunen ado	after being refreshed by the cleansing
ketakar juus uli	after the soul has returned
ketanyak ruo unur	after the essences have turned back
balik oit utut jemu	turn with the smoke of the incense
belisei tanges tutung	turn with the rice tossed over it
bemueng saing tamun	the *agathis* from the top of the mountain
kulat dupa tenung batu	the moss on the stone
gengari datai Tiwei	the *gengari* tree on the banks of the Teweh River
kumpai lati lili lio	the grass by the slippery stones
rukang rukut padang mulir	the *rukang rukut* flower in its garden
bengkiras batang bawo	the *bengkiras* tree with its high trunk
siopot kayun kuleng	the *gaharu* tree of decorations[17]
balik napang olo sulet	turn to where the day breaks

ngelama bulan empet	face the new moon emerging
jadi sepatung ganti	become an effigy of exchange
Ma Renga ganti diri	Ma Renga substituting for the self
gantin tiong pererongo	in exchange for the myna bird struck dumb
walo kali berebalik	eight times turn upside down
sie user berebele	nine turns turn around
napang maten olo sulet	in the direction of the rising sun
ngelama bulan empet	facing the new moon emerging
sulet rengin meroe	there is refreshing coolness arriving
sulet lampung melimei	renewed prosperity coming
sepatung kunen kotek	the wooden effigy is carved properly
bayar bulau kunen polas	the gold which is paid is cut correctly
sedediri kunen urai	the rice paste figurines are rightly formed
kesali kunen tentang	the spirit houses are erected
jadi ganti na gilir	become objects of exchange
timbang na gade	pledges given in return
gantin unuk tiong dongo	substituting for the body of the sick myna
ulun bulau tungke kesong	the poor one with the heavy breathing
uli ujung kerepuru	return through the hole at the back of the head[18]
napang pakang peluke	aim at the openings between the shoulders
uli oit rengin roe	return with cool refreshment
ngangung lampung limei	bring renewed prosperity
oit kosi muan golek	hurry do it fast
torik otau lio toto!	quickly with a clean glance!

As God once failed to make the human-like figures into real human beings, so does Kakah Ramat first fail when he attempts to turn the effigies. Kakah Ramat does so deliberately, though. Turning the figures seven times, toward the setting sun and the waning moon, he is turning them in the direction of death and misfortune—seven is a number which Luangans associate with death, while the setting sun and the waning moon are states associated with danger and misfortune. When he, through his words, lights charred incense wood, pours cloudy oil, smears rotten turmeric, he enacts the wrong-doing and brings it into the domain of the senses, letting it smell, look, and feel wrong. In order to undo the illness he evokes death and adversity, making abstract categories concrete, sensible.[19] It is from this point that Kakah Ramat starts turning things the other way, turning "the sugar cane across the squeezer," moving "the betel quid to the other chin" (the latter one not a far-flung metaphor if we remember that Kakah Ramat has his own mouth full of betel while singing).

Turning the other way, "in the direction of the breaking day," "facing the new moon," Kakah Ramat is turning toward refreshing coolness and renewed prosperity, creating what could be conceived of as transformed prerequisites. With the help of Itak Silu Malik and her companions he turns a bad and inauspicious condition into a space of possibilities. Like bushes hanging heavy with yield or branches weighted down by epiphytic ferns, the figures are tangibly transformed by Kakah Ramat's words; they are forced to turn by the sheer weight of the words. The metaphors in the song can be seen as examples of what Arendt (1973: 19) has referred to as metaphors "in [their] original, nonallegorical sense of *metapherein* (to transfer)," that is, as metaphors establishing connections that are sensuously perceived in their immediacy, rather than constituting cognitive riddles to be solved (cf. Fernandez 1977). Kakah Ramat's words do not just produce change, they also, and perhaps more importantly, bring forth that change corporeally. It is when the words are joined with the smoke of the incense, the rice tossed over it, that the transformation becomes materialized, and hence realized (at this stage Kakah Ramat picks up the censer, holding it in his hands while singing).

An aspect not to forget here is the whisking (*ngaper*), an activity carried out not just "textually," but also physically. At the same time as Kakah Ramat turns the figures with his words, he also confers the transformation on them by slowly whisking and fanning over them with the vaguely fragrant *olung* and *jie* leaves. Whatever disruptive elements there are that might disturb the process, these are swept aside by this action. At the same time, the whisking and fanning movement also quite literally produces a cool and favorable condition. Words and movements work together here, creating a transformation that is sensually perceivable by spirits and human beings.

In the process, the human-like figures become personified and receive a name (Ma Renga). They are thus symbolically recognized as becoming, if not real human beings as God's earthen figures eventually became, then at least empowered representations of human beings. The role of Itak Silu Malik (lit. "Grandmother Silu the Turner") in this process is not just that of spirit assistant; in a way, she *is* the turning. As the verb *malik*, "to turn," suggests, she personifies it—she is the act that she is called upon to perform. Like Kakah Embung Mele (lit. "Grandfather Embung the Turner"), who is never mentioned otherwise than as a sort of appendage to her (*mele* also means "to turn"), she seems to lead no separate existence apart from her ritual function. She is, in other words, what the Luangans refer to as a "true" or "genuine" spirit familiar (*mulung bene*). Rather than Kakah Ramat embodying her, she is the embodiment of the act of turning performed by Kakah Ramat. Empowered by her, Kakah Ramat turns not only the human-like figures, but also the miniature houses, which become dwelling places for the illness-causing spirits, rafts for them to lie down on, places to return to.[20] In a similar way, the animal figures (although not separately mentioned in the song) become livestock for the spirits to breed, the heirloom objects valuables for them to keep, and, not least, the spirit figurines become companions for them to associate with.

Chanting and whisking the figures into being, Kakah Ramat makes them into what Luangans call *ganti diri* or *gantin unuk* ("substitutes for the self" or "substitutes for the person"). The verb *ganti* means "to exchange," "to substitute for," or "to represent." The *ganti diri* figures are a special category of figures distinct from others that are used in *belian* rituals. They are representations of the patient, or of offerings, or spirits, which are used primarily as gifts to spirits (but also, in the case of spirit figurines, as bodies to return to for spirits evicted from the sick person). In different ways, the *ganti diri* figures all stand for the patient. The rice paste figurines (*sedediri*), for example, simultaneously represent and substitute for her (and by extension, all other ritual participants), and they are given to the spirits in exchange for the patient's soul (*juus*), which is thought to have been stolen or disturbed by malevolent or dissatisfied spirits (jointly called *blis*), who thereby have induced her condition. All figures—those representing people, as well as those representing heirlooms, livestock or spirits—constitute gifts, or pledges as they are also referred to in the song. They are exchange objects in a system of "pictorial exchange": objects through which the reciprocity between spirits and human beings is invoked, sustained, and made concrete and through which, if all goes well, the spirits are appeased and pleased, and the relationship between spirits and human beings can be renegotiated.

"The *ganti diri* figures are to human beings what walls are to houses." With these words Ma Dengu, one of Kakah Ramat's neighbors, once described the nature of images like the ones used in this

101

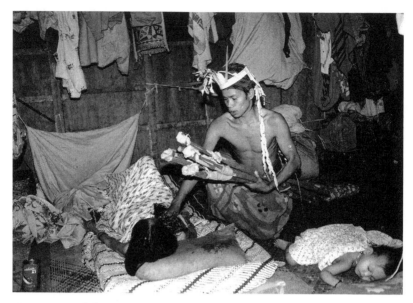

Figure 3.3. A *belian* holding some *ganti diri* sticks while curing a patient

ritual. In an indirect way, the simile says something crucial about what we are dealing with here. It elucidates something important about what is at stake in this process of first making images, and then bringing them into being through singing and whisking. What it points to, as I see it, is the importance of concreteness, of tactility.[21] The *ganti diri* figures offer a form of protection which is not abstract but highly tangible (as walls are). They are sensuously part of what they are protecting. Making copies of something involves coming in contact with that same thing (cf. Taussig 1993: 21). Similarly, in order to make substitutes of the self one has to put something of that self into the substitutes. This brings us back to Kakah Ramat and his performance, since contact is in fact very much what is on his agenda at the moment.

There is one more thing which he has to do with the figures before they can be handed over to the spirits. Kakah Ramat still has to bring them into being for his distracted human audience. He has to make them sensuously part of the world that they represent in still another way. The sleeping persons in Kakah Ramat's audience are woken up and urged to participate at this stage. Kakah Ramat takes some of the carved wooden sticks in his hand and walks over to the patient, holding out the figures in front of her face. Still half asleep, the sick woman leans forward and spits on the effigies. With a fingertip she then takes some saliva from her sleeping children's mouths, and puts it on the roughly carved mouths of the figures. After that Kakah Ramat brings the effigies to her husband, who also spits on them. From him they are then taken to everyone else in the room, and everyone present in turn spits on the images, which so are made, not just into copies, but also, in a more profound way, into part of those that they are made to form substitutes for.

Images for Spirits

> But what pleasure he brings the spirits with his lavish description, bringing them into life!
>
> —Michael Taussig (1993: 111)

Copy and contact, these are the ingredients of James Frazer's (1922) sympathetic magic. The magic used by Kakah Ramat is, however, a magic not so much bound to a law of similarity or a law of contact, as it is a magic evolving from the capacity of representations to simultaneously create and transform what they represent, a magic which Taussig (1993) has labeled "the magic of mimesis." Inspired by Taussig, I argue that what Kakah Ramat does in this ritual is as much to create a reality as it is to change that reality, and his creation of it is, in fact, a precondition for change. It is by making things sensuously real that they become real for those perceiving them. Copy and contact are here elements in a system of knowing which is not primarily based on contemplation, but rather on tactility (cf. Benjamin 1973a).

This is, I believe, how we must look at the images if we are to grasp something of why they are made, and how they function in the ritual. In the process of producing imagery, neither the words, nor the material objects, are enough in themselves; but together, and in combination with such performative actions as the whisking and the spitting, they act upon the world evocatively, bringing forth a vision of it in which change can be not only conceived of, but also perceived. What is at issue for Kakah Ramat is to make his representations of the world as concrete as possible so that human beings and spirits may accept them not only as representations of reality,

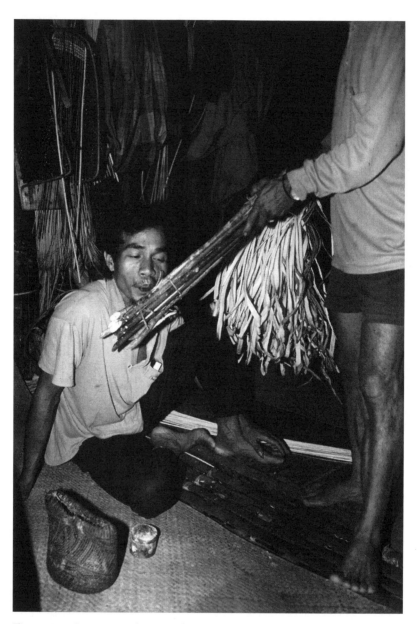

Figure 3.4. Spitting on the *ganti diri* sticks

but also *as* reality. In this process, the figures are not mere details; on the contrary, they can be regarded as essential to what is going on. Representation here is fundamentally about substitution, and it would be hard to conceive of any substitution in the first place without embodiment and materialization.

Contributing to the evocative power of the figures is not just their tangibility but also the complexity that they present. The world evoked through Kakah Ramat's imagery is a world of human beings and spirits, as well as animals, houses and valuables. The different spirits negotiated with in the ritual are presented with a multitude of desirable effigies, many of which are made with a particular spirit in mind. These figures are made of a variety of materials, and in some cases in many different versions, often used simultaneously. *Tentuwaja*, a forest spirit with whom Kakah Ramat negotiates, is, for example, presented with figures representing human beings—some of which are made of rice paste, others of different sorts of wood—and with representations of Chinese jars, pearl necklaces and clothing, as well as with a wooden effigy representing *tentuwaja* itself, a human-like figure with a sharply pointed head.[22] In the same way, *timang*, the tiger or clouded leopard spirit, is also presented with offerings of human beings, animals and valuables, as well as with a wooden figure resembling the spirit itself, a roughly carved cat-like creature with pink dots painted on it. Different spirits are also presented with different houses, taking the shape of longhouses as well as farmhouses: the house with the roof of *topus timang* leaves, which are leaves with reddish dots on them, is intended for *timang*, while the house made of wood and leaves of the *kelewono* tree, which grows in old secondary forest, is intended for *kelelungan*, the refined spirits of dead people, and the *potok pate* house of decayed *potok* wood is made for *keratan*, spirits of old woods and mountains, known for their awesome call and the bad dreams they can invoke.

When a decision has been made to hold a *belian* ritual, the *belian* gives instructions about what kind of figures and decorations are needed in that particular ritual, instructions which are often supplemented later on (the *belian* usually negotiates with many different spirits during a *belian* ritual, and new spirits often enter the scene during the course of events).[23] Some of the figures—the heirloom objects and animal effigies, for example—are used over and over again, and often lent between households, while others, such as the rice paste figurines, and most of the spirit houses, are made anew each time.

A spirit, or rather category of spirits, frequently called upon and depicted in *belian* is the water spirit *juata*, who is thought to cause biting pains in the stomach and so is often associated with diarrhea. *Juata* can be portrayed in a particularly wide range of manifestations—as a crocodile, monitor lizard, snake, turtle, crab, mollusk, water leech etc.—often in all these shapes on the same occasion. The figurines representing *juata* are most often made of rice paste, but they can also be made of sugar palm fibers, coconut leaves, or in the form of cakes (which are eaten by ritual participants at the end of the ritual). *Biang Belau*, a frightening, malevolent bear spirit, is portrayed as a large, dog-sized, wild boar-like statue made of black sugar palm fibers and placed on the ground outside the house. The representation of *Benturan Tana*, an earth spirit who can capture the soul of people who fall to the ground from the house, is similarly placed outside the house, beneath the doorsteps, and represented as a cumbersome clay figure with outstretched arms. During rituals for infants, small animal figurines (*sepatung abei*) carved out of banana trunks are often used; these are representations of animals

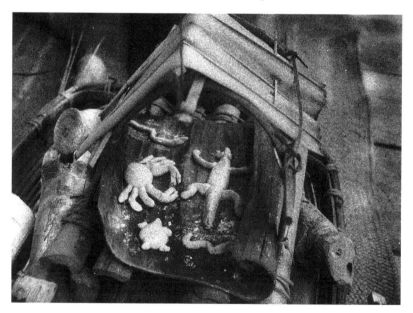

Figure 3.5. Images of *juata*, the water spirit, in its different manifestations

106

(gibbons, monkeys, porcupines, squirrels, deer, civets, mongooses and parrots, to name the most common) in which spirits (*abei*) known to disturb people with "weak souls," such as small children, sometimes reside. When the *belian* negotiates with the *seniang*, who are celestial guardian spirits of the fundamental conditions of nature and society, an image of the sky is constructed; this image consists of small yellow rice paste figurines representing the sun, the moon and the stars, distributed over a circular winnowing-tray.

The houses built for the spirits are as varied as the spirit figures, and are often made of materials which mimic the spirits' appearances or the habitats where they are said to dwell. For example, *timang*, a spirit taking the form of large feline animal, is, as we have seen, given a house with a roof of leaves with reddish dots on them, resembling the spirit's fur. Similarly, *juata* are given houses with roofs of riverside ferns and houses resembling rafts (*juata* are, in fact, also given a whole range of other houses, including both permanent constructions made of ironwood, and temporary constructions made of less durable material).

On some occasions the offerings given to the spirits are not processed materials taken from nature, but living creatures, such as grasshoppers or crabs, representing offerings of chicken and water buffaloes, that is, if translated into a kind of spirit language (cf. Viveiros de Castro 1998). A similar process of translation is performed when the spirits are given "clothes," "gongs," and "Chinese jars," consisting of packs of leaves, coils of liana, and broken-off pieces of termites' nests, respectively.

These various figures used in *belian* all, in one way or another, function as substitutes for the sick person(s); they are exchange objects through which Luangans evoke a world of reciprocity and through which the shamans reach out to and interact with the spirit world. They are not, however, substitutes in the sense that they are used for want of something better, as replacements for the real thing (the spirits are in fact given offerings of "real" things as well; they are, for example, given sacrifices of real animals, beside the figures, but some of them are said to prefer the images, or to want both). Just as God, with the help of Itak Silu Malik, once created human beings out of figures, so *belian* curers make figures when they want to ritually act upon the relationship between human beings and spirits. The making of images is something almost taken for granted, something that is always done in *belian* rituals, and particularly in *luangan* style rituals, where these figures are often particularly abundant. It is as elements in a system of pictorial exchange that the figures must be understood; their attractiveness is tied precisely to their being depictions, images.

The capacity of images to make something concrete and visible, and hence to make "real," is an essential part of what constitutes their effectiveness, I suggest. During another ritual, Kakah Ramat ran around in the house, hiding different sorts of figures all over. When asked to explain his behavior by me, he said that he hid the figures to make them invisible, and so part of the realm of spirits. The running was performed so that the figures would reach the spirit world faster (the journey to the spirits is a long one, Kakah Ramat pointed out). At the same time, the process of traveling to the spirit world was illustrated and—as Luangans commonly explained it— instantiated by rapid drumming. Making the invisible visible—and then invisible again—is very much what this is about. The images are what give the negotiation its tactile quality, its ability to persuade. As Kakah Ramat's ritual has shown us, and as other examples of figures used by Luangans demonstrate, the production and elaboration of ritual imagery is not just an instance in the curing process, but rather a central feature of its curing potential. Producing images is not all that is done in *belian* rituals, or was done in Kakah Ramat's ritual for that matter, but it is an activity of central importance in all *belian* rituals, integral to their structure and to the poetics upon which they are based.

Still, in what has been written about curing in Borneo, there is not much detailed discussion about *ganti diri*-like figures. From the references that there are, one can draw the conclusion that similar figures play a role in the curing rituals of many other Borneo peoples as well, even if not necessarily as central a role as among the Luangans. What role they play and how they function in the rituals is, however, seldom an overt object of investigation. George and Laura Appell (1993: 64) briefly point out that pig effigies made of rice paste are used today by the Bulusu' as a substitute for real pigs, which are no longer killed. Sellato (1989: 40) tells us that unspecified Bornean figurines are offered to spirits in order to distract their attention away from human beings. Similarly, Clifford Sather (2001: 101, 137, 200, 226) describes human effigies used by the Iban to deceive spirits into releasing the captured human soul. Jérôme Rousseau (1998: 255–257) discusses wooden and bamboo figurines used among the Kayan as substitutes for patients in some curing rituals, with the spirits being "satisfied with the simulacrum." In describing *dewa* curing ceremonies among the Meratus, Tsing (1993: 94) mentions a rich variety of offering cakes made in the shape of boats, airplanes, scissors, combs, jewelry, flowers, and lines of uniformed soldiers, presented as gifts to *dewa* spirits. Morris (1997: 81–86) has paid the spirit images of the Melanau some further attention. He tells us that the Melanau make wooden or plaited images of malevolent spirits who have attacked a patient and then spit saliva reddened from chewing betel on them, ordering the spirits to enter the image. He also makes an extensive list of such spirit images, *belum*, which, it should be mentioned, are much more artistically elaborate, "statue-like," than the Luangan images.[24] In his analysis of Taman healing practices, Jay Bernstein (1997: 119–123) provides us with an example of an incantation directed to human-like statues made of sugar cane. This incantation points to similarities in use and function between the Taman and the Luangan figures: the Taman statues are offered to the spirits as substitutes for the sick person, and are said to be attractive to the spirits. Bernstein does not, however, provide further comment, or discuss the question of why the Taman make such figures, or why the embodiment is needed.

The literature on the Luangans, and peoples related to them, is even less informative. In his dissertation on Luangan religion, Weinstock (1983) does not mention the existence of *ganti diri* figures. An article by Mallinckrodt (1974 [1925]) mentions that Lawangans made small rice paste figurines of all villagers during an epidemic, and placed them at the village entrance. P. te Wechel (1915: 43), a captain in the Dutch infantry, paid a little more attention to figures used by the Dusun (who are neighbors of the Luangans). He points out that *ganti diri* figures played an important role in the curing rituals of the Dusun, and then recounts a story about how the bones of the deceased servants of a wealthy man once turned into different sorts of trees, the wood of which has ever since been used to make substitutes for human beings.

For a more detailed discussion of *ganti diri*-like figures we have to move beyond Borneo to Sulawesi, where Eija-Maija Kotilainen, drawing on historical sources, has discussed their use in the central parts of that island (1992: 173–83). Examples and photographs provided by her exhibit a striking similarity to the Luangan material. The Sulawesian figures are also used as substitutes for patients during healing rituals. Kotilainen (1992: 177) points out that these figures cannot be likened to the widespread ancestor images of the Indonesian Archipelago (cf. Feldman 1985). Like the Luangan figures, they are simple, rudely made representations of human beings or animals made of non-durable material which are given as gifts to spirits and are left to decay after the ritual.

When considering this material one cannot avoid feeling that the relative lack of references to *ganti diri*-like figures in the literature on Borneo might not reflect their true importance on the island. Adding further support to this hypothesis is my own data from discussions with Ngaju Dayaks in Palangkaraya. According to this information, rice paste and wooden figurines are essential attributes in the curing practices of the Ngaju as well, and are used in very much the same way as among the Luangans. These data are corroborated by Sian Jay (1989: 40), who indicates their existence in Ngaju curing rituals, and by Schiller (1997: 51) who remarks briefly on their presence in *tiwah* mortuary rituals.

Why then, this general lack of discussion about this kind of figures in the literature? Why has there not been any more detailed analysis of their use and function in the curing practices of many Borneo peoples? A similar silence pertaining to the curing figurines used by Cuna Indians has been noted by Taussig (1993: 9), who finds it strange that the problem of why the figurines exist and are used is not even posed. Kotilainen (1992: 33–36) has commented on the relative neglect of material culture in anthropology until recently, and the difficulties Western scholars have had in accepting information offered by informants in many non-Western societies about material culture. She suggests that an urge to rationalize informants' answers, and an inability to transcend the theories of some of our evolutionist predecessors (i.e., Frazer 1922; Tylor 1871) might have something to do with it. Such primitivist theories could have made it inconvenient for later generations of anthropologists to study such a use of material culture which could seem to correspond to or resemble Tylor's fetishism or Frazer's sympathetic magic. So as not to make the people they have studied appear primitive, they might have chosen to gloss over some of their observations. Some Luangans do, in fact, themselves show anxiety about how the figures might be (mis)understood. For instance, a Luangan leader emphatically pointed out to me that the figures are not used for worship—he had personally been confronted with this view by adherents to world religions—but instead are used just to spit on, after which they are discarded.

Irrespective of what some people might think (or not think) about the figures, Luangan spirits are attracted to them (in theory at least). As Ma Kelamo, a member of Kakah Ramat's audience, framed it, "the spirits like to watch figures, it pleases them." Here the spirit figurines form a special attraction; it is thought to be particularly enjoyable for the spirits to see pictures of themselves, especially as the copies mimetically produce "real" spirits, and so, in the words of Ma Kelamo again, "increase the number of them."[25] An interesting variation on this theme occurs when the death shaman (*wara*) dances with the souls of the deceased during mortuary rituals, wearing a headdress adorned with a mirror in the front. In doing so he pleases them doubly, presenting them with not only his own devoted dancing, but also an image of the souls themselves, dancing with him.

The making of copies is not just a matter of figures, or mirror images, but, as we have seen, also involves the use of poetic language and performative ritual action, adding to the attractiveness of the evocation. Presenting offerings or substitutes to the spirits is not a straightforward business, but an elaborated and condensed act, intended to please the spirits. What the *belian* tries to do is to present the spirits with offerings so numerous and tempting that they are lured by "the feeling of fullness in their stomachs, the pleasant taste in their mouths" (*butung boting, iwei buen*), and become satisfied (*seneng*).

The enticing representations brought forth by Kakah Ramat and other *belian* curers working in the central Luangan region ultimately aim at evoking a relationship of reciprocity between spirits and people. The images, together with the scent of incense, the sounds of drums and singing, the beauty of the decorations, constitute means through which the *belian* attempts to reach out to the spirits and make them act according to principles of reciprocity. Presented with Kakah Ramat's representations, the spirits, if things turn out right, become appeased or even flattered, and so are induced to return the soul of the patient or, at least, be receptive to negotiation. It is hoped that the spirits, having received offerings, will recognize a relationship with their benefactors, and the obligations that go with it.[26] At the very least, it is hoped that the spirits will concede to a formal transaction involving the exchange of the soul for the substitutes provided.

In negotiating with spirits, however, Kakah Ramat cannot be sure of the outcome. He cannot be sure that he will actually be able to restore the soul of the patient. The spirits are, after all, only spirits and as such highly unpredictable. As Lemanius (1996) expresses it: "when talked to [the spirits] do not want to reply, and when called upon, they do not want to answer." Appeasing the spirits is a difficult task, and controlling them is even harder. Control is, in fact, not really what is at issue here. Far from trying to control the world, making images is rather an attempt to utilize its indeterminacy, showing life to be changeable by conjuring alternative scenarios. The gap between the representation and what is represented, the *différance* (Derrida 1982), can here be seen as what enables the transformation through mimetic representations, creating an imaginal space of possibilities. Whether the spirits (or the human beings, for that part) will actually accept Kakah Ramat's representations or not, one can never be sure.

Tactile Knowing

> Tactile appropriation is accomplished not so much by attention as by habit.
>
> —Walter Benjamin (1973a: 233)

There is, it might seem, something of a paradox involved in Kakah Ramat's image making. Striving to make things visible and tangible, why does he, in some respects, act so invisibly? When chanting the figures into being, for instance, why does he sing almost unintelligibly? Or when whisking with the *biyowo* and the *olung* and *jie* leaves—transforming the heat of misfortune and illness into healthy coolness—why are his whisking movements at times so slight, almost imperceptible? Or, to frame the question in a more general way, why is Kakah Ramat's performance so minimalistic, so reticent?

Belian rituals are not, as the curing ritual performed by Tak Dinas in chapter 2 showed us, always this unspectacular or "introverted," and shamans are not always this abstract (however, already being an old man during my fieldwork, Kakah Ramat was seldom up to large gestures anymore). The audience is not always quite as absent-minded as in this particular ritual either, although most *belian* rituals contain their moments of inattentiveness (there are, in fact, quite a few of them in most rituals; see Atkinson 1989: 219 for similar observations among the Wana, and Harris 2001: 138–139 among the Iban). The answer to why it was so in this particular case certainly does not have anything to do with lack of skill, or lack of authority on Kakah Ramat's part—quite the contrary. However, something that could explain it, I believe, is the fact that the patient was not very ill, and that the ritual in question was not a very major one. Should the patient's condition suddenly have worsened, things could have turned out quite differently, and other, more dramatic, ritual strategies might have been employed.

There is more to it than that, however. When Kakah Ramat blows on his whistle, and then starts chanting—swallowing words, rushing on, often pattering out the words rather than singing them, appearing to act almost automatically—he does not do so for some particular reason, but more out of habit (that is, because habit enables it), out of having mastered what he is doing. There is a certain degree of everydayness involved in his actions; he has done all of this before, countless times, and he is acting accordingly. This does not make his actions less efficacious or render his representations less evocative. On the contrary, it might even lend them a certain degree of authority.

There is a suggestive power in the habitual. In a way, Kakah Ramat's representations elude fixation, they press themselves upon their recipients and observers. They *happen to* them, seizing them almost without their knowing it. The aura of familiarity enveloping Kakah Ramat's minimalistic performance establishes what it presents almost in the same instance as it presents it, almost without any effort (i.e., conscious mediation) on the part of the audience (cf. Benjamin 1973a). At the same time it establishes an appearance of control, an appearance of Kakah Ramat being in command of the world he has set out to depict. What this effect is based on is the fact that the copies are copies of copies, and as such part of a tradition of *belian* curing.

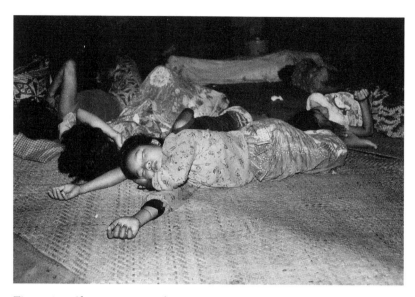

Figure 3.6. Sleeping at a ritual

When the members of Kakah Ramat's human audience lie down to sleep, or when they sit chatting with each other, playing with the kitten, not paying Kakah Ramat much attention, they do so knowing what is going on even without paying any attention to it, they know it almost in their sleep (people who are soundly asleep often wake up precisely at the moments when the drums and other musical instruments, such as gongs or the *kelentangen*, are to be played, or when the ritual paraphernalia should be moved from the center of the room to where the patient is lying and then later back to the center of the room again).[27] A "sleeping person" is, as Robert Barrett has put it in his discussion of audiences at Iban curing rituals (1993: 238), "also an experiencing subject." Or, as Metcalf (1991: 205) has expressed it for Berawan ritual audiences, comparing them to audiences at Southeast Asian traditional drama (see Brandon 1967: 260), "plots are known in advance and ... the attention of audiences is [thus] incomplete." Participating in *belian* rituals is far from unusual for the members of Kakah Ramat's audience, who have taken part in innumerable such rituals during their lifetimes, a great many of which have been conducted by Kakah Ramat.[28] Having heard, seen, smelled, and felt all of this before, the everydayness of Kakah

Ramat's performance might even work reassuringly. Because things are done so obviously according to lived tradition, the participants gain a sense of confidence in Kakah Ramat's *belian*ship.

It is not just in relation to what is happening now, but also in relation to what has happened before, that we must approach Kakah Ramat's somewhat summarized performance. Kakah Ramat can count on the members of his audience to take the hint, that is, he can count on them to fill in the gaps. They know the words of his chanting, not literally or in detail (such knowledge is, supposedly at least, the privileged knowledge of shamans), but in its broad outlines, in its sequences, and in its key metaphors. Although they would not be able to explain or offer an interpretation for every metaphor or expression used by Kakah Ramat—even Kakah Ramat himself was unable to do that—they still have a solid understanding of the contextual workings of the chants, and an intimate sense of their poetics. They can perceive "the silence of the dumb myna," "the darkness of the waning moon," and they can sense the coolness of the turning, the possibility brought forth by Kakah Ramat's words and actions.

The members of Kakah Ramat's audience know *belian*; they know it in their flesh and bones, so to speak. What we are dealing with here is a sort of habitual knowledge which may be largely described as a "knowledge of the body" (cf. Connerton 1989). Spitting on figures is something Luangan children learn how to do even before they learn to walk or talk, and making figurines and constructing ritual paraphernalia is something they put much time and effort into later in their lives. Similarly, playing the drums, chatting with other members of the audience, leaning back on the floor (and occasionally dozing off), preparing the ritual food, and consuming it at the end of the ritual, are all acts closely bound up with one's personal history, firmly incorporated into one's bodily being.

Kakah Ramat's performance can be said to work recollectively. By bringing forth memories of past performances—"embodied cultural memories," as Paul Stoller (1997: 47) would have it—it brings tradition into the realm of experience. It conjures up the past in the present as part of the participants' bodily dispositions, and thus lends tradition the authority of experience. Kakah Ramat does not have to be overtly performative or articulate in his copy making; what is at issue for him is to produce copies that through their distinct

115

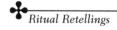

quality as copies (or more precisely, as copies of copies), are able to persuade the ritual participants (both humans and spirits) of the continuity of tradition and of human-spirit interaction.

The past is, as Marcel Proust has expressed it, "somewhere beyond the reach of the intellect, and unmistakably present in some material object (or in the sensation which such an object arouses in us)" (cited in Benjamin 1973b: 155). The taste of Proust's famous *madeleine* pastry, which transports him to his childhood past in the opening pages of *A la Recherche du Temps Perdu* (1913), is of course the paradigmatic example of such "sensuously mediated" recollection (for which Proust introduced the term *mémoire involontaire*). But Kakah Ramat's representations, and other aspects of participation in his ritual, also function somewhat like Proust's pastry: they evoke the past and make tradition palpable. The habitual mode of representation employed by Kakah Ramat brings pastness into juxtaposition with the present; the past is made actual in the present as ancestral tradition (once again) becomes incorporated into the participants' bodily dispositions, becoming, in Paul Connerton's (1989: 72) words, "sedimented in the body." In the ritual, the personal past is connected with the collective past as tradition is passed on as experience. Here it might be illuminating to cite Benjamin, whose discussion of Proust's concept *mémoire involontaire* I have drawn upon above: "Experience is indeed a matter of tradition, in collective existence as well as private life. It is less the product of facts firmly anchored in memory than of a convergence in memory of accumulated and frequently unconscious data" (Benjamin 1973b: 153–154).

It is as copies of copies—that is, as re-presentations of representations—that the images affect their observers. In so obviously conforming to lived tradition, Kakah Ramat's performance can be said to put "the ongoingness of tradition ... on show" (George 1996: 193). To reenact and thus restore tradition is, in fact, a major project not only in this particular ritual, but to some degree in all *belian luangan* rituals. For many Luangans, the *luangan* ritual genre typifies ancestral tradition and what ancestral tradition in its most "local" and "original" form is thought to be.

Belian luangan is regarded (probably correctly) as the oldest style of curing practiced today, as well as the most local one in origin. Whereas *belian bawo* was introduced to the Luangan area from the

Bawo in the Pasir region to the southeast a couple of centuries ago, and *belian sentiu* was introduced from Benuaq Dayaks to the northeast during the twentieth century, *belian luangan* is said to have been created by early mythical Luangan ancestors in the central parts of the Luangan area, in the upper Teweh River region.

Belian luangan is, as I have pointed out before, a style of curing which concentrates on words and images—words and images of the past, in the sense that they are not only seen to be based in ancestral tradition, but also to typify ancestral tradition. The combination of a maximum of words and images, and a minimum of happening (if we conceive of happening as dramatic appearance) is, in fact, very much what distinguishes the *luangan* style of curing from other curing styles. In contrast to *belian sentiu* and *belian bawo*, which are characterized by the use of a special shamanic costume, as well as by distinct music and dancing (melodic in the case of *sentiu*, rhythmic and forceful in the case of *bawo*), and occasionally by trance behavior, the *luangan* style relies almost solely on words (chanting) and objects (figures, ritual paraphernalia) in negotiating with spirits (and it is also herein that the beauty of the genre's aesthetics is seen to reside). Words and objects are, of course, essential attributes of the other curing styles as well, but these styles also have and are generally defined by their "performative elements" (which are largely absent in *belian luangan*), at the same time as the chants and material representations of these styles are not usually as elaborated as in *belian luangan* (the lyrics of these styles are generally described as either shortened or translated versions of *belian luangan* chants).[29] The richness of words and images, and the scarcity of dramatic happenings, is something which can be regarded as quintessentially Luangan, something which in an oblique but simultaneously profound way represents "luanganness" to those Luangans submerged in lived tradition.

Belian luangan rituals are low-key and unspectacular affairs which have to be tactually appropriated to be meaningfully appropriated at all. In their introvertedness they are, at one and the same time, both the least and the most demanding of all *belian* rituals. On the one hand, they do not call for much attention or active involvement on the part of the audience.[30] On the other hand, they very much take things for granted (by presuming habituation and prior experience), and do very little to encourage or aid the audience in appropriating the rituals. Tradition is, in a way, rendered self-evident in *belian luangan*, and it is also largely experienced as such. This taken-for-granted quality of *belian luangan* accounts for some of the strength and persuasiveness of the genre, but it also constitutes a kind of drawback. For those Luangans to whom tradition is not that self-evident—that is, not discernable in the words and images alone—*belian luangan* rituals can be rather difficult to approach, and it might also be that *belian luangan* is losing some of its popularity. Young people seem, as Kakah Ramat once expressed it, more attracted to the dramatic or beautiful dancing of *belian bawo* and *belian sentiu* than to the elaborate words and images of *belian luangan*, and most of the younger people studying to become *belian* today do, in fact, prefer to study *belian bawo* or *sentiu*.[31]

Arranging or participating in *belian luangan* rituals involves embracing a stance of relatively unquestioned disengagement, a mode of apperception characterized by distracted everydayness. It means submitting to a state of being of Luangan everydayness, to a "luanganness" typified by precisely that low-key and introverted character which characterizes the ritual itself. In addition to expressing commitment to the patient and to the *belian* by being present at the ritual (cf. Harris 2001: 139), the sleeping participants during a *belian luangan* ritual at the same time affirm the taken-for-grantedness of tradition, and display trust in ancestral tradition as a force by which the present can be renegotiated.

It is with the authority of the past, of what has been done before, that one negotiates with the spirits in *belian luangan* rituals. The *ganti diri* figures and the familiar phrases in Kakah Ramat's chants derive their power to sensuously evoke the world of human-spirit exchange from having been worn in, so to speak, by tradition. This "power of the past" does not, however, derive from pastness in itself. Neither is it, of course, the purpose of the ritual to reinstigate pastness in the present for its own sake. The past is rather, to use an expression by Nadia Seremetakis, "brought into the present as a transformative and interruptive force" (1994b: 31).[32] Tradition is not just a reminder of what was, but also of what can be. It is not only performed for the sake of repetition; it is also sustained because it contains within it a possibility for change, in this case, a possibility for curing.

In the ritual presented in this chapter, Kakah Ramat is drawing on a history of inter-relation between humans and spirits, a relationship actualized and constructed through words and objects. Regarding this ritual, it is obvious that "the meaning of performance is the imagery that it enacts and evokes" (Palmer and Jankowiak 1996: 229). It is as "indispensable ontological tools," perceived to "provide extra-bodily material forms by means of which nonhuman perspectives can be entertained, and, consequently, the appearances of humans from the point of view of humans as well as non-humans can be altered" (A. Pedersen 2007: 161), that the imagery works. Through the tactile qualities of his representations—through movements, metaphors, and material objects—Kakah Ramat has activated the sensory memories of his human and spirit audiences. Once again he has called on Itak Silu Malik and her companions to turn around the figures, and so brought tradition to bear on yet another instance of disturbance in the human-spirit relationship. Through propitiation and exchange he has then attempted to renegotiate this relationship and retrieve the soul of his grandson's wife, thereby terminating an unfavorable condition (her sleeplessness and general feeling of sickness). Throughout this process, his representations can be said to have occupied center stage, or even to have been its main actors. It is through them that the ritual "drama" has been enacted, and by them that the power of tradition has been sensuously communicated to the ritual participants, whose embodied personal histories have formed the prerequisites of reception and whose corporeal sensibilities, once more, have become recharged.

Thus the copies create tradition at the same time as tradition permeates the copies, and we can see how the process of copying constitutes an activity of central importance in Luangan curing, not an unessential idiosyncrasy marginal to what goes on. I have argued that it is the concrete and sensuous characteristics of representations—their objectness—that account for this importance of image making. Through what I have called the habitual mode of representation and tactile appropriation, words and images in *belian luangan* confer a particular authority on tradition, even though this is often a remarkably introverted and non-spectacular ritual genre, marked by what might be described as a rather abbreviated and condensed style of performance.

Epilogue

Not surprisingly, Kakah Ramat's grandson's wife became well again soon after the ritual was finished (she was not, after all, very ill to begin with). Shortly afterwards, she and her husband and their children moved into Kakah Ramat's son's house (the brother of her husband's deceased father), while Kakah Ramat started to rebuild and enlarge his own house (which was rather crowded at the time of the ritual), so that it would better accommodate his descendants (which included two of his grandsons and their families). Two years later, in August 1998, when I visited Kakah Ramat, he remembered the ritual, but could, perhaps tellingly enough, not recall what had been wrong with his grandson's wife at the time.

Notes

1. This version of the Luangan origin story was written down by Lemanius, a Luangan in his seventies who lived by the upper Teweh River. In 1990 he had a dream in which he was told that he should write down the Luangan origin story and make it into a holy book (like those of the world religions). In order to do so he first had to learn how to write and type, however, which he did on his own, with a little help from his grandchildren. He then wrote this rather amazing book, which contains the "complete" history of the Luangans, from when the earth was created and the first human beings came into existence, through pre-colonial and colonial times, and into the New Order Indonesia, and its politics of religion.

2. "Ill" is perhaps not the term which would most immediately come to most people's minds here. Summoned by Kakah Ramat, who was concerned over the decision of another of his grandsons to move away to another village, Kakah Ramat's grandson had, together with his wife and their children, moved into Kakah Ramat's house only a couple of weeks earlier (before that they had lived in his wife's parents' house in a neighboring village). New in the village and the house, away from her parents, the woman was prone to feelings of discomfort and "soul-loss" (as her sleeplessness suggested).

3. The sharp-edged *biyowo* leaves (*cordyline terminalis*), together with some *ringit* (coconut leaves), serve as the *belian*'s "weapon." The *olung* and *jie* leaves are used by the *belian*, as Lemanius (1996) describes it, "to sweep and chase away what might disturb and disrupt the turning of figures" (*ngapek ngueu pekuyo pekoro ie tau mengganggu pekaur*).

4. *Tiong*, the myna bird, is an excellent singer often heard in Luangan villages. Consequently, according to some of the people I talked to, a dumb myna is a sign of something unnervingly wrong. "The myna bird struck dumb" (*tiong pererongo*) is not just a metaphor for the patient's condition, how-

ever, but what Luangans call a *geler*, that is, a title, for the patient. Such *geler* are usually used much like personal names, denotatively, in the strict sense of the word, with little or no thought of what the words actually mean. The word *pererongo* is used only in ritual language. Etymologically, it is probably derived from the word *dongo* (meaning "sick person") and the image that it evoked for most people was that of a sad and quiet myna bird.

5. Contrary to the Malay healers described by Carol Laderman (1996: 132), "a beautiful voice" is not essential for a *belian*. Many of the most respected *belian* have hoarse voices and sing inarticulately, often with their mouths full of betel like Kakah Ramat.

6. In translating this text I have been forced to take some poetic license. Much of the rhythm and alliteration characterizing the original is unfortunately lost in the translation.

7. These are all (flawed) spirit guides summoned by Kakah Ramat.

8. Luing is the spirit guardian of rice, and the rice paste figurines shaped as human beings are thus "grains of Luing made human beings."

9. According to Lemanius, the Stone of Eternal Fire is located where the sun sets, by the sea. The fire hinders the water of the sea from flooding the earth, while the water simultaneously hinders the fire from burning the earth.

10. The walls of the longhouse are made of the bark from *meranti* (*Shorea* sp.) trees.

11. These are vessels that will freight away the illness.

12. Spirits of different categories have their own "master" or "leader" (*tuhan*).

13. The fern referred to here is an epiphytic fern (*Platycerium* sp.) commonly growing on tree branches; sometimes these ferns grow so large and heavy that the host branches break and fall down to the ground.

14. *Bongai, mulang, blis,* and *setan* are all malevolent spirits (or, rather, categories of malevolent spirits) thought to cause the patient's illness. An Islamization or Christianization of malevolent spirits may be seen in the names of *blis* and *setan*; they are primarily synonyms though, constituting parallel expressions.

15. In making swidden fields Luangans leave groves of particularly large trees untouched, as spirits are supposed to favor such places. Cutting down all big trees close to the village could lead to the spirits coming to the village for refuge, which would be undesirable from the human point of view.

16. I have here translated the Luangan word *ruo* as "essence"; usually this word is only used in association with the word *juus* which I translate as "soul," but it can also occasionally be used in the meaning of "spirit." *Ruo* here replicates *juus*, as in the standard expression *juus jatus, ruo walo*, "a hundred souls, and eight essences," which frequently figures in *belian* chants (parallelisms, of which there are many examples in such chants, including the one reproduced here, are frequently constructed by way of allegedly meaningless duplicate words or sentences). Similarly the numbers "one hundred" and "eight" in this expression are said to be determined not by correspondence to the number of real souls "out there" but

by convention only. In fact, Luangans usually hold that people only have one soul, although no strong opinion or certainty exists with regard to this issue.

17. The trees mentioned here are used for incense.

18. The *belian* returns the errant soul to the body through an invisible hole (*kerepuru*) at the back of the patient's head.

19. As their names (Silu the Dumb One, Lintai the Idiot etc.) suggest, the spirit familiars called upon by Kakah Ramat to enact his wrong-doing are spirit familiars specifically associated with such activities (i.e., "purposively failed or incomplete work"). All these "flawed" spirit familiars are in fact themselves bad or inverse versions of other, "ordinary" or "benevolent" spirit familiars (Silu the Dumb One is Silu's "failed" counterpart, Lintai the Idiot is Lintai's counterpart, etc.).

20. "To return to" (*uli*) here implies going back to their sources, returning home to where they belong. Roseman (1991: 40) shows how the Temiar of peninsular Malaysia use a similar expression in their healing chants.

21. The simile of comparing the *ganti diri* figures with walls may also be seen to point to the importance of boundaries, and of notions of enclosure, of keeping separate, notions which are important in curing practices in many Indo-Malaysian societies, and not least, we may note, because of the typically "sociocentric" and "permeable" selves of their members, which Roseman (1990) argues are central in motivating such notions among the Temiar. If we interpret the simile in this way the *ganti diri* figures can be observed to unsettle the distinction between gift and fetish as conceptualized by Jackson. According to Jackson (1998: 78), "the difference between fetish and gift is that the fetish withholds or prevents communication, sealing self off from other, while the gift opens and mediates communication. The fetish closes gates; the gift opens paths." According to this logic, an amulet, for example, is worn for protection, so as to reinforce the boundaries of the body of its wearer; a gift, on the other hand, such as a sacrifice to the spirits, is presented for contrary purposes, in order to restore the relationship with the receiver, or to ask for favors, both of which amount to increased communication with the other. It seems to me that this distinction is untenable even if it might at first sight appear sensible, or at least it is so with respect to the *ganti diri* figures. It is obvious that *ganti diri* figures, in Jackson's terms, are both gifts and fetishes; they are given to the spirits in order to open a path, to enable negotiation with them. But they are also given with the intention of sealing off the self, in order to reinforce the boundaries of the body of the patient which the spirits have penetrated, and to undo the prevailing connection between the spirits and the patient, to break the relation.

22. Even if *tentuwaja* is seen as an ugly forest creature, it is at the same time considered very human-like, and regarded as a noble (*tatau*), who likes to wear pearls, for example.

23. The *belian* makes the decision about what figures are to be used both with regard to the symptoms of the patient, and with regard to the information

that he gets through a process of exploring the cause of the illness (*pereau*). This process can sometimes be repeated many times during a ritual (the *belian* can never be absolutely sure of who has caused the illness—there might, for example, be several spirits guilty at the same time). Different figures are also favored in different styles of curing.

24. He has also published a similar list made by Lawrence and Hewitt (1908).

25. Being "many" is a value in itself for many Luangans, who feel marginalized by their more populous neighbors, and they consider their spirits to have similar views.

26. The logic here is similar to that of Marcel Mauss' (1925) in his theory of the gift.

27. When Ma Bari, the village head, entered Kakah Ramat's house, he lay down on the floor without saying a word to anyone, and then slept there through the whole evening, waking up just to spit on the figurines, and then again to eat the cakes served at the end of the ritual (after which he went home to his own house to continue his sleep).

28. Participating in *belian* rituals, especially the larger ones, is considered a kin obligation and, because of the inclusive system of bilateral kinship reckoning, this often entails a very high degree of ritual participation. Since there are no clear rules defining exactly when one has to participate and when one does not need to, individual choice still largely determines presence, and so one tends to see some people at rituals much more frequently than others.

29. An additional feature of *belian luangan* which makes it more "local" in comparison with the other curing styles is the fact that the spirits negotiated with in the ritual are mostly local spirits, whereas one also negotiates with different kinds of foreign spirits (in addition to local spirits) in *belian bawo* and especially in *belian sentiu*.

30. They do, however, demand a lot of preparatory work (with offerings, ritual food, figurines, and other ritual paraphernalia).

31. Lack of time or patience to learn the lengthy chants was often suggested as the reason for a diminishing willingness among young *belian* to study *belian luangan*. Engagement in wage labor, uncertain future prospects, and influence from national politics of culture promoting a more performative tradition, should perhaps also be added to the list. A decreasing depth of experience in Benjamin's (1973a) sense, making tactile appropriation increasingly difficult, could also be an important factor, especially among Luangans in downstream areas who live in greater proximity to various aspects of "modernity." Among part of the Benuaq sub-group of the Luangans, *luangan* rituals are rarely performed these days, and they become rarer the further downstream one goes, at the same time as *belian sentiu* becomes more popular. In many Benuaq villages, people say that there are no more *belian* around with a sufficient knowledge of *luangan* curing. On the other hand, *luangan* curing probably never had the same popularity in downstream Benuaq areas that it has had among the central Luangans. Among the latter, several young *belian* whom I talked to claimed

that they were going to study *belian luangan* later, when they were older and would have more time to do so (which my last visit to the area in 2011 proved to be true at least in the case of Mancan, who in the late 1990s practiced only *belian sentiu,* and was now studying to learn how to perform *buntang* rituals, which are performed in the *luangan* style).

32. I am indebted to Seremetakis not only for this particular insight, but also more generally for treating objects and sensory experience as central to the imagination of the past. She understands the relationship between memory and material culture dialectically: "The sensory landscape and its meaning-endowed objects bear within them emotional and historical sedimentation that can provoke and ignite gestures, discourses and acts—acts which open up these objects' stratigraphy" (1994a: 7).

Chapter Four
The Uncertainty of Spirit Negotiation

Somehow the spirits always manage to disconcert

—Michael Lambek (1981: xvi)

"Certainty is not reality," Louis Aragon states in his book *Paris Peasant* (1926). In the realm of ritual representations, it may seem that certainty is at times even less of a reality than at other times. During such occasions the unpredictability of life becomes almost palpable, and forces one to look in new directions, to explore other possibilities that might exist. The possibilities of doing this within the loose confines of an essentially accommodating ritual repertoire are the subject of this chapter.

The chapter deals with a crisis, one which struck the people of Sembulan during a *belian buntang* ritual in July 1996. It is the story of the efforts that were made to cure Ma Bari, the village's unofficial head of customary law (*kepala adat*), when he suddenly fell seriously ill. At the same time it is a story about uncertainty—the uncertainty of representation, and of life represented. Finally, as representation here mainly refers to various forms of ritual action, it is also, to look at it from yet another angle, a story about spirit negotiation—and the bottomlessness of such negotiation.

The story, as I present it here, began late one evening during a *belian buntang*, a "thanksgiving" ritual staged by Ma Dasi and his family in the village longhouse. Ma Dasi had asked Ma Bari, who was the main owner of the longhouse, for permission to conduct the ritual there, as it could accommodate a much larger crowd than his own field house. The ritual was arranged as a farewell gesture aimed at creating "good feelings" (*aseng buen*) among relatives and fellow villagers as Ma Dasi and his family were about to move away to Benangin, his wife's home village. In fact, from the viewpoint of this chapter, the events may be said to have begun already a couple of days earlier when Ma Bari started to have pains in his stomach and decided to spend the night alone in the small, usually uninhabited house that stands next to the longhouse, his usual home. For most participants in the ritual, however, it was only on this evening, the sixth day of the ritual, that they became aware of the seriousness of Ma Bari's condition. As a consequence, this is also the point at which I have chosen to begin my story. Through revised excerpts from field notes, presented chronologically, I will try to evoke what happened, and how. My intention is not to present these happenings in an exhaustive way, accounting for every phase or detail in them—that would be almost impossible, to be sure—but to try to convey them in the elusiveness of the present in which they occurred, subject to the contingencies of life, human finitude and the vicissitudes of inter-action, and human-spirit interaction in particular. This approach reflects my general interest, which is not so much to account for ritual structure as such, as to give a picture of how particular instances of ritual action are affected by the particular contexts in which they are enacted. My objective is, to cite Michel de Certeau (1984: 20), to investigate "the aspects of a society that cannot be … uprooted and transferred to another space: ways of using things or words accord-ing to circumstances." Following de Certeau, I believe that there is "something essential … at work in this everyday *historicity*, which cannot be dissociated from the *existence* of the subjects who are the agents and authors of conjunctural operations" (ibid.). Through the story recounted, I wish to convey that undetachable contextuality, as it appeared during circumstances when it became exceptionally evident. Thereby, it is also my objective to highlight the irreducibility of lived reality to any form of epistemological certainty—indigenous *or* analytic. In other words, I want to explore how the agents' immer-sion in reality, or what Kapferer (2005: 46–47) calls "virtuality," especially in situations when its foundations are shaken, inexorably affects the conditions of representation.

In terms borrowed from Atkinson (1989: 14; see also Sillander 2004: 168), *buntang* rituals are generally "liturgy-centered" rather than "performance-centered." Compared to ordinary curing *belian* rituals, they are much more clearly structured performances follow-

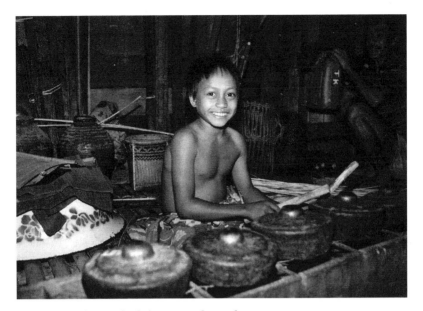

Figure 4.1. Playing the *kelentangen* during *buntang*

ing a predetermined order of procedures, which basically remain the same from ritual to ritual, even if the ordering of these procedures may differ quite significantly between different shamans. It is through a prescribed order of chants and associated activities that a *buntang* is organized (the word *buntang* refers to a melody repeatedly played on the *kelentangen* during the ritual, a melody which, like the "*gombok*" melody played on large gongs during secondary mortuary rituals, is exclusive to this ritual).[1] Still, what happens in between the segments of ritual, and how risk, material happenstances and exterior influences are reflected in them, becomes all the more evident precisely because of this relative structural stability.

Like other genres of Luangan ritual, the organization and timing of a *buntang* is dependent on external circumstances. Decisions regarding rituals are often revised in practice, a fact that I became aware of time after time during my fieldwork. There is an intriguing paradox here, in that ritual, on one level, at least when it comes to *belian* rituals, is contingent upon and significantly shaped by conditions external to the ritual itself, while, on another, an important effect of ritualization is simultaneously, as Bourdieu (1994: 158) phrases it, "that of assigning them a time—i.e., a moment, a tempo,

127

and a duration—which [itself] is relatively independent of external necessities, those of climate, technique, or economy, thereby conferring on them the sort of arbitrary necessity which specifically defines cultural arbitrariness."

Unlike ordinary *belian* curing rituals, which are usually sponsored by conjugal families, *buntang* rituals are arranged by extended families and are not as frequent as the former. They are nevertheless quite common among the central Luangans. During a one-year period in 1996–1997, while I conducted fieldwork in Sembulan, seven *buntang* rituals were arranged, with each extended family sponsoring on average one. In the central Luangan area *buntang* rituals are associated with the *luangan* ritual genre, and they are considered an old form of ritual, which has been practiced for as long as they can remember. In the literature there are references to *buntang* rituals dating back at least to the late nineteenth century (see Grabowsky 1888: 583–584; Knappert 1905: 619).

Although basically constituting "thanksgiving" rituals (Weinstock 1983: 43–46), arranged to pay back debts to the spirits, often in fulfillment of a vow (*niat*) made during an earlier curing ritual, *buntang* rituals always include curing or supplication activities as well, and curing itself is often a principal motive for arranging a *buntang*. There are, in fact, many reasons why a *buntang* may be arranged: the inauguration of new leaders; the reunification of family or village ties (*buntang nuak*); the expulsion of listlessness following death (*buntang moas utas*); the consecration of a new house; the validation of illicit marriages, etc. (see Sillander 2004: 171–173). In the past *buntang* rituals are said to have sometimes included headhunting or the sacrifice of a slave, especially when they were arranged in connection with the death of a person of high status, and the ritual today usually features a mock headhunt during which an old headhunt skull (*utek layau*) is brought to the village from the forest. In many respects the *buntang* is reminiscent of similar rituals among other peoples in Borneo and beyond, such as the *balaku untung* of the Ngaju (personal observation), the Iban *gawai* (Masing 1997), the Toraja *ma'bua'* (Volkman 1985), the Wana *salia* (Atkinson 1989), and the *pangnae* of the Mapparundo (George 1996). As a collective ritual, arranged by an extended family, involving the sacrifice of numerous animals (chicken, pigs, and often water buffaloes), the *buntang* is considered as one of the most powerful *belian* rituals available (only surpassed by the *nalin taun* community ritual) and it represents the standard measure taken when an important elder or leader (*manti*) falls ill.

Negotiating with Spirits

July 1, 1996. It is twelve o'clock at night, the sixth day of Ma Dasi's buntang. Ma Dasi has just returned to Sembulan from a trip to invite some far-away relatives to attend the ritual. A large congregation of relatives and neighbors has now gathered in the house, and the events are picking up speed as Ma Dasi's return has confirmed the ritual schedule. A mock headhunt was staged in the forest during the afternoon, and the headhunt skull has been fed with rice and chicken blood. The longan has been erected as well, and leaves dyed in red and yellow have been suspended on a rattan wire which intersects the length of the large undivided room that makes up the longhouse. Kakah Ramat, Ma Buno and Unsir—the shamans in charge—are now seated on the floor in the middle of the room, chanting, while slowly rocking a suspended ship used for soul search.

It is at this time that a pig is suddenly killed, outside the ritual program. It is not brought into the house for display as sacrificial animals usually are, but is instead slaughtered outside in the dark, beyond sight of the guests. The pig is then brought into the kitchen where it is cut up and cooked, after which it is taken into the longhouse and served, along with rice, to the ritual participants, who were, in fact, served dinner only a couple of hours earlier.

Irregular meals were not unusual during my fieldwork, especially not during rituals, and the unexpected meal served at this stage of Ma Dasi's *buntang* did not attract much attention among the ritual participants (although most people present probably knew why it was being served). In fact, no one even mentioned the killing of the pig, at least not aloud, and consequently the incident passed without much reflection on my part—tired as I was at that moment I did not ponder about why the pig was killed, but regarded it as just another ritual sacrifice. Nor did I reflect much on the fact that Ma Bari was absent from the longhouse at the time, particularly because he often was absent from it, staying in his swidden field from early morning till sunset, and upon coming home he was often so tired that he went almost straight to bed, spending the evening hidden behind his mosquito-net. It was not until the next day, upon the killing of another pig, that I became aware that there was something badly wrong.

July 2, 1996. After a quiet morning, in which the shamans have been sitting by the longan, *silently chanting* tempuun *(origin stories), while all other men in the village have been out in the forest bringing home some heavy ironwood trunks intended to become new house posts in Kakah Ramat's house, Ma Isa, Ma Bari's eldest son, a man in his fifties, suddenly comes walking through the village, dragging a large pig by its feet. He looks angry and walks hurriedly, stopping by a coconut palm in front of the longhouse. Holding the pig by its back feet he smashes it with all his strength against the trunk of the palm. The pig squeals and tries to bite him. Ma Isa grabs it tighter and smashes it once more, this time against the ground. Jube, his sister, who has witnessed the incident, groans: "this is not right, this is not how it should be done."*

Luangans do not usually smash pigs against trees or against the ground, not during rituals, nor at any other time for that matter. Ma Isa was acting in rage here, out of desperation, and this was quite exceptional, since the Luangans I knew, and Ma Isa in particular, rarely showed their feelings publicly, or acted aggressively. Ma Bari was ill, I was now told. He had been having pains in his stomach for many days already, and now he was feeling worse: he had diarrhea, and he was not eating. The pig that was killed the night before had been pointed out by someone in a neighboring village as the possible cause of his illness, and the one killed by Ma Isa just now had been indicated as a suspect by Kakah Ramat.

In the evening the buntang *continues. Kakah Ramat and Unsir are chanting quietly, telling the spirits the news of the ritual proceedings. At the same time Ma Buno begins a* belian bawo *ritual, a continuation and completion of a ritual started six months ago to cure Yan, one of Ma Dasi's sons. At one end of the house there is the quiet, slow beat of the* buntang *as the drummers irregularly slap the drums with the palms of their hands, holding them in their laps; at the other end Ma Buno dances and rattles his* ketang *bracelets while Yan and some other young men play the long upright-turned drums in the* bawo *style, beating them rapidly and loudly with bamboo sticks. The atmosphere is rather chaotic, with the shamans simultaneously singing different songs in different tunes, while the drums are played in different rhythms.*

Ma Bari's condition is not discussed during this evening, and Ma Bari himself is still absent from the house. His illness can be perceived though. It can be seen in the strained faces of his wife and his children, and it can be sensed in their silence, their reserved behavior. It can be tasted in the poor flavor of the food as well, and felt in its scarcity.[2] Most other ritual participants seem to be enjoying themselves, however, talking and laughing, chasing off dogs who are trying to steal some of the offerings.

July 3, 1996. Noon. A belian bawo *is beginning again, this time for Ma Bari, who now physically enters the scene for the first time. He is led into the room by Tak Ningin, his wife, and Jube, his daughter, looking weak and moaning. Ma Buno, who is performing the ritual, is dancing in front of the main door, balancing on his head a small white porcelain bowl containing uncooked rice, plaited coconut leaves and a lit candle. He is holding up a knife-like* biyowo *leaf before his eyes, looking at it as if he was reading, but with closed eyes.*

—A cucumber, he suddenly announces, with a ludicrous voice, a voice of spirits.

— What kind of cucumber?, someone in the audience asks.

— Just a cucumber, a cucumber of the sort that we have here, Ma Buno answers.

— What does it look like, of what pattern is its hair?, someone else asks.

— White feet, white feet—white, an ordinary cucumber (timun bumun), *Ma Buno replies.*

— Catch it, catch it! That's the one that you should chase and run after, that's what you're up to fight and drive away, Tak Ningin, interpreting Ma Buno's words in her capacity of penyempatung *(ritual assistant), urges.*

Pereau (derived from the verb *neau*, to see, meaning to see the cause of the illness, to make it visible) is a diagnostic procedure used at the early stage of most *belian* rituals to search for the cause of an illness. "Reading" the *biyowo* leaf, looking out in different directions, with the surroundings lit up by the candle on his head, Ma Buno here searched for the cause of Ma Bari's illness. And with the help of a spirit familiar he saw a "cucumber," which meant a white pig, as I was to learn later.

Domestic animals are sometimes thought to be entered into or possessed by spirits who trick them into injuring people by, for example, invisibly biting them in their stomachs. In the context of *pereau* these animals are not mentioned by their real names but are discussed in disguised language. A pig is a "cucumber," a cat is a "village tiger," a dog is a "house civet," etc.

There are several ways to "see" the illness or what causes it (the illness and its cause are treated somewhat as synonymous categories by Luangans who talk about *roten*, the illness, as a subject). One way to do so is to spit betel juice in the palm of your hand and then to "read" the reddish saliva; this is what Kakah Ramat and the person in the neighboring village did for Ma Bari. Another common method is to carry a candle on one's head like Ma Buno did here, to enable one to see things in the unseen world; this is a technique employed in particular in the *bawo* style of curing, and it is used not only to identify an animal guilty of causing an illness, but also, and perhaps primarily, to see the place inhabited by the spirit possessing the animal.[3] Having seen the illness, or the one who has caused it, the *belian* informs his audience about it, talking in the voice of his spirit guide(s). If he points out a particular domestic animal, this animal has to be caught and killed as soon as possible.[4] By killing the animal it is assumed that one dispels the illness as well, that is, if it strikes the mark (*aser kune*), if you get the right one.

July 4, 1996. A wedding ceremony between Ma Dasi's daughter Yati and Lodot, a young local man, is staged this afternoon, ending the buntang *ritual, which reached its climax last night with the sacrifice of a pig and some chickens, the blood and meat of which were fed to the spirits of the ancestor skulls, as well as to* naiyu *and* timang *protecting spirits.[5] At this time the white plates that are paid as wages to those involved in the ritual work are distributed as well, and the ritual is officially completed. However, there is a rumor afloat that there will be a new* buntang *ritual starting soon, a* buntang *for Ma Bari this time.*

Late one night during the *buntang* sponsored by Ma Dasi, the wooden ship used for soul search travel (*sampan benawa*) fell down from the ceiling when the rattan cord by which it was suspended snapped, and therefore a *buntang* ritual would now have to be arranged for Ma Bari, it was decided. But the *buntang* would be preceded by an ordinary curing *belian* (as *buntang* rituals usually are), I was told by Ma Dasi. People discussed the matter in whispers, and no one seemed to know exactly what was going to happen. It was rumored by some that the ritual would include the sacrifice of a water buffalo (*buntang mpe kerewau*), but this was denied by others. Ma Bari himself lay concealed beneath his mosquito-net most of the time, sometimes groaning loudly, with either his wife or his daughter sitting by his side.

July 7, 1996. As the three-day pali *(taboo) to enter the longhouse following Ma Dasi's* buntang *is over, all the paraphernalia used during that ritual are thrown out of the house.*[6] *At the same time new ritual paraphernalia are made, this time for a* belian bawo *ritual: carved wooden sticks representing human beings, a variety of spirit houses, bowls and trays filled with flowers, rice, and other offerings. Rice is also pounded, and women gather in the kitchen to prepare cakes for the spirits and food for the ritual guests.*

In the evening the bawo *ritual begins with Ma Kerudot and Kakah Ramat performing as* belian, *the heavy scent of* bemueng *incense wood filling the room. As they dance around to the rapid beat of* bawo *music, the shamans hide* ganti diri *figures all over the longhouse—Ma Kerudot with rattling* ketang *bracelets on his wrists. They search for Ma Bari's soul, grabbing after it again and again with their hands, then putting it in a small plastic box filled with coconut oil (*olau juus *or "soul oil") and eight grains of rice, smearing some of the oil on Ma Bari's forehead. Later a dog is killed by drowning it in the river, having been pointed out by Ma Kerudot in another* pereau *as being responsible for Ma Bari's illness.*

During my fieldwork, Kakah Ramat, the most experienced and respected *belian* in the village, did not usually perform rituals in the *bawo* style any more. He was too old, he said, and not able to dance and rattle the heavy brass bracelets. He made an exception this evening though, dancing with cautious steps, without bracelets. Ma Bari was *payeh*, seriously ill, it was whispered, and that is why exceptions had to be made.

July 8, 1996. The buntang *ritual for Ma Bari is beginning this afternoon, a four-day* buntang *according to present plans. Ritual decorations are again made, some of them identical to those that were thrown out a day ago. The shamans—Kakah Ramat, Ma Buno and Unsir—seat themselves by the* longan teraran: *a conical shaped construction made of* teraran *palm, consisting of four about two meter tall, outward-leaning stalks (use of the* longan teraran *indicates that this is a* buntang *featuring pig and chicken sacrifices only; during* buntang *rituals including sacrifices of water buffaloes the ironwood* longan, longan teluyen, *is used).[7] The shamans inform the spirits about the ritual program by chanting, first next to the* longan, *later near the patient, and finally at the main door, thus initiating the ritual.*

Buntang rituals may last four, six or eight days (or even longer, two times eight days, for example), depending on what sacrifices are made. If only pigs and chickens are sacrificed, they last four or six days, if a water buffalo is slaughtered an eight-day period is the minimum. Except for the opening evening when the coarse, bodily spirits of the dead are sent away, and news of the ritual is told (*mara mansa*) to all categories of spirits, each day begins with the awakening and dressing of Luing (*peruko Luing, nangko Luing*), a female spirit familiar central to the proceedings (usually this is done before dawn, at around half past five in the morning).[8] A number of *tempuun* (origin stories) are then chanted, the order and number of which can vary according to the situation and the *belian* in charge. These *tempuun* minimally include *Tempuun Teraran* and *Tempuun Urei*, which recount the origins of the plants used as paraphernalia in the ritual, and the *tempuun* of chickens and pigs, and, if required, of water buffaloes. These myths, some of which may extend over several days, are chanted by the *longan*—which forms a resting place for spirit guides and protecting spirits during the ritual—to the slow and monotonous beat of the shamans slapping their drums (*betime*), according to a specific rhythm accompanying the chanting of *tempuun*.

Each day of the *buntang* also features the presentation of offerings and rewards to the spirits (*besemah*), in more elaborate and dramatic form toward the end of the ritual, and particularly on the days that animals are sacrificed. Soul-search travel (*berejuus*) is another program activity conducted during most nights of a *buntang*, in which the *belian* search for the souls of their patients among the spirits of dead relatives (*liau* and *kelelungan*), as well as among a varying set of other spirit beings. Besides these activities, *buntang* rituals also include, among other things, the festive hanging up (*nyerewe*) of coconut leaves dyed in red and yellow, the planting and erecting of visible and invisible plant counterparts of human beings (*muat samat, ninek torung*), the smearing of blood on valuable objects inherited from the ancestors (*ngulas pusaka*), the feeding of cooked food to the celestial *seniang* spirits and the *kelelungan* of revered ancestors (*makan aning*), and the feeding of the *naiyu* spirits associated with both the headhunt skull (*utek layau*, a skull usually stored outside the main door of the longhouse and brought into the house during *buntang* rituals), and the ancestor skulls (*utek tuha longan*, skulls which are stored in an ironwood box placed in the rafters above the ironwood *longan*). At the last day of a *buntang*, the members of the sponsoring family "enter the soul house" (*mengket blai juus*), putting their feet on the stairs of a small wooden house, which is then, by being raised up in the rafters, symbolically raised to its location in heaven.

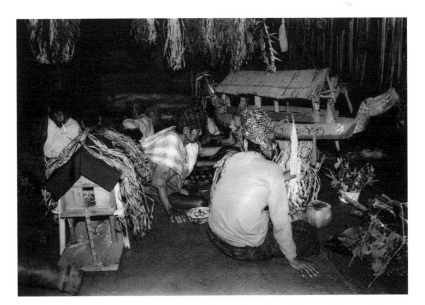

Figure 4.2. Soul search ship (*sampan benawa*) and soul house (*blai juus*)

July 9, 1996. It is ten o'clock in the evening and Kakah Ramat, who has been chanting origin myths the whole day, suddenly performs as belian bawo *again, this time wearing his* ketang *wrist bracelets and a sarong tied around his waist as a skirt. He also wears a "basket" made of* salak *palm stalks full of long, sharp thorns on his bare back. With a rag made of banana leaf shreds he rubs Ma Bari's thin body all over while the drums are beaten rapidly. Then, as he dances, he puts the rag in the thorny basket on his back and runs out of the house, hiding the rag somewhere out in the darkness of the night. After a while he enters the house again, seating himself by the* penyelenteng *and begins to chant, to verbally turn around the* ganti diri *figures, presenting the spirits with substitutes of human beings.*

Some curing (*bekawat*), either restorative or preventive, which typically last only a couple of hours and is usually conducted in the same *luangan* format as the rest of the ritual, is ordinarily carried out during a *buntang*, and is regarded as an integral part of it. Sometimes, however, especially if the patient for whom the ritual is arranged gets worse, *buntang* rituals may also be interspersed with more extensive rituals, conducted in a different ritual format, which are perceived to form separate rituals in their own right. Through different ritual styles different spirits can be contacted and pleased simultaneously (or the same spirits doubly), and the curing effects thus amplified.

Ma Bari was occasionally "losing his breath" at this time, it was whispered, and the situation seemed rather desperate as he appeared to be literally withering away, neither eating nor drinking. The fact that it had been raining for weeks did not make things any better. People were stuck inside the house, the river was flooding, too dirty and fast-flowing even for bathing, and drinking water had to be brought from a small stream in the forest. Rice should have been dried in order to feed ritual guests, but this could not be done due to the incessant raining. Also, decisions should have been made about the ritual schedule, but at the moment no one seemed to know exactly when the ritual would, or could, end.

July 11, 1996. After a quiet day and night of chanting, which has included the killing of Boruk, one of the shaman Ma Buno's dogs, the buntang *finally seems to have reached a turning point today. Colorful banners are raised outside the house as a sign that a sacrifice will be made, red and yellow colored leaves are hung up in the house during yelling and yodeling, plant counterparts of human beings are erected, and the headhunt skull is fed the blood of a chicken.*

At eight o'clock in the evening Kakah Ramat leaves the house, together with Ma Kelamo and Ma Isa, Ma Bari's two sons, who carry kerosene lamps and offering trays. They head for a hill behind the longhouse where a balei, *a temporary ritual shrine, has been built. This construction consists of two spirit houses, both intended for* Bongai tasik *("Bongai from the sea"), one with two small wooden guards holding daggers in their hands in front of its door, the other with an ugly-faced figure made of a banana trunk standing beneath it. Having seated himself by the construction, Kakah Ramat starts yet another* belian *ritual. Chanting in Indonesian he calls out for* Bongai, *"the Lord of* Blis" *(Raja Blis), "the Lord of Satan" (Raja Setan), "the Lord of Iron" (Raja Besi), striking together the blade of an axe and a chisel, asking the spirit to return to where it belongs, with a satisfied heart* (hati senang).

This *belian* ritual, which manifested striking similarities to *belian sentiu* rituals—both because it was sung in Malay/Indonesian (in contrast with the local language used both in the *buntang* and the *bawo* and *luangan* rituals) and because it summoned downriver spirits (from the sea)—was, according to Kakah Ramat, a *"belian dewa."* Contrary to *belian sentiu*, however, according to Kakah Ramat, it represented an old form of curing (he did not practice *belian sentiu*), already developed before he was born. It is not a very common style of curing, however, and it certainly was very different from the curing styles normally employed by Kakah Ramat (*belian luangan* and *bawo*).

July 12, 1996. A balei for juata, the water spirit, is built by the river today. Banners are hung up outside the house again, and a pig is brought into the house for display, its jaws tied together with a rattan strip, not tight enough to prevent it from letting out occasional shrieks though. Guests from neighboring villages arrive in large numbers now as the ritual finally reaches its climax. The belian dress up in the clothes of their spirit familiars: Kakah Ramat in a vest made of bark cloth, Ma Kerudot in a woman's skirt and blouse, carrying a fishing

137

basket under his arm, and Unsir with a rattan basket on his back and a mock spear in his hand. Embodying their spirit familiars they stab at the pig with the spear and shoot at it with a blowpipe. With the fishing basket they scoop for the illness.

Before dinner in the evening, Mancan starts another belian ritual, a belian sentiu this time. He dances wildly, swinging his arms in circular movements, running out of the house, where it is raining heavily, then back in again, soaking wet. The drums and the gongs are played in the melodious rhythms of sentiu curing, faster and faster as Mancan dances toward Ma Bari, the bells around his feet ringing with his steps. He bends down over Ma Bari and sucks all over his body, then runs to the front door and spits, then back to Ma Bari again, and to the front door—over and over again.

Later, in the evening, Kakah Ramat performs yet another belian bawo ritual. He lies face down on the floor, concealed by a tent-like screen made of kajeng leaves, which in turn is covered with a black cloth. Lying there invisible to the audience he sings and rattles his ketang bracelets. Then he suddenly stops chanting. There is almost complete silence in the room as everybody stares at Kakah Ramat's concealed body. A while later, when someone finally lifts the screen, Kakah Ramat lies there motionless on the floor, his body stiff, looking almost dead. Members of the audience hurry to splash water over him and rub his feet. After a while, a rather long time it seems, he gains consciousness again, and continues to chant.

According to then-stated plans, the buntang, which at this point was reaching its conclusion, would end with the sacrifice of a goat by the river the next morning.[9] But the efforts to discover what ailed Ma Bari—who was not feeling any better yet, I was told—continued throughout this last evening, with Mancan searching for Ma Bari's soul among downriver spirits, and trying to suck out the illness, while Kakah Ramat searched among the seniang, the celestial custodians of the cosmos and of life on earth, traveling in the heavens to look up Ma Bari's placenta, his younger "sibling," who held his fate and the key to the origins of his illness (the search thus forming a form of pereau as well, Kakah Ramat told me afterwards).

July 13, 1996. Morning. The belian *sit close to the* longan, *chanting* tempuun, *looking tired, Kakah Ramat singing with a hoarse voice.*

*The sacrifice of the goat down by the river has been postponed, and
the ritual is not ending yet, after all. Most of the ritual guests have left
the longhouse to work in their swidden fields, where trees are felled in
preparation for next year's swiddens, and it is very quiet in the house,
with those still around either resting or sleeping.*

The *buntang* was to include the sacrifice of a water buffalo after
all, and the shamans had decided that the ritual would therefore
have to be prolonged by four more days (the decision was said to be
related to Kakah Ramat's latest *pereau*, but precisely how remained
unclear to me). People discussed the sacrifice of the water buffalo
using sign language, pointing their fingers out at both sides of their
heads to mimic the horns of the animal. There was speculation that
the *buntang* would be extended to a *nalin taun*—a community ritual
which forms the grandest and most expensive of all Luangan rituals,
arranged only at infrequent intervals, every ten years or so—but this
speculation was denied by others.[10] The atmosphere in the longhouse was tense, no one spoke much, and the food consisted of only
boiled rice and ground chili. Ma Bari was still very sick, people told
me reluctantly.

*July 14, 1996. Nen Pare, who has been ill for almost a year now, is
moved into the longhouse, so that she can be cured along with Ma
Bari. She has not eaten anything for fifteen days and is very weak. At
times she loses consciousness, and the children are rushed away in case
she dies. At one end of the longhouse Nen Pare is groaning loudly; at
the other end Ma Bari is breathing heavily. The shamans chant quietly
by the* longan, *telling* tempuun, *while the house slowly fills up with
people again as Nen Pare's family is moving in with her.*

The presence of death could almost be felt in the longhouse at this
time, with worrying parents rushing their children away and listening anxiously for Ma Bari's and Nen Pare's breathing. As the house
became more and more crowded and the food ever scarcer, the
rain still pouring down outside, the tension intensified, with people
getting quiet and irritated with each other.

Ma Bari's illness had forced a number of people into a somewhat
liminal state of being for an indefinite time it seemed, preventing
them from going on with their everyday lives as usual. This concerned

139

not just Ma Bari's own extended family, but also, among others, the members of Ma Dasi's family, who had not been able to move out from the longhouse after their own *buntang* was concluded, but instead had had to stay and help out with the ritual arrangements, and also Ma Buno's family, who lived temporarily in the longhouse before Ma Dasi's *buntang* begun and decided to stay until it ended, but then became stuck in it for a much longer time, as, in fact, did we (at this time Kenneth and I had intended to travel downstream to submit our quarterly report to the Indonesian Institute of Sciences, but could not do so as Ma Bari sent a message that he did not want us to leave the village before the ritual was over).

Some work had to be done in swidden fields and in the village, however, whether there was a ritual going on or not, and therefore it was now decided that the *buntang* would have to be prolonged once again. The incessant raining, which prevented people from drying rice, was another factor influencing this decision. The *buntang* would last eight more days, instead of the four previously estimated, otherwise there would not be enough time to obtain all the food, and construct all the ritual paraphernalia needed to conclude the *buntang*.

July 16, 1996. After a quiet morning when all the men have been out working in their swidden fields—except for the shamans who have been chanting as usual—new ritual decorations are being made again. Another balei, *with three levels, is built on the hill behind the house as well, a* balei *for the* naiyu *spirits this time (this kind of* balei, *"balei naiyu," is used only when water buffalos are sacrificed).*

At this time Mancan brings two new ganti diri *figures to the longhouse. They are strangely shaped wooden effigies with long twisted, moveable arms, seemingly protecting their stiff bodies, and with downcast heads, looking to the side, as if embarrassed, or frightened. The effigies arouse amusement among the ritual participants, some of whom say that they have not seen anything quite like them before.*

Mancan had a vision when he was performing as *belian sentiu* four days earlier, and it is from this vision that he has made these peculiar wooden figures—images of malevolent spirits, as he called them, which were somehow inspired by his own dancing. He had made other more ordinary figures as well, including a water buffalo, a goat

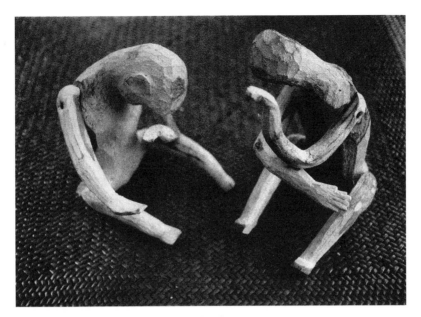

Figure 4.3. Mancan's peculiar *ganti diri* figures

and a gong, and these effigies were added to the old ones in the fishing basket placed by the *longan*. As more and more guests arrived, insinuations were made that Ma Bari might be feeling a little bit better. He had been brought some pills from a doctor in a logging camp some distance away, as well as some kind of "local medicine" (*obat kampung*) from downriver, and he had started to take them.

July 17, 1996. After a day of chanting, including the inauguration of the balei naiyu *through a pig sacrifice, yet another* belian ritual *is beginning this evening, a* belian sentiu *this time. With a shrill and penetrating voice Ma Putup, who is conducting the ritual, calls out for some of his odd spirit familiars: "Raden Muda Kuasa, Pangeran Mas Wali, Tuhan Yesus, Tuhan Perbes, Tuhan Hop, Tuhan Obos, Sum Kua, Sum Hai, Ahdukian, Ahlu, Ban-Ban-Ban-Bah-Ban, Tuhan Mangku Joyo, Karna Biana, Peteri Dori Puti, Sana Mari, Dayung Lisi, Mangku Kerta Joyo, Isa Nabi; [spirit familiars] from the hamlet village island of Melega, from the hamlet village island of Celebes, from the hamlet village island of Pengorep." He chants at a hurried pace in a language unknown to his audience (some say that it is Arabic), jumping up and*

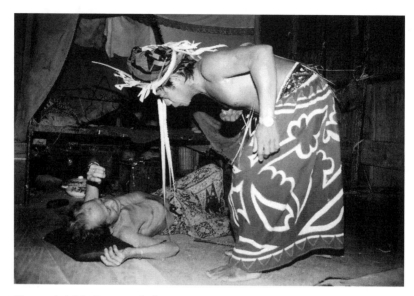

Figure 4.4. Ma Putup as *belian sentiu*

down with both feet together, dressed in a skirt decorated with tiger images and wearing anklets with small silver bangles that ring in time with his steps.

With the help of spirit guides from foreign places, unknown even to Ma Putup himself, he has set out to seize Ma Bari's soul, to buy it back from whomever it is that has taken hold of it. The people in the room look both afraid and amused as they listen to his curious words and watch him jump around, stamping his feet on the floor, rubbing the sweat from his body into his hair, yelling and grunting.

"This is a *buntang* at which souls are bought, a curing *buntang*," Ma Lombang, who had taken charge of most practical arrangements in the village now that Ma Bari was ill, announced in the morning. He then ordered Ma Putup, his son-in-law, to perform another *belian sentiu* ritual. By stressing that this was a "curing *buntang*" he both justified the need for yet another ritual inside the ritual, and distinguished this *buntang* from others less focused on curing. Coming from another village than the majority of his audience (having recently married into Sembulan) and sometimes acting rather loudly and boastfully, Ma Putup was regarded with some ambivalence by his fellow villagers and was mostly employed as *belian* within his own (affinal) family. Even so, most people agreed that he had powerful spirit familiars, of which some claimed to be afraid (see Introduction).

All of a sudden Ma Bari's son, Ma Isa, comes running into the room through the back door, looking absent-minded, laughing and waving his arms. He stops in front of the place where Ma Bari is sleeping and stands there by the mosquito-net, shivering, seemingly lost. Someone in the audience then takes him to the longan where he sits down, while people splash cold water over him. After a while he returns to being his normal self again, asking for something to drink, looking exhausted, talking about the incident as if he had acted totally out of his own control, sounding startled, and a little bit amused.

It was Ma Putup's strange and potentially dangerous spirit guides, concentrated in the room in large numbers, that here possessed not only Ma Putup himself, but also Ma Isa, who suddenly lost control of himself. To some extent Mancan seemed to be affected as well, inasmuch as he sat alone during the whole evening, with vacant eyes, mumbling to himself.

July 18, 1996. Morning. People assemble by the balei *on the hill behind the longhouse. A bamboo chair has been built and placed close to the* balei *and now water is brought in large plastic canisters up to the hill. The ritual participants, who include almost everybody in the village, except for the patients, Ma Bari and Nen Pare, seat themselves in turn on the chair while the shamans, Kakah Ramat, Ma Kerudot and Unsir, who today are joined by Ma Putup, pour water over them with ladles, chanting, asking for good fortune and good health for those that they wash. There is a festive ambience, with people laughing and screaming as they are hit by the cold water. Suddenly, Mancan climbs up to the highest level of the* balei *and starts shouting angrily and loudly about a* nalin taun *and the* seniang *spirits that are summoned during such rituals. He goes on shouting for hours; no one, however, pays much attention to him.*

Mancan had become possessed by an ancestor spirit, the spirit of a *belian* curer, a *belian* from the island of Java, he later told us. The spirit interfered in the *buntang*, questioning its length and ultimate destination, confusing it with a *nalin taun* ritual, thus expressing a confusion that was felt more generally among the ritual participants, but dissipated as the ritual finally reached its closing stage.

Tak Ningin, Ma Bari's wife, smiled for the first time in weeks that morning, and the atmosphere was one of exhilaration, with people getting ritually washed, becoming cleansed from the heat of sickness and worries. Ma Bari was definitely feeling better now I was told; he was eating again, not much, but at least eating. The *buntang* would, at last, be completed tomorrow, with the sacrifice of the water buffalo, even though Ma Lombang still made a last-minute effort to postpone it by one more day, as he had mistakenly invited people from a neighboring village to participate in the conclusion of the *buntang* one day too late. The shamans refused to change the schedule though, and Ma Lombang had to walk back to the village and change the invitation.

July 19, 1996. The twelfth day of the buntang, *the day of the water buffalo sacrifice* (olo kolak, *the final day). It is half past six in the morning and Mancan is performing as* belian sentiu *again, dancing with a bowl containing rice and flowers in his hands, asking the spirit guests to return home, to take the offerings and leave. Food is brought up to the* balei *again as well, and the water buffalo, standing in a cage at the hill, is tied to a carved ironwood pole. Kakah Ramat, Ma Buno, Unsir, and Ma Putup seat themselves by the* balei *and start to chant, presenting food to the spirits, including a pig and some chickens, which are then killed and taken down to the kitchen.*

More and more guests arrive now, and the longhouse is getting crowded. The belian *walk around among these people, smearing lime paste on their foreheads, whisking over them with large bunches of leaves. At this time three large pigs and some chickens are brought into the house and tied to the bamboo slats in the floor by the front door. The ritual participants pluck some hair from the pigs and some feathers from the chickens, holding the hair and feathers above their heads for a few moments, before throwing them into the air.*

At about three o'clock in the afternoon the belian *ascend to the* balei *once more, this time to call down Jarung, a spirit familiar who is summoned when water buffalos are sacrificed. Jarung is embodied by Kakah Ramat, who sits at the highest level of the* balei, *wearing a crown made of palm leaves, dyed in red and yellow. Mancan sits with the other* belian *at a lower level of the* balei, *but does not participate in the chanting (unlike the others he is not competent to perform* buntang *rituals), watching over the events so to speak, dressed in a black velvet* kopiah *(a cap frequently worn by Muslims, but at times also by non-Muslims to symbolize their Indonesian citizenship), appearing overly serious, perhaps representing the Javanese* belian *who has been possessing him.*

It is already dark when the water buffalo is finally killed. After the shamans have presented food and cigarettes to it, asking it to die peacefully and not to hurt people, the cage is opened and the buffalo is allowed to run out, tied only to the blontang *pole with a thick rattan cord. Angrily it tries to gore the group of young men who are encircling it, while they in turn try to stab it with their spears. Badly hurt, the water buffalo then finally falls to the ground.*

At midnight, after hours of waiting, the ritual guests are finally served the buffalo meat, which has been cooked in a sauce and is now served with rice and fried pork on plates arranged in a long row on the longhouse floor. After eating, most of the guests take their torches and jungle knives and walk back to their own houses, some of which are located in a neighboring village some three kilometers away. The shamans go on chanting throughout the night, rocking the wooden ship, returning from their soul-search journey.

Large sacrifices usually draw large audiences, with neighbors and relatives gathering together to make preparations, socialize, and partake in the food served. This last day of Ma Bari's *buntang*, which was to be completed by the sacrifice to *juata* by the river bank the next morning, was no exception. On the contrary, more than one hundred people had gathered in the relatively small longhouse to pay their respects to Ma Bari and enjoy the festivities. Although the sacrifice in itself became something of an anticlimax because it took place so late, after dark, there was a general feeling of relief this evening, born out of endurance and the possibility of break up. Ma Bari remained hidden behind his mosquito-net, but the chance of recovery had become a real possibility now, or at least it was felt to be so.

July 20, 1996. Morning. The buntang *ends with the simultaneous sacrifice of a white pig by the river bank and a bathing ceremony performed outside the longhouse in the flower grove. Together with Ma Dengu and Nen Bai, Mancan pours water over a group of people, who sit in a row under the shrubs, wrapped in sarongs. Mancan is in a good mood, joking. He was again possessed by the Javanese spirit last night, and he stood on this same spot shouting angrily for the whole evening while the* buntang *continued in the longhouse. Kakah Ramat and Ma Buno perform the pig sacrifice to* juata *by the river, collecting the blood of the white pig in a wooden canoe, while gongs and drums are played inside the longhouse. Together with some children, Kakah Ramat and Tak Ramat then wash themselves in the blood, which has been mixed with water, sitting in the shallow canoe as they do so.*

A little while later people enter the longhouse again and white plates paid as wages for the ritual work are distributed to everyone involved, together with pieces of buffalo meat, some cloth and a couple of jungle knives. Kakah Ramat receives the most, but he is closely followed by the other shamans, the penyempatung *assistants, the decoration makers etc. Ma Bari's extended family, including his wife, his two sons and his daughter, as well as their spouses and children, then enter the soul house together, placing their feet on the doorstep of the small wooden house, which the* belian *then verbally make ascend to the heavens.*

Thus twenty-five days of ritual (if we include Ma Dasi's *buntang*) had finally come to an end, at least for the time being, and this was at last the time for dispersal. The shamans left the longhouse with their wages, which were carried by men assigned to do so, while Nen Pare was carried away on a stretcher to her own house. The members of Ma Buno's family departed for their swidden house as well, and Ma Dasi's family started to make preparations to leave, to move to the home village of Ma Dasi's wife, three days away by foot, while Kenneth and I prepared to travel downstream. Besides the water buffalo, eight pigs and dozens of chickens had been sacrificed during the course of the ritual, along with two dogs that had been killed (and two cats I was to discover later), all in the effort to cure Ma Bari, who now sat up for the first time in weeks, although he still looked very weak.

This dispersal was not an end however, but rather a starting-point toward recovery. When I returned to Sembulan three weeks after the *buntang* had ended, I learned that Ma Bari was still feeling unwell and that he had been eating poorly for a long time after the ritual ended. I also learned that his son-in-law (a schoolteacher) had considered it necessary to travel downstream to bring a *menteri* (a male nurse, Kakah Ramat's son's son-in-law) to the village in order to give Ma Bari a series of injections. It still took months before he could leave the longhouse, or walk down to bathe in the river, and even longer before he could again work in his swidden field as he used to. For Nen Pare, however, things did not turn out as well as they eventually did for Ma Bari: she died the day after the *buntang* ended, after not having eaten for twenty-one days.

If it Strikes...

I ask you guests to leave
illnesses with names we do not know
maladies with epithets we do not know

—Excerpt from a *belian sentiu* chant by Mancan

Not to know, not to know for sure: these are the conditions that *belian* curers have to deal with and try to make sense of. Instead of a particular spirit being, or category of spirits, it is often "the illness," *roten*, or *roten saan*, that a *belian* addresses in his chants, asking it to leave the body, to return to where it belongs. He does so because he does not know which particular spirit is guilty of causing the illness, I was told by Kakah Ramat. He also does so, he suggested, because he wants to make sure that all the spirits, not just the one he suspects or "feels" is guilty, are included in his requests (cf. Metcalf 1991: 242 for similar observations among the Berawan).[11]

To play it safe, to prepare for all contingencies: this is the kind of certainty that is on offer in spirit negotiation. Like the Berawan spirit world (Metcalf 1991: 47, 242, 248), the Luangan spirit world is "unbounded" and cannot be fully known or controlled by anybody.[12] There are always other spirits to account for, other spirits that are possibly involved, and possibly with bad intentions. As the story of Ma Bari's illness has shown us, to search for the cause of an illness is not an easy or uncomplicated task, but something that might have to be done over and over again, and once a diagnosis has been reached, this still does not mean that negotiation with spirits other than the one(s) pointed out in the process can be excluded.

147

Belian rituals are "operations ... relative to situations" (de Certeau 1984: 21), in the sense that the decisions made in and through them must attend to the particular circumstances out of which they are born, while also taking into account the unpredictability and opacity of these circumstances through a certain degree of generality or lack of specificity. This entails a balancing act which may sometimes seem rather easy—the *belian* first diagnosing the cause of the illness, then negotiating with a number of spirits—but at other times can become quite a complex process, involving an increasing variety of spirit beings, and including several intermixed styles of negotiation.

When Ma Bari suddenly fell ill during Ma Dasi's *buntang*, no one paid much attention or reflected much on the causes at first— stomach pains are after all not unusual, especially during the larger rituals, when houses tend to get crowded and food has to be cooked long in advance to feed all the guests. However, after a few days had passed without Ma Bari getting any better, some members of his family began to worry, and, as we have seen, first asked a person in a neighboring village, then Kakah Ramat, to diagnose the cause of the illness (this was done outside the context of *belian*). Both pointed out pigs as possible culprits, and these pigs were quickly killed. Ma Bari did not show any signs of recovery, however, and at this stage it was decided that a *belian* ritual would have to be arranged. Acting as *belian bawo*, Ma Buno conducted a *pereau*, and, as in the two previous cases, a pig was pointed out as the probable cause of Ma Bari's biting stomach pains and was thereafter soon killed.

Discovering which particular animal (in this case which pig) is the cause of someone's suffering (assuming that it is an animal, which it does not have to be) is a question of interpretation (and in the context of *belian*, of deciphering the words of the *belian*'s spirit familiars). There is no way to know for sure if the interpretation has struck the mark (if the symptoms disappear one can nevertheless feel quite positive that it has done so), and even if one identifies the right animal, or animals (as there might be many) one still has to consider the fact that it is not the animal itself that is the origin (*asar*) of the illness, but rather a malevolent spirit (*blis*) who has "tricked" (*ngerongo*) the animal into injuring the sick person, and that this spirit (or these spirits) might do it again unless (or even if) precautions are taken. In Ma Bari's case the first killings did not have an immediate effect, and as he rapidly got worse there was no time to wait and see if they would possibly have an effect later. Other measures had to be taken, and fast.

It was at this moment that Ma Buno was asked to perform the *belian bawo* ritual, a ritual which was carried out in the middle of the day—rather than in the evening as is the case with most curing *belian*—because of Ma Bari's rapidly deteriorating condition. In this ritual, Ma Buno set out not only to identify the illness or its perpetrator (although this was perhaps the most important motive for this short, one-hour long ritual, which can be said to have left most of the curing for subsequent rituals), but also to please the spirits through offerings, which were given both to the spirits helping him in this process and to those who were possibly responsible for Ma Bari's illness. These offerings, which, as usual, consisted of both food and ritual decorations, were directed both to spirits generally known to cause stomach aches—such as *juata* and *bansi*—and to spirits identified through the process of *pereau*—in this case *blis simpung*, an unmarked category of spirits from a grove of high trees left uncut in the vicinity of the village.[13]

The issue for Ma Buno was—and is for *belian* in general—to have enough (and the correct) ritual paraphernalia and offerings. There must be enough spirit houses and *ganti diri* figures, among other things, to please not only one of the *blis simpung*, for example, but the whole multitude of spirits counted among them (*tentuwaja, bansi, buta, bongai, naiyu, timang*, etc.). As Kakah Ramat expressed it to me: "You have to negotiate with all of them" (*sentous la kahai dali*), because "you do not know who among them is guilty" (*malum beau tau tudu dali baro*). In a similar vein, he said "you do not know whether it is *bongai*, whether it is *bansi*, or whether it is *tentuwaja*" (*beau tau bongai, beau tau bansi, beau tau tentuwaja*). What matters, according to Kakah Ramat, is "only that there is enough paraphernalia made" (*ede ruye ye sukup*).

The ritual paraphernalia, *ruye*, is what creates the elementary conditions of contact, and thus what enables the negotiation (Luangans accordingly put much time and effort into the fabrication of paraphernalia and decorations, which sometimes are used for only an hour, as they were in Ma Buno's case). The various *ruye* are, as was frequently pointed out to me, the material manifestations of the words chanted by the *belian*. It is through them that human intentions are materialized; and it is also through them that the spirits

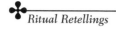

come to recognize themselves as parties (*imang*) in the negotiation, and thus as having ritually prescribed obligations toward the other parties involved. The process referred to by the verb *sentous*—to procure the soul of the sick person through exchange, which is closely bound up with the process of *besemah*, to present offerings and respect to the spirits and thus allure them into participation— implies and presupposes negotiation precisely through both words and objects (with the addition of dancing in *sentiu* and *bawo* curing).

The question, once again, is to denote without excluding, to be specific enough without being too restrictive. When Ma Buno diagnosed the pig as responsible for Ma Bari's illness, he reacted to an immediate situation, attempting to remove Ma Bari's symptoms by dispelling the cause of the illness. However, even in the same ritual, he (and other shamans later) had to consider other possibilities as well, addressing the spirit world in a more inclusive way and directing his words and offerings not only to "identified" spirits but also to spirits or illnesses whose names were not known.

A Falling Vessel

In their very materiality ritual decorations and offerings are prone to vicissitudes; they are, to use a phrase of Keane's (1997: 31), "subject to nonsemiotic happenstances." Things sometimes happen to them, things which cannot be anticipated or foreseen. Their use in social practices, located as they are in the material world, opens them up to risks and possibilities which can destabilize their meanings. Keane (ibid.: 29–33) provides an example of such an unintended event, which altered the interpretation of a representational act (more precisely, the presentation of a gift in Anakalang, Sumba). A valuable textile, which was used as a banner on a tomb, was accidentally torn (by becoming tangled in a tree) while the tomb was dragged to a new location (and as a result the textile was cut down to half its size). When this same piece of cloth was later presented as a gift, without the giver knowing what had happened to it, the receiver, believing that he had been intentionally given an inferior textile, became offended and rejected the gift. As this event illustrates, representations are contingent upon materially conditioned circumstances. But they are not, of course, influenced by material conditions alone.[14] Interpretations are always contextual, and in the case of *belian* rituals, deeply informed by a more general "logic," according to which there are always other possibilities, with the suspension of certainty by inclusiveness constituting the most practical and the safest strategy available.

Late one night during Ma Dasi's *buntang*, the ship used for soul-search travel suddenly fell down from the ceiling while the *belian* were on a soul-search journey. At the time the incident passed without much notice; it was simply attributed to "natural" causes. The cord by which the ship was suspended snapped because it was old and worn out (which is not to say that the possibility that something else could have been involved in the incident did not pass through the minds of those still awake at the time, but just that no one back then found reason to draw public attention to such a possibility). However, as Ma Bari's condition got worse, and as people started to worry—the killings of the pigs not having the desired effect—the incident was reappraised, and the falling of the vessel was interpreted as an "intentional sign," a bearer of "non-natural meaning" (Grice 1957, in Keane 1997: 32). The event was conceived of as an intervention from outside (from ancestors or associated spirits), as a sign that actions had to be taken, and it was specifically interpreted (by the shamans) to mean that a new *buntang* had to be arranged (ships used in *buntang* rituals are reserved exclusively for these occasions, and thus are a kind of indexical token of them).

Ma Bari's involvement in Ma Dasi's *buntang* as the owner of the house in which it was arranged and as a participant in, and initiator of, much of the preparations, as well as his status as the (unofficial) head of customary law and a local leader (*manti*), were also factors that influenced the decision to arrange a *buntang* for him. Because of the former, the sign of the falling vessel was seen as pointing directly at Ma Bari, and because of the latter, Ma Bari's illness and the threat of his imminent death touched upon the village as a whole to a much larger extent than it would have if someone else had fallen ill. Not to take appropriate measures in this situation would have endangered not only Ma Bari's life but also the future of the village and its inhabitants at large. This was partly so because there was no credible candidate to succeed him in office, which along with the village itself lacked official status, and the combination of these two factors meant that his death could have provoked a crisis threatening the unity of the village, and its autonomy. For these reasons alone a *buntang* was an appropriate measure in this instance, particularly because *buntang* rituals are collective rituals, engaging a much larger number of villagers than is normally the case in more family-restricted curing rituals—even if the decision to hold it at such an early stage would have still been unwarranted, if it had not been for the sign of the falling vessel. As it turned out in this case, the decision to arrange the *buntang* was forced by the latter occurrence, before the actual curing had even begun (instead of being arrived at during a preceding curing *belian*, which is the ordinary practice).

Not to arrange a *belian* ritual when circumstances appear to demand one is conceived of as a risky enterprise, not just in this particular case, but more generally. Whereas the risks inherent in ritual activity have been frequently emphasized in the literature (e.g., Howe 2000: 229; Keane 1997; Schieffelin 1996), and whereas it is true that *belian* rituals entail various hazards (spiritual, existential, material and political), it is perhaps not these risks that are seen to constitute the greatest ones among the Luangans, but rather the risks involved in not arranging a *belian*, in not responding to the spirits. *Belian* rituals hence are frequently arranged even when no one seems to be particularly ill, or when the patient has already recovered, and they are often arranged over and over again, even in situations where there is not much hope of a cure (as in Nen Pare's case, see chapter 2).[15] Not to arrange a *belian* ritual is, as the Luangans see it, to refrain from contact, to decline the reciprocity of human and spiritual coexistence, to rashly throw oneself into the uncertainty of life by relinquishing the relative security created by ritual representation and interrelation with spirits.

Ritual failure (or success for that matter) is not usually what is at question in *belian* curing. As I will argue later, there are no clear-cut boundaries between *belian* rituals, and an individual ritual thus cannot be judged as an isolated event, but must be seen rather in relation to both prior and possible future events.[16] To play it safe means to take every chance available, to employ every imaginable option (or at least several realizable ones), instead of being caught in just one mode of representation. When the ship fell down from the ceiling during Ma Dasi's *buntang* the incident was not so much interpreted to mean that something wrong had been done in the ritual as that more had yet to be done, that there were other measures to be taken (Ma Dasi's *buntang* was completed according to the plans, and it was never regarded as a failure in any sense).

As Arendt (1958: 237; ref. Jackson 1998: 204) has argued, "The remedy for unpredictability, for the chaotic uncertainty of the future, is contained in the faculty to make and keep promises." This is also how *belian buntang* rituals function; they are the fulfillment of vows or promises made to the spirits in order to invoke reciprocity and inter-relatedness, and thus to exercise some degree of influence over the future (the spirits are considered to be the siblings of human beings, see chapter 6). The promise here, as always, is seen not only as binding for its maker, but potentially also as affecting its receiver, who, it is hoped, will act in a particular way as a result of it. This is, of course, no less true in cases in which the promise is brought about by direct indication from the spirits, as it was in Ma Bari's case. On the contrary, its making (and swift fulfillment) attained a particular kind of urgency in this case, since a failure to act on the indication would have meant a refusal to respond to the spirits, a refusal to negotiate on their terms and to take the chance given.

Considering the binding character of the promise, not to arrange a *belian* ritual when a promise of one has been enunciated, or even intimated, constitutes a particular risk in spirit negotiation. To create expectations and then not to act on them entails much greater hazards than, for example, doing something wrong or deficiently. This is also one of the reasons why there is so much secrecy, so much silence and whispering surrounding the "not-knowing" that precedes a decision or promise of *belian* curing. Words said out loud produce expectations that must be met so as not to create or aggravate already critical situations.[17] Following a similar line of reasoning, the Luangans often overstate the seriousness of an illness, or rather describe all illnesses as similarly serious, so as not to give the false impression that their intentions (in negotiating with spirits) can be taken lightly. A further example of the risks of enunciation can be seen in the use of cover names during *pereau*, as the uttering of real names might serve to attract unwanted spirits rather than to identify them. The "explicit" here accommodates both danger and potentiality; it creates a demand for realization, but it also engenders possibilities to influence and direct the actions of the spirits.[18]

Extreme Measures

Belian rituals are points of departure rather than ends (cf. Taussig 1992: 161), in the sense that they constitute the prerequisites of curing without ever promising "full restoration of stability" (Seremetakis 1991: 48). *Belian* rituals are followed by other *belian* rituals, often several in a row, and occasionally overlapping each other. The possibilities that are explored and the different measures that are taken in *belian* curing are not ends in themselves but rather constitute new beginnings, which widen the horizons of negotiation. Over the course of a serious illness in particular, digression is the rule rather than the exception; alternative styles of curing are employed as the ritual participants become reminded—in one way or another—of their potentiality, their capacity to reach out in new directions (cf. Tsing 1984: 100). "Afflicted people [thus] 'try out' ... a plan of action to see if it works," to cite Susan Whyte (1997: 23) on the curing practices of the Nyole of Eastern Uganda.

The suddenness of Ma Bari's illness, as well as its rapid course, provoked Ma Bari's family not only to initiate the new *buntang* as soon as Ma Dasi's *buntang* had been completed, but also to introduce other measures, both before and after the *buntang* had begun (the *buntang* can here be regarded as constituting a background against which these other measures took place). Due to the seriousness of Ma Bari's condition and its urgency (resulting not least from the potential repercussions it had for the future of the village and its inhabitants), these different efforts at curing sometimes followed one upon the other at what seemed like a remarkably hurried pace, and took forms that in some instances were rather extreme.

New measures demand new decorations and paraphernalia, and it was with the making of new decorations that the quest(s) to cure Ma Bari began. With the throwing out of the old decorations and the constructing of new ones yet another journey into the spirit realm began.[19] Starting out with a *belian luangan*, which was soon transformed into a *belian bawo*, Kakah Ramat, together with Ma Kerudot, set out to catch Ma Bari's errant soul, a pursuit undertaken not only in these curing *belian*, but also throughout the *buntang*.

By including curing, Ma Bari's *buntang* was by no means unusual, however. On the contrary, *buntang* rituals, as already stated, always contain elements of curing. Souls are searched for (*berejuus*) and snatched (*nakep juus*) in them, and illnesses are wiped off patients' bodies with banana leaf whisks (*nyelolo*). Malevolent spirits are also presented with minor offerings (*besemah*), while being verbally requested to withdraw. This notwithstanding, the Luangans primarily conceptualize *buntang* rituals as "thanksgiving" rituals: as *upah*, "rewards," presented to the spirit guides (*mulung*) for curing the sick, and the protecting spirits (*pengiring*) who continuously guard people and regulate the social and natural order. These rewards can be presented both before or after actual alleviation has been achieved, in return for help already obtained or as advance payments or requests for future help. The spirit guides and protecting spirits (including various *seniang, naiyu, timang, juata* and *tonoi* spirits, as well as *kelelungan*, the refined spirits of the dead) are also the recipients of most of the food and ritual paraphernalia offered in a *buntang*, and it is to them that most invocations are directed (what is asked for in *buntang* rituals, again and again, is a good life: a state in which there are "no illnesses, plenty of rice, plenty of meat, where you live happily, where illnesses pass by, injuries heal, dreams are good dreams, and omens favorable"). Curing (that is, activities directly associated with the removal of illnesses and the retrieval of souls), or at least the initiation of the curing process, is something that is basically seen as belonging to preliminary curing rituals, although the actual curing can be continued and elaborated in *buntang* rituals, which, in contrast to curing *belian*, are regarded as being enacted primarily in order to present offerings, the use of which is authorized through the chanting of *tempuun*.

What distinguished Ma Bari's *buntang* from most other *buntang* rituals then, was not divergence from this order of procedure (according to which a *buntang* should follow on a preceding curing *belian*), but the fact that the curing continued to such a high degree throughout it (while the curing rituals preceding it were relatively short and incomplete), a fact which made Ma Lombang use the expression "curing *buntang*" for this particular ritual. The circumstances surrounding Ma Bari's illness—the falling of the soul-search ship in particular—precipitated the commencement of the *buntang* at the same time that Ma Bari's condition demanded immediate action (i.e., curing), which could not wait until the *buntang* began (the *buntang* could not begin before the three-day *pali* following Ma Dasi's *buntang* was over). Elements of curing and thanksgiving

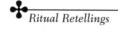

were thus juxtaposed, and a project involving both entreatment and reimbursement was initiated, a project reaching out both toward the malevolent spirits causing the illness and toward the spirit familiars and protector spirits that were summoned to suspend it.

The scene of Kakah Ramat performing as *belian bawo* bears witness to the seriousness of the situation being dealt with here. Due to his old age—he was in his early or mid-eighties at the time of the ritual—Kakah Ramat had not acted as *belian bawo* in years, but had only practiced the much quieter *belian luangan* style that lacks the dancing and spinning characteristic of *belian bawo*. An extreme situation therefore called for extreme measures. Performing as *belian bawo*, Kakah Ramat incorporated both the potency of extraordinary procedures and the authority of his experience in the process of curing, embodying commitment and sincerity as he, dancing on stiff legs, repudiated the perishableness of life.

Grabbing after Ma Bari's soul again and again, Kakah Ramat engaged repetition as a form of security, and in doing so demonstrated a multiplicity of efforts that are typically involved in soul retrieval, a multiplicity that could also be seen in the diversity of curing styles employed in Ma Bari's *buntang* as a whole. Such a multiplicity points to a fundamental evasiveness—of spirits, of souls, and of the present—which shamans continually have to deal with both in curing *belian* and in *buntang* rituals. By resuming the *bawo* curing over and over again (after the *buntang* had already begun), oscillating between the *buntang* and *bawo* rituals, Kakah Ramat confounds any notions we might have of beginnings or ends, or of stability. Alternating between the quiet chanting of the *buntang* and the dramatic summoning of *blis* in the *bawo* inserts, Kakah Ramat, together with Ma Kerudot and Unsir, draws our attention to the potentially diversifying nature of the curing process, which involves pleasing, pleading, trading, expelling, retrieval and repayment, which are not so much different measures aimed at different objectives (e.g. negotiation, curing, reciprocation) as they are parallel strategies to make a general condensed statement about commitment and uncertainty. Whereas, to cite Atkinson (1989: 289) whose observation about Wana curing practices also applies to Luangan curing, "no immediate signs of recovery are expected from a patient at time of treatment," a change for the worse still demands attention, and as Ma Bari's condition got worse, Kakah Ramat reached out in yet another direction, initiating a *belian dewa*. Summoning downriver spirits, "*bongai* from the sea," a spirit category known to cause epidemics among other things, he once again took to the extreme, chanting in Indonesian, a language he did not speak well, performing in a style very different from the ones he usually employed (for example, he used a rather limited vocabulary in this ritual, in contrast to the verbosity which usually characterized his curing).[20] Through this ritual he entered the realm of *sentiu* curing, although not quite, since *belian dewa*, as Kakah Ramat himself emphasized, should not be mixed up with *belian sentiu*—notwithstanding the obvious resemblances—which is of much more recent origin (at most, as he saw it, *belian dewa* may be seen as a precursor of the *sentiu* style). What Kakah Ramat did here was to open the negotiation for yet another possibility, by including "other" spirits this time. As in the case of his *bawo* curing, he responded to a critical situation by engaging tradition in an effort of exploration, drawing on his long experience of *belian* curing and at the same time reappraising his knowing, adjusting to the elusiveness of reality.

A prominent characteristic of Kakah Ramat's *belian dewa* ritual was that he employed a downriver aesthetics in negotiating with (downstream) spirits. The spirits were summoned by the sound of iron tools struck together, indexing the trade relations that have linked upriver and downriver peoples for centuries (cf. Roseman 1996: 244). Iron, in this instance, epitomized foreignness, as well as the power of that foreignness. The "other" was further pleased in a "language of otherness," reduced to its essentials, like the trade Malay used in past contacts with Malay and Buginese traders, and in marked contrast to the elaborated language of *luangan* and *bawo* curing. Kakah Ramat thus stressed distance at the same time that he invoked interdependence in this ritual, pronouncing and dramatizing the foreign, while simultaneously bringing it into the familiar domain, domesticating it through incorporation (cf. Boddy 1995: 19). In this connection it is significant to recall that the rite was performed at the hill behind the longhouse, away from and unlike the other ritual activities (and without much of an audience, except for Ma Bari's two sons, who served as Kakah Ramat's assistants).

Throughout the performance of the *belian dewa*, the *buntang* continued in the longhouse, gradually reaching its climax: the sacrifice of pigs and chickens, the hanging up of *ibus* leaves, and the enacted embodiment of the spirit familiars distributing offerings to spirit guides and protecting spirits. However, since Ma Bari's condition was worsening rather than improving, some last minute efforts to expel the illness were still made. Performing as *belian sentiu*, Mancan, Kakah Ramat's granddaughter's husband, tried to suck out the illness while pleasing the spirits with his graceful dance movements, employing the power of what the villagers perceived to be refined Malay aesthetics (imitating the culture of the royal court of the Kutai Sultanate), to be distinguished from the much coarser style of Kakah Ramat's rather minimalistic negotiation in the *belian dewa*. A more recent variant of curing involving the addressing of downriver spirits was thus performed, initiated by Mancan himself, one of the most ardent advocates of *sentiu* curing in the village. Chanting in a mix of Kutai Malay and Luangan, summoning his *dewa* spirit familiars (not to be confused with the name of Kakah Ramat's preceding ritual), Mancan reached out toward the *bongai* spirits, and in addition toward a category of spirits causing death throes (*blis ene sengkerapei*), thus doing his part in trying to keep death at a distance.[21]

Traveling to the *seniang*, the celestial spirits that regulate the cosmic order, Kakah Ramat—performing as *belian bawo* again—confronted Ma Bari's "fate," looking the possibility of death straight in the eye, so to speak, while he, once again, searched for the origins (*asar*) of Ma Bari's illness (in this case the spirit causing the illness, rather than an animal possessed by it). During this journey, Kakah Ramat looked up Ma Bari's double and "younger sibling" (*ani*)—his placenta—and the *seniang* acting as its guardian—and thus of Ma Bari's "fate"—from which he then received signs regarding Ma Bari's condition. In doing so he took an "ontological risk," the risk of coming up with answers that his audience might not have wanted to know. If the *seniang*, as Kakah Ramat expressed it, had "turned their back" on him during this process, this would have meant, according to his own account, that the possibility of continued life was foreclosed, that there would be nothing else to do (though if this had happened Kakah Ramat would probably not had told his audience). At the same time, however, Kakah Ramat's action also provided an opening for renewed hope—for a good sign—and thus for further action.

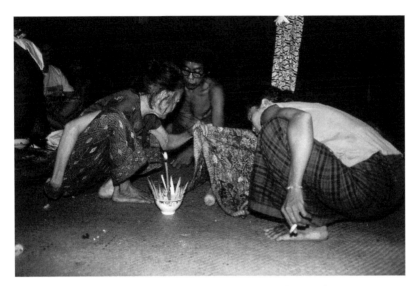

Figure 4.5. Kakah Ramat (beneath sarong cloth) traveling to the *seniang*, confronting Ma Bari's fate

Buntang Again

The *belian* practitioners came and went, one replacing another in swift rotation, but the illness would not disappear. Rather than any signs of improvement, Mukng [a *tatau solai*, or great leader] grew ever thinner and more desiccated. His belly was as hollow as a rice-mortar, his ribs were as the rocks exposed after a landfall, his fingers like sticks of bamboo, his hands like knots on a tree-trunk, his feet like the tangled roots of the bamboo. He was dying but he would not die; he was living but could not get well.

—Excerpt from *Tempuun Bekeleu* (Hopes et al. 1997: 141)

And so *belian* descended, and *belian* ascended. There was a *buntang* including a sacrifice of a water buffalo. Without any signs of recovery, however. And thus there was a new *buntang* again.

—Excerpt from a story told by Kakah Ramat (my translation)

Ends are not always ends, as I hope I have made clear by now. On the fifth and what was meant to be the final day of Ma Bari's *buntang*, a decision (influenced by Kakah Ramat's *pereau*) was made by the shamans, together with Ma Bari's family, to prolong the ritual and to include the sacrifice of a water buffalo. What at first had seemed possible to achieve in four days, turned out to be impossible in such time (a four-day *buntang* in practice usually takes five days, but is still considered a four-day *buntang*, since *buntang* rituals should not last an uneven number of days). The *belian* thus resumed the singing of *tempuun* again, repeating the *tempuun* of chickens and pigs, preparing further sacrifices.

The sacrifice of a water buffalo implies a higher hierarchical level than the sacrifice of a pig, because water buffalos have more economic value, and thus they indicate a higher input. There had been speculations from the very beginning of Ma Bari's *buntang* that it would include the sacrifice of a water buffalo, but these speculations were dismissed, not least because such *buntang* rituals demand plenty of material resources that take time to amass. There has to be enough rice to feed all the ritual guests during every day of a *buntang*, and there has to be enough money to buy the sacrificial animals, including dozens of chickens, several pigs, and the water buffalo itself, in case one does not own one.[22] The water buffalo has to be caught as well, something that may take considerable time, as most water buffalos are allowed to roam free in the forest and have to be caught in cages. Large rituals also demand large wages for the shamans—plates, cloth, rice, meat, and, in downriver Luangan communities, money—and more shamans have to be engaged the larger the ritual is. Considering this fact and the fact that a *buntang* had already been in progress for many days when Ma Bari fell ill, it is not surprising that the people involved were content with a smaller scale *buntang* at this stage, even if Ma Bari's standing in the village caused them to speculate that the sacrifice of a water buffalo might be required.

A prior history of rituals that had been arranged for Ma Bari probably contributed to these speculations: there had been grand rituals arranged before when Ma Bari had been seriously ill. High status and old age often occasion large rituals; sacrifices are regarded as substitutes for sacrificers, and the importance of the person for whom a sacrifice stands should be reflected in the sacrifice. This is, once again, a question of stakes, but also of the seriousness of intentions. Abundance (in the form of offerings and sacrifices) is a strategy to demonstrate commitment and an appropriate sense of proportion, and thus to bring forth transformation. But then again, promises should be actualized, and in this case the promise of an eight-day ritual, including a water buffalo sacrifice, was not made at first in the hope that such a ritual would not be needed after all, and perhaps also out of fear that it could not be implemented on such short notice.

Decisions regarding the length or scope of rituals are never totally fixed in advance, but depend on circumstances or external factors: the weather, the possibility of getting people in time to do the work that is needed (rituals are frequently extended for this reason), the arrival of guests, delays in the ritual program, and the development of a patient's condition. Hence, revisions of decisions regarding rituals are frequent, especially in the form of extensions and complementary additions. In fact, decisions have often to be reached during the process of ritualization, rather than before the ritual's implementation, as it is often not possible to know in advance how serious the condition is, and how soon the necessary practicalities can be carried out.

"Although ritual creates its own time out of time, it is also part of the ongoing temporal world" (Coville 1989: 119). I would argue that this is very much the case with *belian* and *buntang* rituals. People walk in and out of rituals, and rituals often have to be adjusted to their movements (which does not mean that it does not work the other way round as well, as I have already shown in this chapter). Because not all the preparations required for the sacrifice of the water buffalo in Ma Bari's *buntang* could be made in time—in as much as the rain prohibited the drying of rice and people had to work in their swidden fields, for instance—the ritual was extended not once but twice. Beginning as a four-day ritual, it was first extended to eight days, and then, finally, to twelve days (including the curing of Nen Pare). This apparent flexibility undeniably served its purpose, but it also caused tension and exhaustion among the ritual participants, who did not know what to expect next in the ritual, or how long it would last.

The not-knowing (and constant revisions) surrounding Ma Bari's *buntang* provoked speculations that it might be extended to a *nalin taun*. While these speculations were eventually quashed by the *belian* (*nalin taun* rituals are not normally arranged without careful planning in advance, and seldom just for an individual patient), they still say something about how deeply a large number of people were involved in this ritual, and how much it had become a communal affair, affecting not only Ma Bari's immediate family, but also almost every person in the village. A *nalin taun* ritual would have been *the* ultimate action. Normally extending over at least sixteen days, involving all villagers and a large number of invited non-villagers, reaching out toward the *seniang* spirits who protect the basic order of life on earth, and including the recitation of the myths of origin of heaven and earth and of humankind, a *nalin taun* ritual, by invoking the very foundations of human existence, is the most powerful ritual available to Luangans.[23] On the other hand, a *nalin taun* would have demanded a considerable amount of preparatory work, which would have been especially demanding for the villagers considering how much ritual work had already been done. Moreover, it would have also constituted a somewhat ambiguous affair, since there was no prior history of arranging a *nalin taun* for the curing of "ordinary" illnesses (its arrangement would have seemed much more appropriate if Ma Bari's illness had been caused by incest or illicit sexual relations, *bunsung sumbang*).

Although *buntang* rituals are not as wide in scope as *nalin taun* rituals, they are, as I have pointed out before, collective rituals, involving a large number of people, particularly toward their conclusions. In Ma Bari's case this became exceptionally clear as practically everyone in the village took part in the ritual at some stage, and as guests arrived in large numbers from neighboring villages as well. The twice-extended *buntang* became almost as imposing as a *nalin taun*, and it drew almost as many participants. It was with a seemingly unified force that the spirit familiars were credited here, with people collectively partaking in the sacrifices by throwing chicken feathers and pig bristles over their heads (*mesik merik*), by spitting on *ganti diri* figurines, and by participating in the fabrication of ritual preparations. A collective anxiety was thus attended to by collective efforts, with people participating out of respect for Ma Bari, but also out of personal concern for the future, and how it might unfold.

Lying beneath his mosquito-net in an enclosed corner of the room, Ma Bari remained invisible throughout all of this. He was the main character, the one who most of the action centered around, but he was an invisible main character (as patients often are). His authority was not absent, however, but rather took concrete shape through the actions of others. It was out of respect and the perceived need for his office and knowledge that people acted here, trying out every possibility at hand. And this is very much the kind of authority that Ma Bari held, even when he was well: an authority based on the power to stir people without much direct intervention, an almost invisible influence, which nevertheless was felt to be incontestable. Ma Bari's authority was one based on tradition, and the knowledge of tradition. It was an authority inherited from the ancestors, but brought into the present and people's everyday lives by his experienced leadership in *adat* law negotiations, his quiet but dignified person, and his extensive kin networks, linking him to most persons in the village and many of them to each other.

Extending the *buntang* again and again so that *buntang* followed on *buntang*, Ma Bari's family and fellow-villagers followed a tradition of intervention: they did what had been done before, in stories and in real life (if we can separate these categories) when leaders had fallen ill, and when the future had been at stake (cf. the quotations above). Chanting by the ancestor skulls and smearing blood on the inherited valuables and the headhunt skull, the *belian* called on the power of the ancestors and ancestral tradition, expounding tradition itself as a powerful agency capable of influencing human concerns. The elongation of the ritual, and the commitment-signifying-endurance which it implied, was a means not only toward enabling Ma Bari's recovery, but also one toward the re-creation and re-enactment of procedures applied previously in similar circumstances (i.e., rituals arranged for important persons). Arranging *buntang* on *buntang* was thus an appropriate measure, and at the same time was born out of practical demands. In this sense Ma Bari's status and position in the village was of central importance for the complexity of this ritual, even if it cannot be said to have been its only motive.

Speaking from the Outside

Possessed by a Javanese *belian* (said to be an ancestor spirit), Mancan—standing on the *balei* built for the *naiyu* spirits and interrupting the *buntang* by shouting about a *nalin taun*—serves as yet another reminder of the uncertainty and complexity of spirit negotiation, and of authority. Ancestors, apparently, may come from

163

many different directions and hold varying understandings of what
is right, of what should be done (*nalin taun* rituals were brought
into the Luangan region as a result of contacts with the Sultanate
of Kutai toward the end of the nineteenth century, at the time
the Luangans settled in villages; see chapter 6). Dressed in the
black *kopiah* (signifying progress and cosmopolitan national culture), Mancan represented another aspect of tradition, a tradition
marked by development as he explained it, comparing Java, where
"the ancestors already have become developed by the government,"
with Kalimantan, where they were "not yet perfect." Exactly what
the spirit possessing Mancan wanted remained unclear to most of us
participating in the ritual, but through its confused utterances the
spirit did express concerns and uncertainties felt more widely during
the *buntang*, even if its political agenda seemed somewhat out of
place (as did, more particularly, its timing).

Bathing the ritual participants, and later, sitting at the highest
level of the three-storied *balei naiyu*, wearing a crown made of palm
leaves (thus personifying another kind of tradition)—embodying
Jarung, a spirit familiar originating as a local leader who is always
invited to partake of water buffalo sacrifices—Kakah Ramat did not
pay Mancan much attention. Neither did the other *belian*, nor for
that matter did anybody else in the audience, except for Ma Dengu
and his wife Nen Bai (both of whom shared Mancan's fascination
with "the outside world," and like him were ardent advocates of
sentiu curing); assisting Mancan in fulfilling the spirit's requests
they washed the headhunt skull and replaced the dried leaves that
covered it with fresh ones. Through his possession Mancan introduced another voice, but a voice speaking mostly for itself, not relating to the other people present or to the activities going on at that
moment. This was particularly evident when late at night Mancan
stood shouting beneath the flower shrubs (*baang bunge*) outside
the longhouse, while the *buntang* continued inside it, with no one
seemingly paying him any attention. In a way then—embodying the
Javanese *belian*—Mancan fought a one man's fight against disorder,
a fight brought about probably as much by his own involvement
in Tak Dinas' *belian sentiu* (or *belian dewa-dewa* as she preferred
to call it), as by Ma Bari's condition (this is, of course, not to say
that he was not as deeply concerned about Ma Bari as most other
people were).[24] Mancan's somewhat perplexing behavior, and the

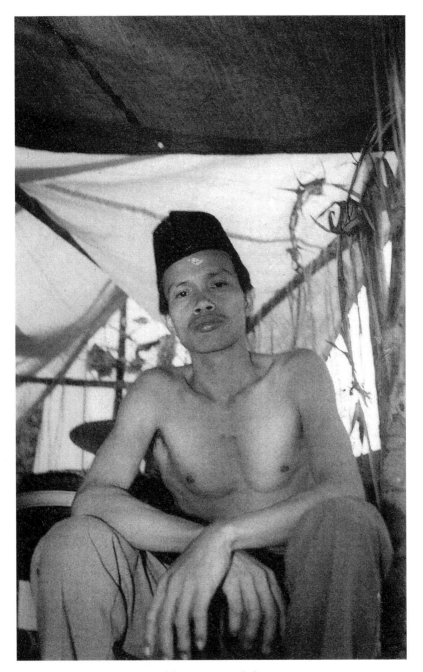

Figure 4.6. Mancan possessed by a Javanese *belian*

lack of response he got, may be seen as a rather striking image of the ambiguity involved in Luangan relations with powerful outsiders, of the more disconcerting side of outside intervention (Mancan was a respected and regularly appointed *belian* curer, as well a skilled carpenter, and was in no ways marginalized within his community, although some people considered some of his behavior somewhat strange). It was only later, when Mancan "transformed" his possession into *belian* curing and acted as *belian sentiu* (three times in all), or when he gave his "visions" (received during the possession) concrete shape by constructing his peculiar *ganti diri* figurines—thus "articulating inspiration through tradition" (Tsing 1993: 238)—that his project became an integral part of the larger project going on at that moment and thence managed to gain relevancy for other people as well.

It was not just Mancan who became possessed during these last days of the *buntang*, however. As Ma Putup, performing as *belian sentiu*, called down his peculiar spirit guides, and as they arrived in great numbers from all over the archipelago (Celebes and Melega in the spirit world are not necessarily the Celebes and Malacca of this world, though, as Ma Putup pointed out), Ma Isa, Ma Bari's son, lost control and suddenly rushed into the ritual arena, shivering and laughing uncontrollably, standing by his father's mattress. What overwhelmed Ma Isa here, and in a way Mancan as well, I think, was the condensed atmosphere, or as the Luangans would have it, the concentration of spirits (both local and foreign), or in yet other terms developed here, the empowerment of possibilities (but also the indeterminacy of life). It was only when Ma Isa was made to sit down by the *longan*, and cold water was splashed on him, that he became his normal self again, keeping his emotions in control.[25]

By summoning spirit guides, some of them previously unheard of and others presumably associated with downriver sultanates (Raden Muda Kuasa, Pangeran Mas Wali), Muslims or Christians (Nabi Isa, Tuhan Yesus—although Ma Putup argued that Tuhan Yesus in this case was not the same person as the Christian Jesus), Chinese (Sum Kua, Sum Hai), or Arabs (Ahdukian, Ahlu), Ma Putup convened a spirit congregation powerful enough both to frighten and to impress, leaving no one unaffected. It was, generally speaking, in situations like this (that is, when spirits were conjured in large numbers, and when their presence could be felt particularly clearly

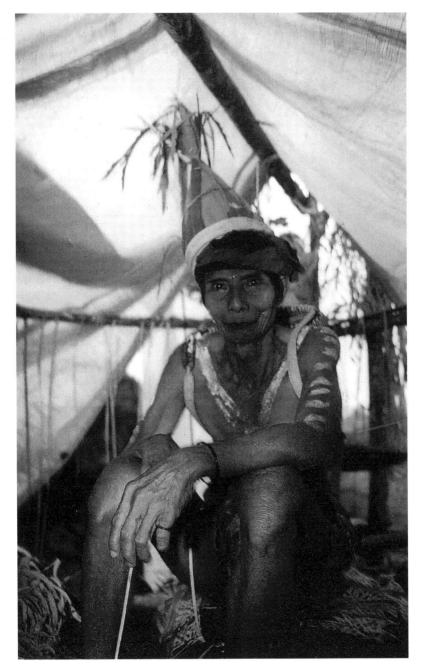

Figure 4.7. Kakah Ramat embodying Jarung

167

through the words and actions of the *belian*) that possession by spirits tended to occur among the ritual participants during my fieldwork, often among close relatives of a patient (such as Ma Isa, for example) or people particularly susceptible to spirits (such as Mancan, who often became possessed during grand rituals).[26] In Ma Isa's case, I would argue, it was both the power of the multitude of spirits summoned through Ma Putup's evocation, and the urgency of the situation itself, that caused the possession, bringing the invisible into the realm of experience, and experience (i.e., emotions) into action.

When Ma Lombang asked Ma Putup to contribute to the curing he did so in order to introduce Ma Putup's "inspirational curing" as yet another option. But he did so also, I would say (judging from his behavior in general), because of his own kin relation to Ma Putup and in order to facilitate the latter's integration in the village and to give credit to his knowledge and experience as a *belian*. Ma Putup, who was in his sixties at the time of the ritual, had worked as a shaman for more than thirty years, and he was, in fact, the only *belian* in the village who knew *belian luangan, belian bawo,* and *belian sentiu*, besides which he was also a *wara*, or death shaman. Despite this, and the fact that he was a highly valued shaman in his home village, he was not a particularly well esteemed *belian* in Sembulan, probably partly due to his lack of an established kin network there, and partly because of his extraordinary curing performances, which the villagers tended to regard with some degree of suspicion (or fear). In a way then, Ma Putup—an outsider summoning foreign spirit guides—spoke from the outside in a double sense in this ritual, and he may also be said to have had a double agenda, curing Ma Bari at the same time that he was asserting his own social position and authority as a curer in the village (with the crucial help of Ma Lombang).

Existential and socio-political motives were thus indistinguishable in this case, as they usually are in spirit negotiation. As I have argued before, a *belian*'s reputation as a curer is created and recreated through his or her ability to draw both a spirit and a human audience. For Mancan, as for Ma Putup (and even for Kakah Ramat), convening a human and spirit audience is just as important as the curing itself, and it is, in a way, a presupposition for it. Ritual authority results from an ability to act at the right moment, and in a proper way (as others see it). In this sense authority is not fixed, but rather has to be reconstructed over and over again. In bringing in the authority of foreign spirits, Ma Putup and Mancan brought in their visions of what authority might be like—with varying success. Speaking from the outside—acting through "other" agents—Mancan and Ma Putup, and in a more indirect way Ma Isa as well, unsettled any assumptions we might have about agency and authorship. Acting according to their own motivations, they spoke with the voices of someone else. Like Kakah Ramat in the case of his *dewa* ritual, they brought the foreign into the local. Whereas Kakah Ramat did so with the double intention of "borrowing" its power (Tsing 1993) while domesticating it, Mancan acted more ambiguously, being "consumed" by an otherness that he struggled to control. For Ma Putup the otherness and strangeness of his spirit guides served as a form of empowerment, allowing him to reach out, to "yield into" the realm of the unknown. At the same time, however, his actions seemed frightening to some members of his audience, with the foreignness evoked during the ritual being a little too overwhelming.

All these (foreign) voices added to the diversity of curing efforts employed during the *buntang,* and clearly demonstrate the often multi-purpose character that the loosely concerted efforts they and many of the other curing attempts in the ritual constituted. The complexity of Ma Bari's *buntang* thus resulted, at least in part, from the political agenda that lay behind the acts of its participants in this seriously existential project.

Uncertainty and Representation

> But in every human society concepts such as fate, history, evolution, God, chance, and even the weather signify forces of otherness that one cannot fully fathom and over which one can expect to exercise little or no ultimate control. These forces are given; they are in the nature of things. In spite of this, human beings countermand and transform these forces by dint of their imagination and will so that, in every society, it is possible to outline a domain of action and understanding in which people expect to be able to grasp, manipulate, and master their own fate.
>
> —Michael Jackson (1998: 19)

I will end this seemingly endless story where we began, with the scene of Ma Isa brutally smashing the pig suspected of causing his father's illness against the trunk of the coconut palm. In doing so, I want to draw attention to the existential apprehension with which representations are associated, as well as to point to the power that circumstances have over deeds. Ma Isa did not act according to any carefully prepared plan here, but was overwhelmed by his own anger and anxiety, as well as by what one might call the elusiveness of the present. Attempting to get rid of the cause of the illness, as quickly as possible, before more damage was done, he forgot discretion, killing the pig without compassion, almost out of revenge. Innocent in itself, but thought to be possessed by a malevolent spirit, the pig became a symbol of adversity, a symbol for what Ma Isa wanted to do away with before it could hurt his father even more.

By recalling this scene with Ma Isa I also want to conjure all those other moments when uncertainty came to the fore in the story. There was not just one pig killed during the course of Ma Bari's illness, but several, together with a number of other animals. And there was always more than one possibility for action open (cf. Whyte 1997: 83), forcing people to make conscious decisions about the most appropriate one. In fact the whole endeavor of curing Ma Bari was constituted by flashes of excitement, resolution and climax, interspersed with moments of slowness, not-knowing, and doubt. Grasping, manipulating and mastering one's own fate, or that of someone close, is not always an easy task, or one that can be achieved according to predetermined schemes. From time to time, decisions have to be reassessed, and on some occasions tradition itself has to be stretched in various directions.

In this context we have to take into consideration the socio-political context as well. For it matters who the patient is when decisions about *belian* curing are made, not necessarily so that authoritative persons automatically get larger scale rituals—even though they generally do tend to both get and sponsor large rituals—but in the sense that the illness of an important person or elder concerns more people directly than that of a child or a young person. There is a special kind of urgency involved when leaders (or important shamans) fall ill, forcing people to get involved, urging them to do their utmost, even when they feel that they do not have the time or the resources to do so.

What distinguished the curing of Ma Bari from the curing of other people was not merely the large number of measures taken, but the accumulation and condensation of different measures, following one after another or on top of one another. It is often the case that a variety of measures are taken when someone falls seriously ill, but the pace whereby they are taken is not usually as hurried as it was in Ma Bari's case. During Nen Pare's illness, for example, over fifteen rituals were arranged, some of them lasting for over eight days, but these were arranged over the course of one year, not one after another in quick succession as they were during Ma Bari's illness, and they were not initiated by the shamans themselves, as some of the rituals conducted for Ma Bari were.

The imminent threat of Ma Bari's death was too serious a matter for people to delay their attempts at counteraction, and the uncertainty of reality—the unpredictability of illness, people and spirits—was thus countered with redoubling and condensation. "[T]rafficking in human possibilities rather than in settled certainties" (Bruner 1986: 26; cf. Whyte 1997: 24), Ma Bari's family and neighbors reinforced the power of evocation, trying out different measures—often simultaneously—in a joint effort to influence reality through negotiation with a multitude of spirits. To give priority to one or more of these measures would, as I see it, be to misrepresent the whole enterprise. It was essentially in combination with one another that the different styles of curing worked, in an effort to rework the relationship between human beings and spirits.

As Keane (1997: 179) observes, "public, formal action is neither spontaneous nor the mechanical enactment of cultural imperatives." Through fragments of events, I have tried to convey the happenings surrounding Ma Bari's illness in all their ambiguity, accounting for both the doubt and the hope that decisions in and of *belian* curing can comprise. Looking at the different measures as "*operations* of speakers in particular situations of time, place, and competition" (de Certeau 1984: 20), while at the same time questioning the meaning of concepts such as agency and authorship, I have attempted to illustrate both the difficulty and the potentiality of *belian* curing. Spirits sometimes evade negotiation (besides that they are unseen, which makes the monitoring and interpretation of their wishes and actions difficult), material representations are subject to "nonsemiotic happenstances," patients get worse in spite of all efforts to

171

cure them, curers at times work for personal motives as much as for curative ends, and ritual action itself occasionally breeds a need for further action. But then again, the openness between reality and representation also constitutes possibilities—for transformation, and for re-creation (cf. chapter 2).

Ma Bari did get well in the end, not as a result of one of the measures that were taken here, but perhaps by their accumulation (in combination with the medicines brought from downriver). Ritual plausibility was not primarily a question of success or failure, however, but one of trying, and of acting. To play it safe is, as I have argued, to try out every possibility when so needed, to be specific enough, without excluding. The result of this highly experimental even though significantly conventional activity is something of which you can never be sure. But on the other hand, as Atkinson (1989: 290) notes for Wana shamanism: "the idea of having a loved one die without the care of a powerful shaman is grievous ... Engaging the talents of a renowned shaman validates the outcome of an illness, be it life or death."

Ritual representations, as I have tried to show, are "tied to circumstances of instantiation" (Hayles 1992: 9). But they are also grounded in prior action, and in conceptions of proper action. What we might call the socio-political significance of the ritual analyzed here derived not only from the personal, but no less socially embedded, authority-pursuing projects of individual *belian* curers, but also from the generally shared aspiration to reconstruct tradition in accordance with notions of precedence and correctness, motivated both by the specific case at hand, and by more general, if less existentially urgent, cultural concerns. *Buntang* rituals, which are part of the *belian luangan* tradition, represent Luangan culture to Luangans and performing them obviously prompts reflection and concern regarding their value and meaning as cultural statements. This was vividly seen in the case of Mancan whose involvement in the ritual (particularly in his capacity as Javanese ancestor) appeared to be more marked by such concerns (for example, about aligning Luangan tradition with Indonesian government conceptions of cultural order) than by his worries about Ma Bari, even though these concerns might well have been brought about by these worries (as so often, the existential and political domains seemed virtually indistinguishable). More specifically, *buntang* rituals are also commemorative rituals bringing to life not only Luangan culture but ancestral tradition, and therefore represent emotionally strongly charged obligations of maintaining that heritage in a form corresponding to, or at least, compatible with, the desires of those venerated forebears who established it or handed it over. Hence the significance of notions of prior and proper action which constrain every instantiation, even as the latter is never reducible to a "mechanical enactment of cultural imperatives" (Keane 1997: 179), shaped as it is, inescapably, by the situational conditions—practical, material, existential, and political—that are tied to every instantiation. In *buntang* rituals such notions of precedence and correctness take on an even more immediate relevance than otherwise, since *buntang* rituals, more than other rituals, directly address spirits (e.g. *naiyu, timang*) associated with the ancestors and, through the chanting of *tempuun* origin myths, invoke the origins of ritual practices, and the powerful *seniang* spirits who are charged with regulating the socio-cosmic order.

Notes

1. This melody is played at irregular intervals by someone in the audience who does so spontaneously. During *gombok* someone may shout out the word "*gombok*" and then proceed to play the melody, independently of what the shamans are up to.
2. Luangans often seemed to express their discontent with something through the food that they served, which tended to become scarcer and less tasty the more dissatisfied they were.
3. In *belian bawo* rituals *pereau* is also conducted when the *belian* spins around rapidly for a while before he reads the leaf, thus attaining a trance-like state.
4. This means that you sometimes have to kill animals that you dearly love, or that your neighbors love (your best hunting dog, for example, or a favorite cat).
5. This was, in fact, Lodot's and Yati's second wedding ceremony, arranged at this point because there were relatives and friends attending the *buntang* who were not around during their first wedding; that one had been held two months earlier, arranged by the groom's family, whereas this one was arranged by the bride's family.
6. After a ritual finishes there is always a state of *pali* (taboo or restriction) in the house, during which people who did not participate in the ritual cannot enter (an areca palm inflorescence is hung by the door as a sign of this). The patient is not allowed to leave the house during this time either. The concept of *pali* is complex and includes restrictions of different sorts, which may be temporary or lasting, such as on eating certain foods,

173

entering houses or swiddens, etc. The breaking of *pali* may result in soul-loss and misfortune.

7. Whereas the *longan teluyen* is a permanent structure and part of village longhouses (*lou solai*) and some long-lasting extended family houses (*lou*), the *longan teraran* is rebuilt for every ritual and discarded afterwards. Both represent the focus of many important ritual activities in the rituals in which they are used as well as a place where spirits are said to gather during them. The *longan teluyen* is additionally associated with spiritual potency (*kekuasaan*) on a more permanent basis, being inhabited by *naiyu* spirits as a result of having been recurrently anointed with blood (*ngulas*) in previous rituals. It is a place where you may go to cool down if you are possessed by spirits, for instance, or where you might bring a dying child, etc.

8. Luing, the female spirit of rice, is the leading spirit familiar of the *belian* and is summoned during all rituals to negotiate with other spirits. She appears in three different manifestations. During ordinary curing rituals, Luing Boias (Luing of Rice) is called to summon the *mulung* (spirit familiars) and lead their negotiation with malevolent spirits (*blis*); during *buntang* rituals, Luing Ayang (Noble Luing) is called to negotiate with *naiyu* spirits; and during death rituals, Lolang Luing (Beautiful Luing) is called to negotiate with *kelelungan* and *liau* (the spirits of the dead).

9. According to some Luangans, *juata*, for whom the goat was intended, comes from downriver and therefore does not eat pork (it is implied that *juata* is Muslim); in Sembulan, however, offerings to *juata* were often complemented by the sacrifice of a white pig, or consisted of only the pig if a goat could not be obtained (people did not keep goats in the village so a goat had to be bought from another village when needed).

10. A *nalin taun* is a kind of extended *buntang* ritual that usually takes about sixteen days to perform among the central Luangans (longer among the Benuaq of East Kalimantan) and contains some additional program, including, most notably, the chanting of the origin stories of the sky and earth, and of mankind (*Tempuun Langit Tana, Tempuun Senaring*).

11. According to Kakah Ramat and other *belian* I talked to, the spirit(s) guilty of causing an illness are recognized by a "burning" or "stinging" (*mensereu*) sensation in their bodies, often in their ears.

12. Morris (1993: 105) makes a similar observation for the Oya Melanau: "No Melanau doubts the existence of spirits, but if asked about them says, 'They are things which cannot be seen; how can we be sure what they are like?'"

13. Around many Luangan villages a number of small groves of tall trees (*simpung*), believed to be the residences of several different sorts of spirits, are spared during swidden cultivation, out of respect for their inhabitants. Like the *blis sopan*, malevolent (or more correctly, potentially malevolent) spirits inhabiting marshy areas or areas surrounding water holes used by animals, *blis simpung*, "the spirits from forest groves," are sometimes known to trick pigs and other domestic animals that are foraging in or near their territory into hurting people.

14. Keane, who is well aware of this, uses the word "*under*determination" (my italics) when talking about the "possible interpretations of objects," as well as the condition that "meanings and values are not inherent in objects," while at the same time "objects are not open to any arbitrarily imposed set of meanings" (1997a: 32).

15. Janet Hoskins (1996: 272) describes a similar case among the Kodi of West Sumba, among whom "public performances may be undertaken for patients who are already well on the road to recovery, or who are in fact mortally ill, and die soon after the proceedings."

16. When a patient dies during the process of curing this is considered dangerous for the curer, and such situations are thus avoided (though not always successfully), but this still does not mean that the ritual in question is judged a failure. Life sometimes simply eludes ritualization (and representation more generally), which does not mean that there is no use in trying to act upon it.

17. The Luangans, of course, do not always whisper when they talk about *buntang* (or other *belian* rituals). They do so in situations when the arranging of a *buntang* can be seen as being called for, or when spirits are assumed to be around (e.g. during *buntang* rituals in which they are invited to participate). This again reminds us of the fact that interpretations (and actions resulting from them) are contextually determined. To refer back to the case of the falling vessel again, this sign would probably not have been seen as pointing to Ma Bari if it had not been for some combination of the following facts: that Ma Bari was a) seriously ill, b) deeply involved in Ma Dasi's *buntang*, and c) the owner of the house in which the event occurred.

18. Roseman (1991: 28–29) makes a somewhat similar observation for the Temiars, who by naming illness agents may activate "their potential to cause illness," but who may also, by the controlled uttering of names, startle them into departing.

19. Among the Luangans, walking is a prominent metaphor, and rituals are pictured as paths along which offerings are brought to the spirits in exchange for health and good luck.

20. *Bongai* is one of the types of spirits most frequently negotiated with in *belian* rituals. In fact, there are many different sorts of *bongai*, some of them downriver spirits, others upriver. They are described as human-like creatures, with red skin, known to indulge in headhunting (*perbala*) and to carry blowpipes. *Bongai* typically attack their victims by shooting small blowpipe darts (*sipet bongai*) that penetrate the victim's skin, and some *sentiu* shamans are said to have the ability to extract such darts from their patients, by sucking them out, for example. According to Kakah Ramat, attacks from downriver *bongai* have become much more common these days, and this is, in his opinion, an important factor contributing to the increasing popularity of *belian sentiu*. Epidemics (*repa*), which were especially devastating in the early twentieth century, are almost invariably attributed to downriver *bongai*.

21. If one has a weak soul and accidentally happens to watch an animal being killed, there is the possibility of losing one's soul through what is described

175

as a process of mimetization: one is made, by *abei* spirits, to copy the animal in question in its death-throes. Epilepsy, for example, is said to have this etiology, as are (potentially) other types of convulsions. Other symptoms, less severe, which are associated with convulsions, such as loss of consciousness, are also sometimes seen as implying *sengkerapei*, which is the term used to describe these symptoms and the accompanying soul loss. *Sengkerapei* often happens to small children, who are believed to have weak souls. Sick people, who by definition also have weak souls, are subject to the same danger. Weakened by a prolonged illness and having "lost his breath," Ma Bari was thus quite naturally seen as a potential victim of *abei* attack. It is worth pointing out here that a person can also be affected by *sengkerapei* if someone close to the person watches an animal die (small children, who are usually protected from watching dying animals, are usually affected as a result of their parents' actions, even if they have been performed before the birth of the child, during pregnancy). When souls are purchased from the *abei*, a large number of small *ganti diri* figures representing the various animals which have potentially been seen dying are made.

22. Even if one does own a water buffalo one might not want to sacrifice the animal, especially if it is young, for example, or if one expects to get a good price for it in the future, or if it is pregnant at the time one needs it. Water buffalos are thus often procured from close kin or neighbors or bought from more distantly related or unrelated people, in some cases for considerable prices, and sometimes from quite some distance away.

23. In *buntang* rituals that include the sacrifice of a water buffalo, a special ritual construction (*balei naiyu*) is built for the *naiyu* (and other) protecting spirits that receive offerings in the ritual. In a *nalin taun* an additional construction (*balei taun*) is built for the *seniang*, which are not "called down" (*pedolui*) to partake of ritual offerings otherwise (even if they are occasionally contacted and presented with offerings in other rituals, during *pereau*, for instance).

24. Conceptions of order are central in Indonesian nationalist rhetoric. Progress is associated with the regularization and compartmentalization of social and cultural life, and marginal swidden cultivators like the Luangans, who lack a "great" cultural tradition and are characterized by a semi-mobile and dispersed settlement, are hence regarded as particularly unordered and form a favorite target for government criticism. Some Luangans, like Mancan, have largely appropriated these government conceptions, and with them an aspiration to order their own cultural tradition.

25. When Ma Isa was made to sit down by the *longan* it was hoped that the protecting and cooling influence associated with it (which results from the "house" or "ancestral" spirits residing there and in the nearby placed ancestor skulls and valuables) would help him regain his balance.

26. Ma Putup often boasted about how tens of people (mostly women) would become possessed during *belian* performances that he conducted in his home village in his youth.

Chapter Five
So that Steam Rises
Ritual Bathing as Depersonalization

And there was an obligation for the descendants: if there is a child crying, if the child is thin and skinny, frail and faint, has diarrhea, then you should bring a *belian*, you should tell the *tempuun* and perform a bathing ceremony—and thus the child will recover!

—Excerpt from *Tempuun Ngenus*, the origin story of bathing, as told
by Ma Keket (my translation)

This chapter is about ritual bathing (*tota, ngenus*), a basic element of many curing rituals, particularly curing rituals in the *belian sentiu* style and rituals dealing with small children.[1] From a theoretical vantage point, it is a chapter about the embodied experience of being cooled, and the almost tangible power of words—combined with water—to influence the present by integrating it with the past and collective tradition. In more concrete terms, it is a chapter about the transformation brought upon people by *belian* curers pouring water over them, repeating the chants and actions of other *belian*, of other times, thus trying to expel individual heat and misfortune (*layeng lihang*) and create a state of healthy, refreshing coolness (*rengin roe*). In this process of mimetic representation the bathing *belian* evoke the past, I argue, with the effect of "de-personalizing" the subjects of bathing (cf. Deren 1965). As Rachel Moore (2000: 6) expresses it, commenting on film maker Maya Deren's reflections on ritual, "the depersonalized quality of ritual extends the individual into a larger sphere of significance." "The intent of such depersonalization is not," to cite Deren (1965: 20) "the destruction of the individual; on the contrary, it enlarges him beyond the personal dimension and frees him from the specializations and confines of 'personality.'" When it comes to ritual bathing, this is a process which involves both remembering and forgetting as myths are lived and as lives perish.

"Memory," in Seremetakis' words, "cannot be confined to a purely mentalist or subjective sphere. It is a culturally mediated material practice that is activated by embodied acts and semantically dense objects" (1994a: 9). This holds true also for bathing rituals which essentially work by way of integrating the participants with a sensuously experienced collective tradition. The chants, the music, the decorations, and the act and sensation of bathing itself, evoke embodied memories of past rituals for participants who are habituated to ritual bathing as a way to remember the past and a strategy to influence the present. As instances of what Stanley Tambiah (1985: 132) calls "conventionalized behavior," designed not to "express the intentions, emotions and states of mind of individuals in a direct, spontaneous and 'natural' way," but, as the Luangans would put it, in ancestral language (*basa tuha one*), bathing rituals have a "distancing" effect, allowing participants, like Sumbanese ritual speech in Keane's (2007: 182) interpretation, "to lay claim to a form of agency that transcends the spatial and temporal limits of the individual, mortal body." In this chapter I examine the distancing, depersonalizing effect of bathing rituals in terms of how it enables them to serve as strategies of coping with personal adversities, such as the loss associated with infant death.

The exploration of ritual bathing that I will pursue here is based on three cases in which small children and their relatives were bathed ritually. The children involved in these cases were all born during a four-month period between September 1996 and January 1997 in the "village longhouse" (*lou solai*) of Sembulan.[2] I have chosen to base my analysis on these three cases—here presented as separate but partly overlapping stories—rather than on just one of them, because they reveal something important about each other. Taken together, they can be said to bring out the historicity of rituals and the unboundedness of events. Read intertextually, they show how meaning is shaped in the interface between utterances, texts, or events (cf. Briggs and Bauman 1992). No single bathing ritual is, of course, unique. Bathing rituals have been performed and experienced innumerable times—which indeed is largely the point of them—and every ritual should be seen in relation to other rituals, both prior and future (cf. Howe 2000: 66–67). But at the same time every bathing ritual is also always in a sense new, performed for particular individuals, and for particular purposes. Because of this "double historicity" of ritual, I have chosen not to generalize in the sense of condensing the different stories into a general description of bathing rituals: doing so would mean that much of the urgency involved, much of what is at stake in the rituals for the participants, would remain uninvoked. As Patricia Spyer (2000: 214) notes with regard to annual performances (however, her statement is also applicable to non-calendrical performances): "what might seem repetitive and predictable to an outsider is quite varied and different for those who participate year after year … , both personally for individual men, women, and children and more collectively with respect to the larger social processes that are played out."

In bathing small children the stakes are high indeed. It is often the life or death of these children which is at stake. Consequently, this chapter is about the circumstances that call forth these rituals and the strategies of coping employed, as much as it is about the bathing as such. Infant mortality is notably high among central Luangans. Although there are no statistics available for the central Luangan area, my own rough estimates suggest that infant mortality (including perinatal death) may well exceed 30 percent in many villages, some of which still received little professional medical care in the late 1990s. Such a figure—the result of malaria and gastrointestinal diseases, among other things—would by no means be exceptional in the light of documented historical infant mortality rates for Borneo (see Freeman 1967: 318; Knapen 2001: 160–161).[3] The risks involved in bringing up small children are hence an inevitable fact of Luangan life, often present even when not talked about, a silent possibility at the back of the mind.

Scene One: Following the Work of Itak Pantak

Wet bodies, hair that smears against heads, sarongs that cling to the skin, water in the eyes. Laughter and shivering. *Belian* curers with ladles in their hands, pouring scented water from large buckets: river water mixed with fragrant red and yellow flowers (*bungen dusun, telase*). People sitting in a row on an ironwood bench beneath

179

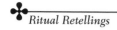

the flower shrubs, coconut palms, and areca palms, being bathed simultaneously by Itak Pantak, Silu and Lintai, mythical female *belian*, and by Mancan and Nen Bai, their shaman representatives and apprentices here today. Bathed in the village flower grove (*baang bunge*), beside the longhouse, just like the mythical Buah Ore Ani, "the crocodile that failed to become a younger sister," once was, before she ascended to the sky.

This is the conclusion of a six-day *belian sentiu* ritual arranged in October 1996 for Liman, a one-year-old boy, who, according to Ma Bari, the owner of the longhouse and the brother of Liman's great-grandmother Tak Rosa, had been crying a lot since his little sister was born two weeks earlier. According to Ma Bari, a *belian* ritual should be arranged for this reason, but also because plans had been made to hold one six months earlier, at a time when Liman was ill, plans that were not implemented then. Liman's parents are not completely happy with Ma Bari's decision as they feel that they are lacking in economic and material resources, having just finished the "birth ritual" (*ngebidan*) for Liman's sister. They do not have much choice but to agree, however. Promises about rituals should be implemented, sooner or later, because of the threat of retribution from offended spirits. Moreover, Ma Bari is an authoritative person whose words are not easily contested and whose motives are known not to be thoughtless.

Now, on this last morning of the ritual, people take turns to be bathed on the bench in the flower grove. Children run back and forth to the river, filling the buckets with more water. Mancan, one of the officiating *belian*, and Nen Bai, his bathing assistant, both look concentrated, bathing the participants in silence: these are Liman's father Ma Denia, his grandfather Ma Pija, and a number of friends and neighbors of the family. There is a sweet scent of flowers enclosing the bathers, mixed with the smell of mud from the wet, slippery ground. A plaited tray (*ansak*) containing small portions of rice is hung up on a branch in the flower bushes and a couple of anthropomorphically carved sticks (*ganti diri*) stand leaning against a palm trunk.

Simultaneously, just inside the longhouse, a special bathing chair (*panti penota*) made of yellow bamboo has been placed in front of the open door. Large plastic buckets are placed next to the chair and are filled with river water brought to the house by some children.

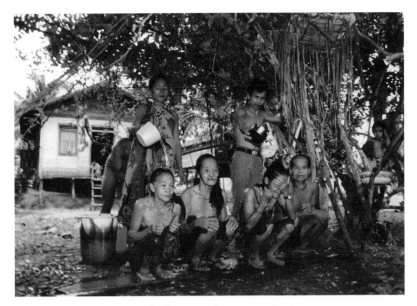

Figure 5.1. Participants in bathing ritual seated in the flower grove (*baang bunge*) of Sembulan

Instructed by Ma Dengu, a *belian* aged around sixty who is specialized in children's rituals and *sentiu* curing, Rosa, Liman's mother, wrapped in a sarong, seats herself on the chair, with Liman in her lap. Tak Rosa, her grandmother, holding the newborn baby in her arms, sits down on the floor in front of the chair. While Mancan and Nen Bai wash people outside in the flower grove, in sight of those at the doorway, Ma Dengu starts to bathe the women and children inside. He pours water over the heads of Rosa and Tak Rosa while chanting in a loud, lingering voice. With an areca palm twig he then splashes water on the children. The baby cries as she is hit by the cold water. Liman rubs his eyes, shivering. Tak Rosa talks to both of them in a comforting voice. After a while she calls out for someone to bring them a towel.

The ritual to cure Liman has been a rather low-profile affair, with relatively few people attending (a result, in part, of the scarcity of the food served), except for the night before, when a large pig was sacrificed, and this morning, which concludes the ritual. It has been a ritual involving a lot of bathing, not only of Liman and his parents, grand- and great-grandparents, but also of Ena and Mohar, a young couple who have just lost their own baby (I will return to them later in this chapter), as well as of Ma Bari and Tak Ningin, Ena's grand-parents who are the owners of the longhouse in which the ritual has been performed (Ma Bari is, as already mentioned, also Liman's great-grandmother Tak Rosa's brother, while Tak Ningin, his wife, is the village midwife who assisted during the births of Rosa's and Ma Denia's children, as well as Ena's and Mohar's child, facts which motivated Ma Bari's and Tak Ningin's participation in the bathing activities). The ritual has, in fact, turned out to be something of an extended bathing ritual, including a lot of bathing only loosely inte-grated with the ritual's other activities. During each evening of the ritual, often as a conclusion to the day's other ritual work, buckets have been filled with water and all volunteers have been bathed by Ma Dengu or Mancan, assisted by Nen Bai. Still, this last morning forms a culmination, with the simultaneous bathing outside and inside the longhouse, in the flower grove, and on the bathing chair, involving a large number of villagers, as well as, for the first time, Liman's newborn sister.

"This is the real way to bathe" (*sarat bene nota*), Ma Dengu declares as he instructs Rosa and Tak Rosa on how to be seated during the bathing, implying that this is the proper way in which the procedure should be carried out according to tradition. This is also in some important respects what is at issue in this bathing ritual: the observance of a perceived tradition, the reproduction of what has been done in the past, and the mythical past in particu-lar. When bathing people outside in the flower grove, Mancan and Nen Bai overtly declare that they do so because this is what was done in the origin myth of bathing (*Tempuun Ngenus*). Furthermore, Mancan has himself constructed the bench on which the bathing is performed as a result of a revelation that he had during Ma Bari's *buntang* (see chapter 4), and in the hope of thus improving the conditions for recurrent ritual bathing (something which he has a particular interest in as he is a *belian sentiu* specialized in ritual bathing). Similarly, Ma Dengu, in his bathing chant, repeatedly points out that he is "following" or "joining in" (*nyang, numun*) the work of his *belian* predecessors, Itak Pantak, Silu and her daughter Lintai, mythical shamans who, as we shall see below, performed the first bathing ritual in order to cure the child Edau who became ill because she was bitten in the stomach by her crocodile sister.

According to the origin myth of ritual bathing, as told by Ma Keket, and repeatedly alluded to in Ma Dengu's chant, Kesiring Bungkong, the crocodile spirit of the Pond of the Sky, once dropped an egg which fell right into the *belian* Itak Pantak's basket of ritual equipment (*tayung pemura*). Itak Pantak was pregnant with Edau at the time, ready to give birth. But the child would not be born. *Belian* rituals were arranged, one after another, but to no avail. At last the great *belian* Silu Nanang Luang Olo was called down from the Door of the Heavens. On the request of Silu, who perceived the cause of the problem, the bag was opened and the small crocodile that had been hatched inside it was released. At the same time Edau was born. Edau and the crocodile, Buah Ore Ani ("The Crocodile who Failed to Become a Little Sister"), were raised as sisters. Growing bigger and bigger, the crocodile brought larger and larger prey to the house, while Tatau Dahur Langit, Edau's father, grew richer and richer. At that time, a woman called Lingan Ayang, who had heard about the affluence of the family, came by to ask for some meat. But she was only offered hard skin and dry bones. Furious, she set fire to all "forbidden" things (*ye tau busa pali*) beneath Tatau Dahur Tuha's house (she had herself once been married to the crocodile spirit of the sea which is why she possessed powerful magic). At that moment Buah Ore Ani started to bite around frantically, and Edau started to cry from stomach ache. She cried and cried. *Belian* rituals were arranged, one after another, until all the family's riches were gone (having been converted into ritual offerings), but Edau just cried. At last Jaweng Pager, the *belian* Silu's husband, was called. He ordered the family to bring cold water for the child to bath in, and for Edau, as well as her crocodile sister, to be sent downstream to look for cold water. Thus they, together with Edau's older sister, also called Silu, went to the sea, the source of all waters. There Buah Ore Ani plunged directly into the sea while some rituals were performed for Edau by local *belian*. When Buah Ore Ani reappeared from the water she stopped biting around and Edau ceased crying. On their way back to Mount Soai they stopped at every river mouth to take some cold water with them (while Buah Ore Ani, who had married the crocodile spirit of the sea during the visit, laid an egg at each river mouth on her way). Back at home, Buah Ore Ani waited outside the longhouse, in the flower grove. A bathing ritual was then performed for both children by Itak Pantak and the other *belian* (in the flower grove as well as in the longhouse) after which Buah Ore Ani was sent off, back to the Pond in the Sky from where she had originally come.

"Hence it came that one bathes up to this very day," Ma Keket, who told this particular version of the myth, declared, thus expressing something important not only about the rationale of ritual bathing, but indirectly also about the workings of the institution. Bathing is, as both Mancan and Ma Dengu in their respective ways pointed out in their chants, an act of re-enactment, both physically and verbally. In bathing people, and in simultaneously bathing them inside and outside the longhouse, Mancan and Ma Dengu repeat acts (and words, as we shall see in a moment) of the past, giving them a certain "presentness" again (Connerton 1989: 63). It is also very much, I argue, by way of evoking a mythical past and making it bodily present among the bathers, that "refreshing coolness" (*rengin roe*), that is, the ultimate general goal of the ritual as expressed in ritual chants, is sought to be achieved. But why this need to copy and to put so much emphasis on the copying? Why all the repetition, what is it that makes it so powerful?

These are questions which obviously have complex answers, one of which is undoubtedly the simple fact that what has proven effective in the past may well do so again in the future. With the aim of identifying some other, perhaps less obvious, answers we shall now return to the particular ritual that I have been discussing and attend more carefully to Ma Dengu's chant, which, as he so tellingly declares, sets out to "trace the origins, the tradition from olden times."

Ma Dengu begins his chant by calling Itak Pantak, Silu and Lintai, as well as the other mythical shamans (Tungkis Bawo Langit, Tatau Dahur Tuha, etc.) who performed the first bathing ritual and who are now called in their capacity as spirit familiars. He then introduces the protagonists of the event: the child Edau (who was bathed in the myth of origin of bathing), on the one hand, and Liman and his baby sister, his patients today (the latter metaphorically referred to as "the bamboo shoot," "the young shrimp," "the *bentas* twig from the flower grove"), on the other.

TOTA	SONG OF BATHING
Dinga ko bawe Silu Itak Lintai Ine	Listen you women, Grandmother Silu, Mother Lintai
tempue punsu ure	prows, young termite nests [i.e., leaders]

Tungkis Bawo Langit	Tungkis Bawo Langit
Itak Pantak Langai Soai	Grandmother Pantak of Mount Soai
bero Tatau Dahur Tuha	with Tatau Dahur Tuha
rarak sensuren one	tracing the origins
tengka lelasa nahaa	the tradition from olden times
bawe Silu bero Lintai	the women Silu and Lintai
Tungkis Bawo Langit	Tungkis Bawo Langit
Itak Uan Bawo Langit	Itak Uan Bawo Langit
Edos bawo Bawui Bayuh	Edos from Mount Bawui Bayuh
ngenus tian Edau	bathing the child Edau
batu baras papan	on the flat bathing stone
be lemoong Pantak	at Pantak's well
be usuk Langai Soai	on top of Mount Soai
Guru Delonong Olo	Guru Delonong Olo [title for Mount Soai]
sekarang olo itu pita oho	now today this morning
ngenus basung urang ure	bathing the shoot, the young shrimp [the baby]
sorok bentas baang bunge	the *bentas* sprout from the flower grove [the baby]
batang unuk laki Liman	the body, the trunk of Liman
bero basung urang ure	with the shoot, the young shrimp
sorok bentas baang bunge	the *bentas* sprout from the flower grove
be munan panti penota	on the bathing chair
be batu baras papan	on the flat bathing stone
bele jaa Sembulan	even though the village is Sembulan
numun awing Pantak Itak	[we're] following the work of Grandmother Pantak
nyang awing Silu Itak bero Lintai Ine	heeding the work of Grandmother Silu and Mother Lintai
puai pererangan datai	the *puai* plant thrives on the plain
be batang olo ehe	on this very day
ulun ngerima basung ure	the people are receiving a new shoot
nyenkalu mamai pinang	welcoming an areca palm inflorescence
nota Ine Memea	bathing the Mother who Feeds
nota Uma Memayor	bathing the Father who Provides
jelen opet tela bene	entering first of all
tengau senseng boa bane	appearing at the opening of the bamboo
tota bawe Pantak Itak	bathe woman Grandmother Pantak
bero Tatau Dahur Tuha	and Tatau Dahur Tuha
walo belian upo	the eight *belian* youngsters
tempue Juring Olo	Juring Olo their prow
sie belian bawe	the nine female *belian*
kepala Pantak Itak	Grandmother Pantak their head [all mythical *belian*]

After that Ma Dengu initiates the bathing, following the standard two-phase *belian* procedure of *pejiak pejiau* (cf. chapter 3), which in this case consists of first undoing or averting bad influences and conditions and then attracting favorable ones. Thus Ma Dengu, and Itak Pantak etc. through him, first bathes towards "the setting sun," "the waning moon," symbolizing undesirable conditions. In a way he, to cite Keane (2010: 198), constructs "the very difficulties ... [his words are] ... designed to overcome." In this phase of the bathing, children's diseases are called up and washed off along with other potential disadvantageous conditions of children, the sick children here metaphorically being referred to as "wilted bamboos," "unripe durians" and "fruit for the caterpillars."

tota napang maten olo tonep	bathe toward the setting sun
ngelama bulan punus	in the direction of the waning moon
nota basung urang ure	bathing the shoot, the young shrimp
sorok bentas baang bunge	the *bentas* sprout from the flower grove
ngoding dero inus mea biwi	avert the sickness of red lips
ngoding busang mea boa	avert the illness of red mouths [children's diseases]
botung jereken bekuan jerengen	sickly bamboos, wilted bamboos
layung riai duyan riai	unripe *layung* fruits, unripe durian fruits
gelaning pepei yei	fruit for the caterpillars
bemulin pupuk Ayus	fruit with no filling
ngoding ara bua ore	throw away the *ara* fruit that failed to ripen
kelumpang bua arang	fruit without pulp
ayak bua lonu	fruit with mashy flesh
turu pejahuran lopa	seven hard rainstorms
tenapik dolek balik	turn away the gale
eke basung urang ure	from the shoot, the young shrimp
sorok bentas baang bunge	the *bentas* sprout from the flower grove
ke Ine Petete	from the Mother who Breast-feeds

Turning around (*berebalik*), Ma Dengu then bathes towards "the rising sun" and "the new moon" which, in turn, symbolize favorable conditions. Bathing towards the iron pillar of the sky, the pillar of rain, the flower grove of Sembulan, there is "refreshing coolness" arriving: "the refreshing coolness of river mouths," "the renewed prosperity of deep pools." There is the coolness of a future, one in which "the *peko* bird betokens the sun," and "the *leliak* bird betokens the stars," both birds being what Luangans call *pempulun taun*, "birds of the year," birds that announce the arrival of the seasons of the year (and thus, in this case, represent desired transition). Applying yellow turmeric and white rice paste—both cooling substances—on the foreheads of the bathers, Ma Dengu finishes the purification. As a last venture, he presents his spirit familiars with some offerings and then returns the bathing chair to its owners on Mount Soai, while also catching the souls of the bathers, which might have got lost in the bathing process. Counting to eight, a number which symbolizes life, completeness, and fortuity, he finishes the bathing.

Biyayung Uma Malik	Biyayung, Father of Transformation
Bensiang Uma Muser	Bensiang, Father of Metamorphosis
berebalik nema oli	turn around once again
tota napang olo sulet	bathe towards the rising sun
ngelangkep bulan empet	face the new moon
be batu baras papan	on the flat bathing stone
tota Itak Pantak Langai Soai	bathe Grandmother Pantak of Mount Soai
tota napang usuk Purei	bathe towards Mount Purei
tota Itak Ratu Manak	bathe Grandmother Queen Manak
Aji Rajan Nungkum	Aji King Nungkum [mythological bathing *belian*]
ujur besi orin langit	head for the iron pillar that supports the sky[4]
durut dotan orin uran	approach the pillar of rain
ori besi beau daki	the iron pillar will not rust
durut olau nyui Purei	applying coconut oil of the coconut palm of Purei
nyui Purei beau tempong	the coconut palm of Purei cannot fall over
ujur besi orin langit	along the iron pillar that supports the sky
ujur dotan orin uran	along the pillar of rain
lisat eta lai lola	said with the tip of the tongue
tota napang baang bunge	bathe toward the flower grove
entep ekang rakun kemang	in between the rain cloud flowers
be baang bunge Sembulan	in the flower grove of Sembulan
nyempitai nyui umur	beneath the aged coconut palm
nenkujur pinang tuah	under the old areca palm
nyui umur ulun deo	the aged coconut of many people
pinang tuah ulun wahai	the fortune areca palms of a mass of people
erai due tolu opat	one two three four
lime onum turu walo	five six seven eight

walo rengin meroe	eight—refreshing coolness
sepuluh lampung limei	ten—renewed prosperity
tuak wat siwo ngado basung ure	so that the young sprout becomes fine and healthy
siwo upo sungkai solai	the *siwo* tree comes of age, the *sungkai* tree grows tall
siwo upo nyang olo	the young *siwo* follows the day
sungkai solai nyang bulan	the large *sungkai* follows the moon[5]
puti jaji lomu tau	the *puti* tree becomes strong, the *lomu* tree bears fruit[6]
rima kunen telingkes	receive and receive again
langkep kunen telungku	grasp and grasp again
rengin roe oleng sungei	the refreshing coolness of the river mouth
lampung limei loyu takei	the renewed prosperity of the deep pool
due kali kulek walo	say two times eight
walo melio ke olo	eight clearer than the day
melintai neke bulan	unclouded before the moon
penatik jomit lemit	put on the yellow turmeric
senua burei bura	apply the white rice paste
peko nana olo	the *peko* bird betokens the sun
leliak nana bintang	the *leliak* bird betokens the stars
sentaran bilas ngeras	the ground is cleared around the *bilas* tree
be batang pita ehe	this very morning
adi olo ditan bernang	so that the sun can be seen clearly
bulan ditan bernang	the moon can be seen clearly
ditan Naiyu Jaweng Langit	can be seen by Naiyu of the Door of Heaven
ditan Timang Unsok Liang	can be seen by Timang of the Corner of the Cave
puti ngasi basung ure	cleanse purify the young sprout
ngado bokang mamai pinang	enhance the areca palm flower bud
erai due tolu opat	one two three four
lime onum turu walo	five six seven eight
sie sepuluh ngasi	nine ten—cleanse!
kerek juus bulau june	catch the precious souls
nangkar batu baras papan	from around the flat bathing stone
nangkar lemoong Pantak	from around Pantak's well
adi juus uli ruo unur	so that the souls return, the life forces come back
la Punen Senaring	to Punen Senaring [human being]
apu solung kain penyerungan	now we are already finished
ngenus basung ure	bathing the young sprout
ngeresui mamai pinang	washing the areca palm inflorescence

ulun belian deo jerungan wahai	many *belian*, manifold denominations
ilak okan penyewaka	we are presenting food offerings
bukun kanen penyewayung	various ritual foods
tetap beremana simpen beremanen	the preparations are complete, nothing's lacking
tinek bawe Pantak Itak	set out for the woman Grandmother Pantak
teree oit panti penota	now take back the bathing chair
uli usuk Langai Soai	return it to Mount Soai
Guru Delonong Olo	Guru Delonong Olo
gengeng upa bulau pala	together with the precious rewards
gengeng pasuk bulau pinang	together with fine, selected betel nuts
be batang olo itu	on this very day
tanda awing lelutung solung	as a sign that the work is finished
koe tengkurek sunek	the labor truly completed
erai due tolu opat	one two three four
lime onum turu walo	five six seven eight

In Ma Dengu's chant, to "turn around" or to "transform" (*berebalik*) reality is to turn back, to become one with what lies behind. The repetition of past acts generates prospects for the future by blurring the boundaries between now and then, between the present-day ritual participants and their mythological predecessors. Ma Dengu verbally traverses time and space in the chant, building a bridge between what takes place here and now, and what took place in mythical times. Oscillating between what had been done before and what is done at this moment, fusing time planes, he takes us into a mythical space in which bodies merge, united by the cold water, and the words of his chanting. We are at Pantak's well, at the flat bathing stone on Mount Soai, and in the same breath, at the bathing chair, in the flower grove of Sembulan. There is the mythical child Edau and there is Liman and his baby sister, bathed side by side, by Ma Dengu and by Itak Pantak and her companions. Thus the individual and the collective become fused while history and myth are embodied and the present is integrated with the past.

To be cooled is to become part of something else, to be "reminded" of one's place in a larger context. Liman *is*, in a sense, the child Edau, just as his sister *is* "the shoot, the young shrimp, the *bentas* sprout from the flower grove." It is in their connection to a past and to what they have in common with other human beings that the coolness and prosperity desired in the chant may potentially be obtained.

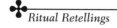

It may be pertinent here to speak of what linguistic anthropologists have called "entextualization" (e.g., see Bauman and Briggs 1990: 73; Keane 1997: 133; Kuipers 1990: 4–7; Silverstein and Urban 1996). This concept refers to a process whereby a particular speech act or segment of discourse is transformed into a "text," that is, a relatively autonomous and repeatable unit that can be detached from the concrete setting in which it is presented (Bauman and Briggs 1990: 73). The desired result of this process is often an identification of this text as an "authoritative version of one that existed before" (Kuipers 1990: 4). In Keane's words, the process "seeks to produce something like a timeless text, whose linguistic forms imply that its sources and meanings lie beyond the realm of particular speakers, circumstances, and interests" (1997: 133).

Entextualization thus at once involves both "decontextualization" and "recontextualization," and it parallels in this respect the process of depersonalization which the participants in the bathing ritual presented here go through, and which, I argue, is much the point of it, or at least an essential aspect of how it is supposed to work. Depersonalization is indeed partly facilitated by formal elements of the chants, such as linguistic devices like parallelism, which have the effect of entextualizing it, making it identifiable as *belian* language and part of ritual tradition. Decontextualization thus works in tandem with the processes whereby ritual participants (and the ritual experts) become associated with an encompassing and contextually transcendent order (e.g., tradition, or the ancestors) such as the identification or association of them with the mythological characters in the chant or the juxtaposition of past and present ritual acts that are described in, and simultaneously occur, within it.

Illustrating this process of depersonalization, in the chant Liman's mother and father become Ine Memea, Uma Memayor, "the Mother who Feeds," "the Father who Provides" (and later, the mother also becomes Ine Petete, "the Mother who Breast-feeds"), thus becoming both anonymized and reduced to a function of a role (i.e., their role as nurturers, providers of life). Still later in the chant, they, and all other bathers with them, are simply referred to as Punen Senaring, "human beings" (according to the myth of origin of humankind, *Tempuun Senaring*, Punen was the first real human being and for this reason the expression Punen senaring, "Punen human being," may

190

be used as a designation for the whole of humankind, particularly in ritual discourse).

What this process of entextualization and depersonalization ideally accomplishes for the bathers is an integration with a community transcending time and space. By bathing "in the flower grove of Sembulan, beneath the aged coconut palm, the old areca palm, the aged coconut palm of many people, the fortune areca palm of a mass of people," the participants are bathing at a place connecting generations through plants (e.g. coconut and areca palms, banana trees, Chinese Hibiscus bushes) referred to as *samat*, which are planted in connection with a child's birth ritual (*ngebidan*) in order to promote the child's growth and improve its fate and fortune (with the child's soul growing strong as the trees and bushes grow).[7] This is a place of significant ritual importance, a place where the fates and life-spans of generations are symbolized by the tall stalks of the palms and the intertwined branches of the flower bushes, and a place from which much ritual material is brought (flowers, banana leaves, coconuts, betel nuts). Similarly, heading toward "the iron pillar that supports the sky," and "the coconut palm of Mount Purei," the shamans are approaching another location representing continuity, or perhaps more to the point, eternity and permanence. Hence the lines: "the iron pillar will not rust," "the coconut palm of Purei cannot fall over." What is referred to this time is Mount Purei, a physically rather small and insignificant mountain which is thought to hold the now invisible iron pillar which once connected the earth and the sky. Like Mount Soai, Mount Purei is also a place where an (invisible) pool can be found in which the souls of death shamans and ritual participants are sometimes bathed by their mythological guardians, and on which an imperishable coconut palm grows, the oil of which is claimed to be used in rituals.

As among the Iban, who perform bathing rituals at points of ontological change in the human life cycle—birth and death, for example—"points of disjunction" which threaten the cohesion of the community, bathing among the Luangans can be seen as "a precursor to re-integration and renewed sociality" (Sather 2001: 77).[8] At least in the Luangan case, the bathing should, as I have argued, be seen as a precursor to a re-integration and a renewed sociality which stretches over generations of bathers, embracing both ancestors and descendants (a chant provided by Sather [1988: 173]

191

suggests similarities in this respect as well between the Iban and the Luangans). "Receiving a new shoot, welcoming an areca palm inflorescence" is thus an expression that can be said to refer not only to the welcoming of Liman's sister into the community of the living but also into a community including those who came before, the shoot and the inflorescence growing out of plants planted in the mythical past.

"The healthy body," to borrow a phrase by Tsing, "incorporates others in its own definition" (1993: 191). Among the Meratus studied by Tsing, as well as among the Luangans, health, and well-being more generally, including fortune and prosperity, is a function of social connection, of attachment to a collectivity, whereas illness and misfortune are functions of isolation, of breaks in the connections. The Meratus use the term *kapuhun* for "isolating oneself from others or from one's environment" (ibid.: 189), whereas the Luangan equivalent is *tapen*, a word which like *kapuhun* implies a failure to involve in social interaction, resulting in a "weakened soul" (*lome juus*) for the offender and the offended, making them vulnerable to spirit attack. For example, by refusing offered food one exposes oneself, and the one offering the food, to the danger of accidents such as snake bites, and to illnesses. "Self-isolation and alienation," however, are, as Tsing (ibid.: 191) expresses it, "unavoidable features of daily life," just as illness is considered "an ordinary human occurrence" (by the Meratus and by Luangans), and the shaman's task is thus "to reconnect people to health-maintaining social and cosmic networks." Seen is this light, the objective of ritual bathing in this case is to reconnect people, to make them part of and remind them of networks that extended the "particularity of both persons and circumstances" (Keane 1997: 114). It is by opening up or enlarging the individual "beyond the personal dimension," freeing him from "the specialisations and confines of personality" (Deren 1965: 20), that Ma Dengu attempts to turn the sometimes overwhelming "heat" of the present into a healthy coolness.

This is not just a semantic project but also a sensuous one. To sit closely together on the bench in the flower grove, surrounded by the scent of sweet-smelling flowers, showered by cold water, or at the bathing chair, encircled by Ma Dengu's lingering voice and the sound of bells jingling as he moves, water dripping in the eyes, is an embodied experience for the participants, and whatever sense of togetherness and collectivity that may be achieved through the bathing results from bodily experience as much as from intellectual understanding of the words of the chant or knowledge of the myth that lies behind them (even if it, of course, is closely bound up with an idea of coolness as something desirable). In fact, the significance of Luangan words is bound to their physical properties, as is their ability to evoke and thus transform reality. Ma Dengu's words are felt almost as much as they are comprehended. They have, to cite Kathryn Geurts, a "physical force which operates not only at the site of the ear and mind but throughout the entire body" (2005: 176). The language of his chant is an embodied language, a language experienced almost palpably as it gushes over the ritual participants. Rich in alliteration, rhyme and parallelism, full of so-called blind dyads (see Metcalf 1989: 41), words that only receive their meaning from words they are coupled with (and typically rhyme with), the language of ritual bathing (and of *belian* curing in general) prominently displays its own materiality. Its form is as important as its content; in fact, the form of the language (i.e., its acoustic qualities) is at times inseparable from its referential meaning.

What we are dealing with here could be described as a language which is in a sense lacking in arbitrariness, a language whose qualities of sound and rhythm are intrinsic to its purpose, inseparable from its performance. There is, for example, no easy way to separate the meaning of "rengin roe, lampung limei" (here somewhat awkwardly translated into "refreshing coolness, renewed prosperity") from the materiality of the words describing it. *Roe* and *limei*, which are incomprehensible words on their own that cannot be used outside these expressions, are essential parts of the expression, of what we might call its "illocutionary force" (Austin 1962). Worn in by use, the components of such expressions are irreplaceable, in the sense, for example, that they cannot be replaced by synonyms and retain the same relationship to sensuous experience. Meaning here, to cite Charles Bernstein (1998: 17), "is not something that accompanies the word, but is performed by it." Stylistic devises such as alliteration and parallelism are to an important degree what marks the language as ritual language, and what gives it its power to sensuously evoke reality, rather than just invoke it. For many Luangans it is also this physical aspect of the language that they seem to value most in *belian* chants: its poeticity, the way it "tastes," so to speak, an opinion all the more understandable as the precise semantic meaning of words or expressions is not always clear, either because it is lacking, as in the blind dyads, or because it is archaic, foreign, or known only to *belian* (see Metcalf 1989 for similar observations in respect to Berawan chants). This is an aspect of language which, at least to some degree, is unavoidably lost in the process of translation and therefore, in order to convey both the sensuousness and the meaning of Ma Dengu's words, I have presented both a transcription and a translation of the chant.

Another, closely related, and in this respect critically import-ant aspect of Ma Dengu's words is that, through their poetic materiality—that is, through such features as assonance, alliteration and parallelism but also through such formal qualities as meta-phor—they index ancestral tradition. That is to say that these are precisely the characteristics that are commonly associated with the "language of the ancestors" (*basa ulun tuha one*)—the ancestors are said to have been particularly apt at using assonance, parallelism and metaphor in their speech—and that these features, therefore, have the effect of establishing a connection between the ancestors and their descendants. The pertinence of Ma Dengu's words—their "lack of arbitrariness"—therefore not only springs from their per-ceived poetic qualities but also from how they are thought to have been used. The fact that ancestral speech in itself is often attributed with extraordinary powers only adds to this pertinence, in the sense of making the chants more authoritative.

As this indicates, repetition, in this case, is not just about reproduction, but also about construction. It works, as Keane has observed for Sumbanese ritual speech, "to fit events into a preexist-ing template ... [as well as] to *construct* in concrete forms the very ancestral order that it appears to *reproduce*" (1997: 96, original ital-ics). In bathing rituals, this mediation between the past and present is to an important extent sensuous. To repeat words and acts of the past is to make these words and acts corporeally alive among the audience, and to make the audience sensuously part of the ances-tral order which is thought to have produced these words and acts. When Ma Bari decided that Liman's crying demanded ritualized action he did so as a preventive step, he saw the "alienating" effect that the birth of Liman's sister might have had on Liman and the potential dangers involved in that alienation.[9] Ma Bari thus initiated a process of (re)integrating Liman and his sister into a community of bathers (encompassing past and present members) at the same time as that community was reconstructed by the "habituation" of the children into what it is constructed of (i.e., the bathing, or, ritualization). Moreover, the ritual provided an opportunity for other community members to be bathed as well, some of them for reasons that, although not directly related to Liman, still contributed to the sense of urgency that caused Ma Bari to insist on a ritual in the first place.

To cool is to "clear the ground around the *bilas* tree," to remove weeds and competing growth so that the tree can grow unimpeded. Ritual cooling is about providing conditions for growth and the progression of a good or at least tolerable life, to eliminate, or perhaps more to the point, to dissipate the conditions which hinder such a development, particularly such conditions which Luangans think of in terms of heat and adversity (*layeng lihang*). The concepts of heat and coolness, as used by central Luangans, are generalized categories, not so much part of a system of humoral classification which dichotomizes foods, medicines, or illnesses into "hot" or "cold" categories (cf. Golomb 1985; Laderman 1983), as generalized metaphors used along with other similar metaphors in ritual language to describe the process of transforming something bad into something good (*pejiak pejiau*).

However, such development, if achieved, is seldom lasting or comprehensive—and may not, with the passing of time, be unequivocally interpreted (rituals are, in fact, as I have pointed out before, seldom judged on the basis of "results," and they are never deemed failures on this basis alone). Coolness, then, is a relative concept. Luangan bathing, which unlike its Iban counterpart is not primarily performed at points of ontological change in the life cycle, seldom achieves unambiguously, and is seldom associated with unequivocal expectations of achieving, the "comfortable, peaceful, and ordered state" associated with Iban cooling (Sather 2001: 77; see also Barrett and Lucas 1993: 578). What is at issue in bathing is typically not so much establishing an "ordered" state as establishing preconditions for continuing life, or making an uncomfortable or undesirable condition bearable (and maintaining relations with spirits, as always in *belian* curing). After all, weeds often grow violently, and as the two cases that I will present next will show, things do not always turn out as one would hope (which does not diminish the motivations for bathing, as I hope to show). As for Liman, he did gradually stop crying (he was not crying very much in the first place, as far as I could judge) and grew into a healthy little boy, who, together with his mother, father, and sister, moved away to his father's home village sometime after the ritual was finished, being dearly missed by his great-grandmother, who stayed behind.[10]

Scene Two: Fruit for the Caterpillars

Among those bathed during each evening of the ritual arranged to cure Liman and his baby sister were Ena and Mohar, a young couple who, together with Ena's parents, were living temporarily in the longhouse where the ritual was performed. At this moment we shall move back in time to events taking place a few weeks before the ritual for Liman took place. This is the story of Ena and Mohar and their baby, but it is also the story of events that in an unspoken way informed the events surrounding the bathing of Liman four weeks later.

In August 1996, about a year after they were married, Ena and Mohar were expecting their first child. This was Ena's second marriage; her first, very short, marriage was arranged by her parents against her will to a much older schoolteacher who they thought would be a good match, presumably because of his secured income. Ena, however, resisted all attempts to live a married life with the teacher (who had a rather bad reputation because of his numerous affairs with women, including six earlier marriages) and they were soon divorced. Ena's second marriage was initiated by the couple themselves and was very much based on mutual attraction. Following customary practice, Ena and Mohar were at this point living with Ena's parents, and helping out in their swidden field. Ena and Mohar led what seemed like quite a happy and heedless life, watching television whenever there was an opportunity, dreaming about clothes and pop music, spoiling a cute little puppy.

In the beginning of September that year, Ena gave birth to a baby girl, perhaps a bit prematurely (she was just barely visibly pregnant at the time). The child nevertheless seemed healthy and everything went fine. Ena, who together with her husband and parents had moved into the longhouse (owned by her grandparents, Ma Bari and Tak Ningin) for the birth, spent almost all her time with the baby, as is customary, breast-feeding, leaving the house just to take quick baths in the river. At times she received visits from friends who stopped by to chat, but most of the time she was alone in the house with the baby and either her mother or grandmother. Mohar went on with his life pretty much as before, hunting and farming, the only exception being that he had to wash cloth diapers in the mornings before going to the swidden or to the forest (in answer to a question about what had happened in the village while we were away on a short break, he only mentioned that he had been slashing his field, but did not mention that his first child had been born).

Two weeks after the baby's birth, Nen Tampung, Ena's maternal aunt from a neighboring village, visited and it was decided that a *belian* ritual was to be arranged for the newborn baby girl, not because she was ill, but "so that the baby would grow fat and healthy," as the aunt who would perform the ritual expressed it. Another ritual assignment came in between, however, and the ritual was postponed (at one moment it was even said that it would be cancelled). At about this time Ma Bari, Ena's grandfather, saw fit to give a formal speech to Ena and Mohar about the responsibilities of parenthood, emphasizing the work required and making frequent references to "the ancestors" (*ulun tuha one*). At this same time, Ena suffered from blisters in her mouth, making it hard for her to eat, and some smaller rites (*semur*) were held during which Nen Alam (Liman's father's mother who was visiting the village at that time) blew on Ena and recited some spells.[11]

Finally, a "bathing *belian*," as Nen Tampung, now returned, called it, was arranged. Decorations were made by Mohar and Ena's father Ma Kelamo. A small *nansang kapoi* tree was brought in and placed upright in a large jar, its trunk wrapped in white cloth and decorated with red and yellow flowers and small packages of sticky rice wrapped in banana leaf. "A *lomu* tree, full of fruit" (the fruit represented by the flowers and the rice packages), "for the baby, to grow with," as Nen Tampung expressed it (the *lomu* tree, *canarium decomanum*, one of the tallest trees growing in the area, is one of the trees that attract honey-producing bees and it is for that reason always left standing in swidden fields). Together with Nen Bola, her sister and another of Ena's aunts, Nen Tampung then started the ritual. Sitting on the floor by the tree they took turns chanting, calling their spirit familiars (*mulung*). The ritual attracted a predominantly female audience, who sat close to the shamans, listening carefully to what was sung; Nen Tampung, an apprentice of Tak Dinas', was the only female *belian* in the neighborhood who could "stand as *belian*" (*jakat belian*) on her own and for that reason drew attention to this otherwise rather small event.[12]

The bathing then began. Two plastic barrels placed by the front door were filled with water which was brought up from the river. The water was mixed with the usual areca palm twigs and sweet smelling flowers (*telase, bungen dusun*). People gathered around the barrels, wrapped in sarongs or dressed in shorts, among them Mohar and Ena. Chanting, Nen Tampung and Nen Bola, together with Nen Bai who had joined in, poured water over the people who sat on their heels close together on the split bamboo floor. Ena massaged her hair as she was washed by Nen Bola, while Nen Tampung poured a bucket full of water over Mohar's head. Last of all the baby girl was brought forth by her grandmother and water was sprinkled on her with an areca palm stalk. The ritual was finished by eleven in the evening and rice flour cakes were served to the participants.

A couple of days later Mohar complained that the baby had not been sleeping during the night and that she suffered from constipation. At this time I was leaving the village temporarily but I was later told that the *belian* ritual was resumed, unsuccessfully. The baby died a few days later. A couple of weeks later when I returned to the village, life went on pretty much as normal, with Ena and Mohar seeming to be cheerful enough, and no one mentioning the baby. Ena still wanted the pictures she had asked me to take of the baby before I traveled downstream though (she had ordered ten copies), as well as the feeding bottle she had asked me to buy.

The ritual arranged for Ena's and Mohar's baby did not start out as a regular curing ritual although the circumstances made it end as one. It was initiated by a close relative—a maternal aunt is called "mother" by her sister's child—in order to strengthen the soul of the child. The bathing served to integrate and welcome as much as to cool and purify the child, who was especially welcome as neither of Ena's two aunts had children or grandchildren of their own. In this sense they were not bathing just any child here, but a child of their own "daughter" (Ena lived with her aunt Nen Tampung when she was younger and attended school in the neighboring village where her aunt lived, as did her younger sister Lida at the time of the ritual, see introduction). The ritual clearly served other agendas as well, however. It most notably formed an arena in which female curing was encouraged, the child providing an opportunity for Nen Tampung and Nen Bola to perform a ritual in the village (in which neither of them lived and which neither of them visited frequently at the time) and to convene an audience of apprentices and other interested persons, among them many women (and some men) with an apparent interest in the *sentiu* style of curing and ritual bathing. For many of those present the ritual represented an opportunity to, figuratively speaking, follow in the footsteps of Itak Pantak: to take up through *belian sentiu* what women at some point along the way had given over to men (until recently female curing had been declining rapidly whereas it was said to have been much more common in the past). *Belian sentiu,* and especially the *belian dewa-dewa* style of *sentiu* curing which was introduced to the village in which this ritual took place by Tak Dinas (see chapter 2), and which here was resumed by Nen Tampung and Nen Bola (whose brother was married to Tak Dinas' daughter and who both had studied to become *belian* with Tak Dinas), has provided a new path towards female *belian*ship and female control over the mythical past, a path in which ritual bathing takes a central position.

In a way *belian sentiu,* with its strong emphasis on downriver aesthetics and downriver language (Kutai Malay)—neither of which, however, were that prominent in this particular ritual, which mainly focused on bathing—has provided a perfect ground for the growing popularity of ritual bathing. Ritual bathing, after all, also had its origins downriver, if we are to believe the myth of its origin, and it was first performed by female shamans, which might add to its appeal for women. Besides, during the trip to the sea to seek a cure for Edau, Buah Ore Ani married the crocodile spirit of the sea, Tatau Tempuk Gelung, and laid an egg at every river mouth on her way home, thus creating a spiritual link between the upriver and downriver realms. *Juata,* the water spirit (which has numerous manifestations, some of which reside in river mouths and whirlpools, while others reside in the sea and in the sky), is also commonly said to be a Muslim and is therefore frequently offered goats instead of pigs during rituals, a fact which might make *belian sentiu* appear an especially suitable forum for negotiating with the spirit. Although *juata* can be approached in other styles of curing than *belian sentiu,* it is not uncommon to mix curing styles and add a sequence of *belian sentiu* to other styles of curing whenever the spirit is given special attention. And albeit ritual bathing is included in other styles of curing, it is particularly prominent in *sentiu* curing, and especially in the curing performed by Tak Dinas and her disciples (among them Mancan, Nen Tampung, Nen Bola, as well as a number of women who "follow," *nuing*, them in the capacity as co-*belian*). As always when Tak Dinas was involved, there was an intriguing mix of the old and the new here, of the autochthonous and the foreign.

But let us return to Ena and Mohar. In spite of all the efforts made their first-born baby passed away at only four weeks old. To see this as a failure on Nen Tampung's and Nen Bola's part would be less than fair, however. Fruit sometimes fail to ripen; the shamans' task is to clear the ground around the tree, to provide the conditions for growth, but this is nevertheless not always enough. When I asked Luangan women how many children they had I was often given the number of living children, and another of children that *boreng*, that is, that literally "did not become," that died during birth or in infancy. This is part of most women's experience and so common that it appears almost inescapable. From my experience, it seems to be especially the first child who runs a risk of dying prematurely. In such cases, the "entextualization" of ritual bathing works somewhat differently than it does under ideal circumstances, I suggest. The embracing of an infant into a community of past and present members does not always strengthen the soul of the child or reinforce the community, but, through the depersonalization of the participants, it nevertheless distances them—more or less lastingly—from the immediate conditions of their individual fates; this promotes a broader view according to which what happens can be seen to belong to human experience as inevitably as, to borrow metaphors from Ma Dengu's chant, "the sun sets" and "the moon wanes" (both unlucky but unavoidable conditions), a factor which may ease some of the pain experienced in the case of infant death, for example. Not talking about, or avoiding paying attention to such uncontrollable events, is, as I shall show shortly, another "strategy" employed by Luangans in order to avoid the alienating effects that such events may cause.

Ena and Mohar showed no overt feelings of distress two weeks after the death of their baby. Like other young, newly wed couples they were not unambiguously enthusiastic about having children so soon (caring for young children limits the everyday life especially of women who are prevented from, among other things, participating fully in farm work and visiting relatives etc.; see Tsing 1993: 113 for similar observations among the Meratus). This is not to say that the child was unwanted. The slight indifference that could be detected in Mohar's behavior after the birth of the child (which probably caused Ma Bari to give his speech about his and Ena's new responsibilities as parents), was in no ways exceptional and could also be interpreted as an emotional strategy to deal with the very real risks infants face. Infants frequently arouse a certain amount of ambivalence: they are enjoyed and treasured but at the same time one keeps a certain distance to them while they are very small (one indication of this is the fact that one does not give them a name). What we are dealing with here could perhaps be described as what Tsing (1993: 115), recounting a story of how a prematurely born baby was left to die unattended by Meratus Dayak women—perhaps unwanted by its teenage mother, perhaps just not considered salvable—has referred to as "an area of inchoate understandings without fully developed, public articulations." This is an area "at the edge between silence and speech" (1993: 115), an area of marked ambivalence in which cause and effect are hardly separable categories (a parallel can be drawn here to the discussion among social historians of whether the indifference observed by mothers to their infants in the early modern period was a cause or an effect of high infant mortality, see Schepher-Hughes 1992: 356).

In a way, the photograph Ena wanted me to take of the baby, and the circumstances surrounding the photographing itself, says more about the feelings involved in Ena's and Mohar's case than any words (which anyhow were not uttered). Time and again the photographing was postponed by Ena and Mohar in order to let the baby grow a little larger, until it could not be delayed because of my journey downstream. Standing stiff and upright in the picture, Ena and Mohar are dressed in their best, looking serious, with the small sleeping baby in Mohar's arms, pale against his sunburnt hands, for the first time dressed in socks and a white shirt. I do not know what Ena did with her ten copies of the picture, whether she put them away or shared them among the members of her family. Somehow though the picture—as much because of what it does *not* show, as

because of what it shows—materializes "what did not become"; similarly, Ena and Mohar frequently asked me to take their photograph,
always dressed up in fancy clothes which I never saw them wear
otherwise, the pictures then collected in an album portraying a life
not quite theirs.

It was only two weeks after the death of Ena's and Mohar's baby
that Liman's sister (bathed together with her brother Liman in the
case first presented in this chapter) was born in the same longhouse.
This was in itself a little disturbing: for many people to enter a house
where someone has just died is *pali*, taboo, and during the birth
ritual for Liman's sister, many women with a history of ill health
were for this reason restricted to the kitchen at the back of the
house (where they were helping out with the cooking).[13] Although
no one made an overt connection between the two cases (no one
spoke about Ena's baby at all), I would argue that the happenings at
least partly affected Ma Bari in his decision to insist on a ritual for
Liman, not so much because of the uniqueness or rarity of what had
happened, but because of the frequency of such events. The happenings, in a most concrete way, reminded everyone of the risks that
infants are subjected to, risks that most people have personal experience of. Evidence of a connection and continuation perceived to
exist between the events could be seen in Ma Bari's and Tak Ningin's
own participation in the bathing during Liman's ritual (Ma Bari,
in particular, did not usually participate actively in bathing rites,
preferring to stay more in the background of events). It could also
be seen in Ena's and Mohar's continual participation in the bathing
during the ritual. The death of Ena's child was present in a silent but
perceivable way throughout the bathing ritual for Liman: a reminder
of what might happen if things turn out wrong.

This did not, however, mean that it visibly influenced people in
the sense that they appeared depressed or frightened. It was only
in the need to be cooled that the "heat" could be sensed, in the
multiple bathing rites, instigated not only by the shamans, Mancan
and Ma Dengu, but often by someone in the audience asking to be
bathed. In a way then the ritual served not only to cure Liman but to
cool down after what had happened before as well (there were also,
as usual, people wanting to be bathed for other reasons, because of
their own illnesses, for example). In any case, the ritual for Liman
did form a turning point for Ena and Mohar in the sense that its end

formed an end to their stay in the longhouse: the day after the ritual was finished they, together with Ena's parents, moved back to their own single-family house. When I visited them a year and a half later they were the happy parents of a lively and somewhat spoilt little boy.

To be cooled involves a movement between self and group; it represents an integration, but it would be ineffective if it did not resonate in personal experience. It is in the tension between individual fates and the human condition that the bathing rituals receive their meaning for the participants. In order to understand what goes on in bathing rituals we have to see how "what happens" is related to "what has happened" as well as to "what might happen." Rituals and extra-ritual events alike are always situated. Past experiences and expectations about what is possible condition present-day events. However, the experiences and dispositions that these give rise to also mediate and create the significance of tradition and the past. The past is, as Michael Lambek (2007: 21) has expressed it, "continuously realized—made real—by the work of the present." The impact of the past is always mediated by the experiences and present-day conditions of those concerned, and what urgency there is in rituals for the participants derives from the tension between past and present experience. Rituals cannot thus be treated as closed units, as universes unto themselves. Hence, although the case that I will present next is not directly connected to the two already discussed, it will shed light on these two as well, both through what they have in common, and through what is unique in it.

Scene Three: So that the Sun Can Be Seen Clearly

It is still dark outside when Monyeng enters the longhouse at half past five one morning in early January 1997. In her arms she carries her daughter Juni's and her son-in-law Ma Bubu's newborn baby boy, wrapped in a white cloth. She brings the baby to the *longan* near the center of the longhouse, close to the back wall where I am still lying half-asleep on my sleeping mat. She attaches a mosquito-net to the roof so that it covers the baby who she puts down on the floor. She then sits down on the floor herself, telling me that the baby is *payeh* (mortally ill). The day before, while Ma Bubu was away at an old farm house quite some distance away, bringing home rice that he

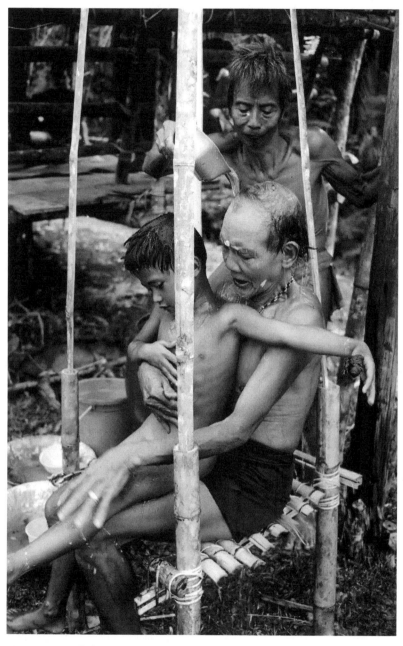

Figure 5.2. Kakah Ramat bathing people outdoors at *balei naiyu* during *buntang* for Ma Bari

still stored there for the birth ritual that was planned to be arranged a few days later, the baby had begun to cry and would not stop, no matter what was done. Mancan was called to *nyemur*, to blow air on the baby and recite some spells, as was Ma Dengu and later Kakah Ramat. Tak Ningin, the village midwife, visited the house to look at the baby as well, while Tak Lodot, Juni's grandmother, also tried to *nyemur*. But the baby just cried, refusing to accept Juni's milk.

The family has had no sleep during the night and the baby has not been eating since yesterday, I am told by Monyeng. The baby has stopped crying now; only a faint whimper can occasionally be heard from under the mosquito-net where he is lying. At times Monyeng lifts up the net and looks at the baby but she does not touch him. Visitors come by, among them Ena, Ma Bari, Nen Wase, Tak Hai, sitting down for a while to talk to Monyeng, but no one looks at the baby. Some time later Ma Pile, Ma Bubu's father and the baby's grandfather, comes by to *nyemur* with a black cloth on his head. The baby's stomach is hard and swollen, I am told. I am also told that the illness is due to Ma Bubu having seen a dog kill two of its puppies during Juni's pregnancy (it is considered dangerous for parents expecting a child to see animals get killed as the child might start to emulate the death-throes of the animal). Juni and Ma Bubu now enter the longhouse as well, together with their two older children, but they do not come close to the baby. Lunch is served and eaten and the people present in the longhouse sit talking together or continue with their normal chores.

Without consulting anyone, Ma Lombang (the husband of Tak Lodot, Juni's grandmother) decides that a *belian* ritual should be arranged and gives order for those present to gather the *ruye*, the required offerings and other material paraphernalia. He asks Kakah Ramat to perform the ritual. People seem skeptical but no one raises any objections and some *biyowo* leaves and *dusun* flowers are eventually brought in for the ritual. As the afternoon advances Monyeng wonders whether one should try to nurse the baby or not and calls for Tak Ningin for advice (she even discusses the matter with me and I try to persuade her that one should, feeling helpless and uncomfortable to just sit and watch the baby's condition worsening). Reluctantly Tak Ningin comes by and looks at the baby. Laughing apologetically she tells Monyeng that she does not know. Kakah Ramat is then called for. He blows on the baby and announces that perhaps there are those who might know, but he does not. He also makes clear that he does not want to perform a *belian* ritual. Ma Lombang points out that he cannot force him to do so and the plans are put off. The baby boy still lies under the mosquito-net, with his eyes closed. His breathing is getting heavier now and his chins are flushed. Monyeng strokes some water over his face but does not pick him up even when he occasionally cries.

More people enter the house during the evening, among them Rawen, Ma Bubu's brother, who lives some fifteen kilometers away at a settlement that has developed adjacent to a transmigration camp. The general ambience is cheerful even if somewhat uncanny. Tak Ningin and Ma Bari (who are the owners of the house) seem to be in an unusually cheerful mood, laughing and joking excessively (which is quite unusual as both are normally rather serious-minded), while more and more people assemble in the house. Ma Buno, who has been away on a trip to a downstream administrative center to get some money for a government financed village development project, happens to come home at this time as well, and the discussion focuses on the money. Big projects are planned and Ma Buno describes his trip in detail. At this time Ma Lombang quietly brings in an old suitcase which I am told is intended to serve as a coffin. Kakah Ramat also comes by briefly and asks Monyeng to move the baby away from the *longan* (he does not like the idea of the baby dying by the *longan* because of the *pali* the death would cause). The baby is moved a few meters to the side and a sheet is hung up as a shield so that Juni and Ma Bubu cannot see him. Monyeng still sits by the baby. At ten o' clock in the evening she announces that the baby has stopped breathing.

After the death is announced, Ma Lombang, who is a death shaman (*wara*), wipes the baby with a wet rag and wraps him in a white cloth and puts him in the coffin. Rawen fabricates two small human-like statues (*sepatung lusan*) of bamboo, which are placed next to the coffin together with a small lighted kerosene lamp. Monyeng, who feels uncomfortable sitting alone by the dead body, asks Mompun, a mentally handicapped woman who lives in the house and who at times helps out with minor chores, to come and sit with her by the coffin. Later during the night, Ma Lombang strikes two knives together, first seven times, then eight, and calls for the *liau* and the *kelelungan* (the body and the head soul) of the dead child's already dead relatives to come and bring his souls to the death realms of Lumut and Tenangkai, respectively (children who die before having begun to eat solid food are not guided to these realms by death shamans, *wara*, as adults are, but are brought there by their dead relatives who are called on for this purpose). Ma Bubu, the father, comes forward and briefly sits down by the coffin at this moment. Most of the other people present sit talking, not paying the event any attention. Ma Lombang even has to instruct Ma Buno, who is a *belian*, to leave the house while he is washing the corpse (as this could affect Ma Buno's *belian*ship adversely), as Ma Buno himself does not seem to notice what is going on.

The next morning Ma Lombang decides that the funeral will take place first and after that there will be a *belian* arranged in order to *ngaper* (whisk over, and thus purify and cool down) the next of kin. People arrive at the longhouse again. Some chickens are slaughtered and a meal is served. The coffin is then carried out of the house, through a side opening instead of the front door, together with the bamboo cane filled with Juni's breast milk, and the two bamboo figures, which represent substitutes for the baby's mother and father (*gantin ine uma*). Most villagers, including Ma Bubu but not Juni, follow in a procession to the graveyard where a grave has already been dug. The coffin is put into the grave and each person throws a handful of earth on it. The grave is covered and the figures, together with the milk cane, are put on it, while Ma Lombang recites a few words and strikes the knives together again. Shortly after, all people return to the house.

A bathing ritual is now performed at the spot where the baby died. Juni, Ma Bubu, Monyeng, Ma Lombang as well as Tak Ningin are bathed by Ma Dengu who pours water over their heads from a large bucket. Chanting, he calls for some spirit familiars and cools down the heat of death and adversity. He then whisks with some leaves over the heads of all people present in the house. The ritual is rather short and people seem relieved rather than sad. Plates are finally distributed as a reward (*temai*) to those who have helped out with the baby, after which most people leave the longhouse, among them Monyeng, Juni, Ma Bubu and their older children, who move back to their own house.

When Monyeng came in with the baby early that morning she already knew that he was dying, according to Jonjong, who discussed

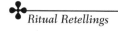

the matter with Tak Hai and me afterwards. According to Ma Bari, on the other hand, she brought the baby close to the *longan* to see if that would help, to give him another chance: the *longan* is an abode for *pengiring*, protecting spirits, and is as such considered to accommodate a concentration of propitious spiritual power. Both were probably correct, Jonjong in announcing what everyone knew but would not say out loud, and Ma Bari in refusing that kind of closure, wanting to emphasize what little hope there still was. To watch someone die is dangerous, as Jonjong put it, it might cause *sengker- apei* (a condition in which death throes are mimetically imitated), and therefore the family did not want the baby to die in their own house, she concluded (especially as Tak Lodot, Juni's grandmother, had been ill recently, which also explains why she never entered the longhouse during the events). According to Jonjong and Tak Hai, the baby boy became ill because he was taken out of the house in which he was born (or literally because he "stepped on the ground," *najek tana*, as he was carried to Ma Lombang's house by Juni) before the birth ritual was held and the child had been ceremoniously welcomed.[14] This caused *tonoi* (the spirits of the earth) to take him back. As they also pointed out, the tradition in Benangin from where Monyeng, Juni's mother, originates, allows such a procedure, but that tradition is not necessarily applicable in Sembulan, they remarked. Jonjong and Tak Hai also told me that Tak Ningin had had a dream in which she dreamt that she killed a monkey, a dream that was interpreted as meaning that the baby would die.

In a way, then, the baby was predetermined to die (whether Tak Ningin had told about her dream at the time or only did so after- wards is unclear, often facts such as these are brought to light only after the fact, so to speak). A "mantle of social death," to borrow an expression by Nancy Scheper-Hughes (1992: 385), had already begun to envelop the baby when he was brought into the longhouse that morning. In removing the baby from his parents, not trying to feed him or rock him anymore, the family, represented by Monyeng, had given up on him, at least to a certain extent (and to a very real extent in that the baby could not survive very long without fluid). At the same time the baby was largely ignored by the other people present in the longhouse, some of whom took great effort not to become emotionally involved in the case (such as Tak Ningin and Ma Bari who seemed almost overly cheerful). Juni's and Ma Bubu's baby was thus basically left to die alone under the mosquito-net (with Monyeng, his grandmother, by his side, but yet at a distance with the mosquito-net between them). It is true that some did try to intervene; Ma Lombang, for example, who tried to arrange a *belian* ritual, and Monyeng herself, at times struck by doubt, wondering whether one still should try to feed the baby or not. The response they got from other people did not support any further measures, however. Instead their initiatives were met with silence, excuses, and claims of ignorance.

Yet, had we been dealing with an adult, or an older child, a number of measures would probably have been taken even after one had lost hope of probable or even possible recovery: *belian* rituals following on *belian* rituals. This also very much points to what is at the heart of the matter: infants die whether we want it or not, their "souls" (*juus*) are still "weak" (*lome*), and as both Kakah Ramat and Tak Ningin (who should be the utmost experts on these matters, Kakah Ramat in the capacity as a highly experienced *belian* and Tak Ningin as the village midwife) readily admitted, they did not know what to do in cases such as this (or did not consider it worthwhile to do anything). Infants simply have a loose grip on life, their "souls" are easily frightened and they are highly vulnerable to spirit attack. There are a number of preventive steps that can be taken, to be sure; the bathing ritual performed for Ena's child constituted one example of such a "soul-strengthening" enterprise, but when death strikes this early in life it is widely agreed that there is not much that one can do (at least not without worsening the case for those around).[15]

The vulnerability of small children is reflected in the Luangan naming practice as well (see Sillander 2010 for a more thorough description of this practice). Infants are not given a name until several months or even a year after birth but are instead referred to as *tia mea* (red children). This can be seen as a form of "delayed anthropomorphization" (Schepher-Hughes 1992: 413), serving to protect the child from spirit attack, but also to protect parents and other members of the family from the "heat" and alienation caused by potential loss. By not having a name and thereby an individual and social identity, the baby becomes more easily replaceable. As is well-known among many Borneo peoples, children are often called by names such as "rubbish," "soot," "latrine" or "larvae" (Rousseau 1998: 276; Metcalf 1991: 257; Sather, personal communication) so as to divert the attention of potentially malevolent spirits. Among Luangans, a boy might be called *semeritek* (meaning "willie," referring to his male genitalia), a name which not only deindividuates him (recognizing only his sex), but which also, as with other such names, excludes him (or perhaps rather his parents) from definition through social relationships: Luangan parents are typically called by teknonyms such as "mother of x" or "father of x," something which cannot be initiated before the child is given a personal name. In a society in which a person is very much "a complex of social relationships" (Radcliffe-Brown 1940: 193), refraining to designate such a relationship might work to enable an easier termination of it. Or, in M. W. de Vries' (1987: 173–174) words: "In societies where infant mortality is a regular and common occurrence, late naming may help individual mothers manage their grief reactions."

In any case, keeping a certain distance was an explicitly expressed strategy employed in order to protect Juni and Ma Bubu when their baby fell mortally ill. When they eventually entered the longhouse that morning they never approached the baby or looked in his direction; in fact, a sheet was, as already remarked, suspended so that they would not be able to see him even by accident. Similarly, it was over and over again expressed to me that the reason why no further effort was made to nurse the baby was that one wanted to prevent the parents from becoming too upset or sad. In its own way, Tak Ningin's and Ma Bari's overly cheerful behavior also worked to distract the parents from what was happening (at the same time as it served to protect Tak Ningin and Ma Bari themselves), as did the indifference shown by most people present in the house. Physical and emotional distancing worked here not so much to repress or suppress negative feelings as to actively keep them away, not allowing them to take over in the first place. Reference can here be made to Unni Wikan's discussion of Balinese among whom the "forgetting" of sadness means "not to think" about it, and "thus not feel it" (1990: 157). Another parallel can be made to a case described by Laderman (1983: 164) in which Malays present at the birth of a still-born child repeatedly commented on it by the phrase: "Tak apa-apa" ("It's nothing, it's all right"). *Iklas*, the feeling of "willed affectlessness" and "not caring" produced by Javanese funerals represents a further parallel (Geertz 1973b: 153; cf. also Siegel 1983). To be overcome by sadness is, for Luangans, to put not only your own health at risk, but also that of

210

your relatives (health being seen, as I have pointed out before, as a function of social connection) and thus the distancing worked here to facilitate a (collective) giving up of what could not be retained.

Death in itself is considered a "hot" condition which might prove dangerous not only for persons with a "weak" soul, but for anyone. If a patient dies during a *belian* curing ritual, for example, the *belian* curer has to go through a process of purification before he can resume his curing practice. Similarly, listening to tape recordings of *gombok* chants (i.e., death ritual chants) during the progression of *belian* rituals (life rituals) is, as I was informed when I made that mistake, considered dangerous. Apart from the direct danger involved, something which was at question in both these cases is what some Luangans described as a "mixing of *pali*" (*sampur pali*), that is a mixing up of life and death regulations or taboos. Jonjong, for example, described how she had her sister Nen Pare taken out of the longhouse in which she was cured along with Ma Bari when her life was drawing to an end, so that Nen Pare's death would not interfere with Ma Bari's recovery. Death might in itself cause more death, or ill-health, as when a child imitates the death throes of an animal that the child, or the child's parents, has witnessed being killed.

When Ma Dengu bathed Juni and Ma Bubu, together with various relatives of theirs (including Tak Ningin) at the spot where the baby had just died, he did so in order to wash away the negative influences or to reduce the "heat" which inevitably and in spite of all precautions follows death. However, the attempt at cooling in this case was not one of "exposing what has been hidden from the senses," as Joel Kuipers (1990: 98) describes the function of cooling efforts in similar circumstances among the Weyewa of Sumba, who, he contends, experience when struck by misfortune a "psychic numbing," which is negatively valued and must be overcome. On the contrary, the bathing, in this case, served to sensuously and collectively detach the bathers from the experience of death, to release them from the "physical" and "social" dangers that it entails. In this respect, the bathing worked to erase the experience from the mind and body of those involved, rather than to expose them to hidden or denied sensory experience. This does not mean that the event as such was wiped from memory, however. Luangans do remember their dead children and, as already mentioned, they often provided me with figures for the number of their infants who had died (*boreng*)—Juni, for example, on her own initiative told me about her firstborn child who also died in infancy. Instead, what is involved here is rather an erasure in the sense that the uniqueness of the experience is denied: a "forgetting" which allows the experience to become a collective, rather than purely individual matter.

Bathing the participants, and whisking over them with a bunch of leaves, Ma Dengu washed away the individualized, embodied memory of death. Contrary to Western psychological theories of mourning, which emphasize the need to grieve a dead infant in a "healthy" way in order to prevent various pathologies from developing (this, they advise, is attained through, among other things, the holding, touching, naming and weeping over a dead newborn; see Nancy Schepher-Hughes 1992: 426–428 for a critical discussion of such theories), Luangans cannot afford to lose themselves in individualized pain and grief, especially not when it comes to infants who demonstrably hold a very loose grip on life.[16] "To see clearly," to borrow a metaphor from Ma Dengu's chant of bathing, is to see past individual experience. The coolness of a future is the coolness obtained through what I, following Deren (1965), have called de-personalization, a coolness which "contextualizes the individual death within a transcendental order" (Seremetakis 1991: 225). Through a process of entextualization and recontextualization, ritual bathing, as I have interpreted it here, works to "translate individual experience into cosmological generality" (ibid.: 238), and thus to reduce some of the heat caused by such sometimes inevitable misfortune as infant death.

* * *

Ritual bathing is an element of complex Luangan curing rituals, particularly of the *belian sentiu* variety. In recent decades both ritual bathing and *belian sentiu* have become increasingly popular among East Kalimantan Luangans. This growing popularity may be seen as an outcome of a number of related factors: the increasing impingement upon the upriver realm by the downriver world; the relative approachability and sensuous appeal of ritual bathing and *belian sentiu* for the audience in comparison with more liturgical and less participant-focused ritual practices and formats (which makes them especially attractive to younger people); and the resurgence of female *belian*ship for which ritual bathing and *belian sentiu* are the principal vehicles. Notwithstanding this association of ritual bathing with the downriver world and recent developments, present-day *belian* curers keenly emphasize that the foundation of ritual bathing was laid in the remote mythical and ancestral past. Its efficacy, they claim, derives from its original performances and their continuous re-enactments through ancestral tradition.

In this chapter I have studied how ritual bathing, an instance of *pejiak pejiau*—the standardized two-phased ritual formula of enacting or dramatizing a transformation of something bad into something good—serves to wash off "debilitating heat" (*layeng lihang*) and establish a condition of "refreshing coolness" (*rengin roe*), a state of generalized well-being. As a particular method of curing, one of many employed in Luangan curing rituals, ritual bathing serves to achieve this double end by way of water and words, which mediate the potency of earlier bathing rituals performed by the mythological heroes and ancestors. Curing in this case, I have argued, is above all a means whereby the personal suffering and potential alienation of ritual participants may be overcome through their "depersonalization." Through integration with ancestral tradition and a collectivity of living and dead bathers the ritual participants are distanced from the potentially dangerous and sometimes overwhelming particularities of the present and presented with the assurance of what has been done before. This is a sensuous project, and the appeal of bathing for the participants, gushed by the cold and scented water, may partly be explained by the immediate sense of refreshment which it brings about. However, at the same time, the experience is subtly and tacitly conditioned by the embodied and tactile memories of the ritual participants to whom the words and the water speak with the authority of the self-evident.

Bathing rituals are not, as I have tried to show, isolated events. It is in the conjunction between the past and the present that I have analyzed bathing rituals: as a practice which serves to readjust the relationship of the participants with the present through invocation of local tradition and the authoritative mythological past. But bathing rituals must also be contextualized in the material and historical circumstances of their instantiation. By presenting and juxtaposing three interrelated instances of ritual bathing, largely involving the same protagonists and taking place shortly after each other in the same location, I have explored what is at stake for particular participants in particular circumstances, situating these participants and circumstances in a history of ritual performances, a history with both personal and mythological bearings. Performances are, in Leo Howe's words (2000: 67), "never isolated activities; they are always in relation to or against previous performances which act as remembered precedents." In this sense ritual performances are, as Margaret Drewal (1992: 3) has pointed out, "by [their] very nature intertextual." Moreover, it is only if we see the bathing of small children in relation to the fact that so many of them die so early in life that we can appreciate the importance these rituals have for individual participants. What is not said in bathing rituals, in means of contextual inducement, is still very much part of their performative potency, their faculty to act upon their participants' experience of the world. It is, I argue, in the interplay of repetition and transformation that the possibilities of establishing a refreshing coolness emerge in ritual bathing. To cool "so that steam rises," to borrow a metaphor used by Ma Dengu as he explained his chant of bathing to me, is to follow in the footsteps of Itak Pantak, while attending to the needs and conditions of present-day bathers. Were it not for this openness of *belian,* and ritual bathing as part of it, to the particularity of circumstances it would not, I suggest, be as effective in transcending these circumstances.

Notes

1. *Tota* refers to bathing performed inside the house, whereas *ngenus* refers to bathing performed outside.
2. Or to be exact, they were born, as is customary, on a special, temporarily constructed covered platform, *blai sawo,* attached to the back of the longhouse.
3. Early historical figures on infant mortality on Borneo are lacking. P.J. Koblenzer and N.H. Carrier (1959–1960: 275) have presented some data for the 1950s, indicating a child mortality rate of 33 percent among the Dusun of Sabah. G.J. Reibel (1976: 93, 149, 174) reports child mortality rates of 21–29 percent, and infant mortality rates of 11–15 percent in three Mentaya (Ngaju) villages with access to medical care; whereas H.F. Tillema (1939: 231) reports a child mortality of 50 percent among East Bornean Punan groups in the early twentieth century (in Knapen 2001: 160–161). Derek Freeman, in his famous study of the Iban (1967: 318fn), in 1949–1951 calculated the rate of stillbirth and childhood mortality among the Baleh Iban of Sungai Sut at 47 percent.

4. Luangans conceive that there are iron pillars that support the sky on many mountain tops in the central Luangan area, which were once visible, but have now became invisible. The one on Mount Purei, in the subdistrict of Gunung Purei in Central Kalimantan, is particularly important mythologically, and is sometimes referred to as *the* iron pillar of the sky (see Endicott 1979: 42–48 for beliefs about similar stone pillars among the Batek).

5. *Siwo* and *sungkai* are trees which grow large extremely fast, almost overnight, and here function as metaphors for the child who one wishes will grow as fast as they do.

6. *Puti* (*Koompassia excelsa*) and *lomu* (*Canarium decumanum*) are among the largest trees in the area; both carry honey and the *lomu* also bears fruit.

7. There are multiple examples of counterparts or doubles of the self recognized by Luangans, the most prominent being the soul (*juus*) and the spirits of the dead (*liau* and *kelelungan*). In addition to the *samat* plants planted during *ngebidan* rituals, other types of *samat* include the invisible plant counterparts planted during *buntang* rituals described in chapter 4. Yet another example of counterpart of the self described in chapter 4 is the placenta (*juma*)—looked up by Kakah Ramat in the heavens in the *buntang* for Ma Bari—which is described as a person's younger sibling. All these plant counterparts and the placenta, all symbolic of a person's well-being and fate, are believed to be guarded by the *seniang* in heaven, at a place called Datai Leok Langit, as is the soul, or perhaps more correctly, a manifestation of it (also called *juus*) that stays there in a house of which the soul house (*blai juus*), which it enters along with those of its family members at the conclusion of a *buntang*, is the visible counterpart.

8. In contrast to the Saribas Iban, the central Luangans do not perform bathing rituals at predetermined points in the life cycle such as at birth or death. There is, for example, no prescribed ritual except the *ngebidan* birth ritual (which does not include bathing) for a newborn child. Bathing rituals are arranged when circumstances so demand, or as preventive steps in order to strengthen the "soul" of a child or an adult.

9. It is worth noting that having children with such short intervals between them as between Liman and his sister is considered undesirable by most Luangans, both because of the burden it places on the mother who has to breast-feed and take care of two small children at a time, and because of the risk that the milk of the mother will not be sufficient to feed them both.

10. The custom of post-marital residence prescribes that the couple stays with the bride's family for about three years after which they stay with the groom's family for approximately another three years, after which they can either move back to the bride's parents or form a household of their own. This is not an absolute system and in this case Ma Bari tried to prevent Alam and Rosa from moving as he claimed that Alam's work effort was essential for many villagers (Alam was a very skilled hunter), but due to various circumstances (a prolonged rainy season, among other things, which prevented Alam from making a swidden that year) they eventually went ahead with the move anyway.

215

11. *Semur* is a minor curing practice that in contrast to *belian* can be performed by almost anyone and consists of reciting some spells and blowing on the patient.
12. The expression "to stand as *belian*" is used for the performance of *belian bawo* and *belian sentiu* rituals, whereas Luangans use the phrase "to sit as belian" (*tuwet belian*) in respect of the performance of *belian luangan* rituals.
13. This particularly concerns people who have been sick and for whom "death" has been interpreted to be harmful by a *belian*. "To enter a house with a dead person in it" (*letep blai mate*) was one of the things Kakah Ramat, for example, considered dangerous but which he as a *belian* obviously could not avoid and thus had to be cured or cooled from.
14. The birth ritual (*ngebidan*) is held on the fourth or eighth day after a child's birth. It is a one-day ritual during which *samat* plants are planted for the child and during which relatives congregate for a common meal.
15. This does not mean that Luangans are unaware or uncritical of unequal social and economic conditions; Luangan women often admired the chubby and, as they saw it, healthy babies in Indonesian commercials and advertisements and complained about their unequal opportunities to raise such healthy children (because of lack of health-care, food and vitamins, etc.).
16. When it comes to older children or adults, Luangans do openly grieve dead relatives. However, even then this happens mostly in a ritualized way (for example, they often cry heavily at certain points in mortuary rituals), and excessive grieving outside ritual is certainly not encouraged.

Chapter Six

It Comes Down to One Origin
Reenacting Mythology and the Human-Spirit Relationship in Ritual

Mythmaking is the backbone of culture, the fundamental means by which human beings demarcate, that is to say, create, human being.

—Elizabeth Baeten (1996: 20)

You ask what they "mean" … ? I'll tell them to you again.

—Michel de Certeau (1984: 80)

In September 1996 it had been raining for months in the central Luangan area. The fields were already slashed and everybody was waiting for a chance to burn. But it just kept on raining. People were depressed as the rain kept them inside, the river flowing over, the water becoming brown and dirty, the ground muddy and slippery. Finally then there were a few days of sunshine, and those who had cleared their swiddens in secondary forest took the opportunity to burn. The burning was not good, but good enough if smaller fires were lit later on. For those that were going to make swiddens in primary rainforest things were not looking as well, however. In order to burn a field in primary forest at least a week of full sunshine was needed. Time was running out, the position of the moon telling them that it would soon be too late to burn for a successful harvest to be possible.

At this time the people of Jelmu Sibak decided to arrange a *ngeraya* ritual to ask for "heat" (*langet*), for dry weather. *Ngeraya* are two days and one night long rituals in which the *seniang*, the god-like celestial spirits who regulate the social, natural and cosmic order, are presented with offerings and asked to provide a good harvest alongside other things required for a good, prosperous life. A *ngeraya* is only a prelude to a much larger ritual, the *nalin taun*. *Nalin taun* rituals are large community rituals which, as their name suggests, are held in order to "treat" (*nalin*) the year (*taun*), that is, to affect the natural cycles favorably, so that rice grows and fruits and game abound. Such rituals may be held either out of gratitude for good yields or as a reaction to unfavorable natural conditions (e.g., drought, rains) threatening poor yields. The principal purpose of a *ngeraya* is to make a vow (*niat*) to the spirits, promising them that a *nalin taun* will be implemented at some point in the future if the spirits provide what they are asked of (including enough rice to enable the staging of the ritual). *Nalin taun* rituals are only rarely held, perhaps once in ten or fifteen years. Together with larger secondary mortuary rituals (*gombok empe selimat*), they are the grandest rituals performed by the central Luangans and the only occasion during which the whole community has to gather. Like the *nulang* rituals performed by the Berawan (Metcalf 1991: 155), the *nalin taun* is a somewhat "paradoxical institution" in that it is "sociologically crucial yet rarely held." A *nalin taun* is also the only forum in which all the origin myths of the Luangans are chanted. At the same time it is a relatively new form of ritual, which spread to the central Luangan area as a result of tributary contacts with the Sultanate of Kutai in the latter part of the nineteenth century (Sillander 2006).

Somewhat like the *ngeraya*, in which the *nalin taun* figures as a physically absent presence—its anticipated completion—this chapter deals with a finality that always seems to be in some sense displaced, remaining beyond reach. The chapter is built around beginnings of different sorts. It is a chapter about the *ngeraya* as a prelude to the *nalin taun*, but also about how ordinary *belian* rituals through invocation and allusion conjure origin myths (*tempuun*), which in the case of the origin myths of heaven and earth (*Tempuun Langit Tana*), and of human beings (*Tempuun Senaring*), can be performed ritually only in the *nalin taun*. The chapter also includes an account of the *tempuun* of human origins itself and shows how the myth forms a beginning, in the sense that it points to what for the Luangans is conceived of as a process of continued human-spirit interaction.

In his study of Sakalava mythopraxis, Lambek (2007: 21) distinguishes between "origins" and "beginnings": origins are events that imply extra-human forces, often situated "in a pre-temporal or pre-historical horizon," whereas beginnings "emerge against what precedes them," are "humanly made" and "located in time and in society." If we follow this distinction this chapter can be said to deal with both origins and beginnings, since it is concerned both with origin stories, representing "origins" in this sense, and with the ways in which these stories are used as "beginnings," with how they are brought to bear on human life at particular times and places. However, the primary significance of *tempuun* is as beginnings, as with how they are used in ritual. As Lambek (2007: 21) observes for the Sakalava, "myth is living or lived," and cannot adequately be understood as "sacred narrative abstracted from its content." Even though Luangan myths are occasionally narrated as stories (for recreation, or for the authorization of particular conditions or courses of action), they are primarily performed as ritual actions, as part of rituals for whose efficiency they are deemed essential. It is in this context, Luangans often told me, that they really matter, and it is here that the most authoritative versions of them are seen to be recounted. This chapter then is about the ongoing practice of Luangan mythmaking, about how origin myths are presented and invoked in particular circumstances, and about how the world is created for and by human beings through them, especially in relation to spirits. Looked at from another angle, the chapter deals with the precariousness of the human condition, and the salience of contingency in it—and in the ritual enterprise—in the form of spirits, the weather, and other forces beyond human control. The relevance of *tempuun,* and especially the need to recite them in ritual, is triggered by developments which bring these aspects of human life to the fore, typically in association with spirits.

Like the *nalin taun,* a *ngeraya* is a community ritual, sponsored by an entire community, rather than by an individual household or extended family as other *belian* rituals are. The *ngeraya* that was performed in Jelmu Sibak in 1996 was held on the initiative of the village's *kepala adat,* a Christian and highly controversial person who had sold village land to the nearby logging company for his own profit, infuriating many villagers, including his own brother who refused to have anything to do with him and did not attend the ritual, even though he, unlike his brother, had not converted to Christianity. The inhabitants of Sembulan, which officially is a hamlet (*dusun*) of Jelmu Sibak, were invited to attend the ritual as well, but, except for Ma Lombang, no one came (jokingly they said that it was good that Kenneth and I attended and thus represented Sembulan).

Despite all of this, the *ngeraya* was a festive event, with crowds of people gathering in a large modern-style multifamily house (which was used instead of the principal longhouse of the village, because of the unwillingness to be involved of the *kepala adat*'s brother, who was the custodian of the longhouse). In this house, the ritual activities centered around a two-storey platform in the rafters of the house, to which a bamboo ladder led up from the floor, a construction representing the "great meeting hall" of the *seniang* in heaven (*Langit Balai Solai*), where the *seniang* are negotiated with during some rituals such as this. Holding offerings dedicated to the *seniang* in their hands while chanting, the shamans climbed up the ladder, ascending one step at first, then descending one step, then taking two steps up, and then backing one step down again, and so on, until they finally reached *Langit Balai Solai*. Approaching the *seniang* in this way, they acted according to an idiom of respectful "indirect" (*mengkelotes*) behavior generally employed in rituals and for interaction with persons of high status, as well as to symbolize and mark the fact that they were climbing all the way up to *Langit Balai Solai* (Ma Geneng, one of the *belian* performing in the ritual, mistakenly climbed all the way up right away, but was corrected by the other *belian*).

At this moment I will leave the *belian* chanting at the *balei* for a while, and go back in time to the era of the first human beings. Somewhat like the *belian* when they stepped up the ladder, I will take one step forward, just to take one back again in this chapter. It is like "slices in time laid on top of one another—a now overlaid by a back then" (Taussig 2009: 198) that I have tried to compose the chapter, so as to convey the ongoingness of the process of myth-making. There is, in a way, no finality in the process whereby myths are put to use, only beginnings, and new beginnings. Hence, I have chosen to organize the chapter around what could be described as variations on a theme: myths, ritual accounts, and excerpts from ritual chants that are in some sense telling us—more or less—the same thing, although in different forms, media and contexts.

By exploring the importance of the Luangan origin myths here, close to the end of the book instead of at its beginning, I have wanted to foreground a view of myths and rituals as "complex commentaries on one another," over a view of myth as an explanation of ritual (Gibson 2005: 28–29). As in Kapferer's understanding, with whom I share a view of myth and ritual as united, myths "do not constitute a closed circle of interpretational possibility but are continually open to new meaning and import derived in the contexts in which they are reiterated," an "openness" which he suggests is crucial for their continuing contextual relevance (1997: 62). Rather than representations, myths are better seen as actions, as "instruments through which dimensions of human actualities are enframed and grasped" (ibid.). They are, however, "less paradigms for rites than their residue, which, when separated from their ritual context, assume the character as stories, the tales that people tell" (Kapferer 1997: 82). From the Luangan point of view, it is crucially in and through ritual performance that the origin stories are thought to receive their world-molding potency and become myths proper (*tempuun*), instead of "just stories" (*kesah bene*).

The Myth of Human Origins

It is to the myth of origin of human beings, *Tempuun Senaring*, as told by Kakah Ramat to me and Kenneth during the first weeks of our fieldwork in 1996, that I now turn. Kakah Ramat made us a proposition when we first came to Sembulan that year: for the price of five *tulang antang* (Chinese ceramic jars, or alternatively, 50.000 Indonesian rupiah) he would tell us all the *tempuun*, all the origin myths, beginning with the *Tempuun* of heaven and earth, followed by that of human beings, and then the ones about the origins of houses, water, rice, pigs, chickens, water buffaloes, ritual paraphernalia, and so on (there is no exact number of existing *tempuun*, but a number of *tempuun* used more or less regularly in rituals and *belian* always seemed to be on the search for further stories). This was half the price a *belian* would have to pay for the stories, he told us, offering us a discount since we were not going to use these stories for ritual purposes, that is, present them as chants addressed to the spirits during major rituals. This was the beginning of a long

221

process of telling and re-telling *tempuun*. Kakah Ramat told the stories—which we recorded—sometimes in great detail and with great insight, sometimes hurriedly, giving us mere contours. Other shamans came along, and other versions of the stories were told and recorded. Toward the end of our fieldwork Kakah Ramat gave us another proposition: he offered to help us write down some of his stories in exchange for photocopies of them, photocopies that we would make while in town and that he would be able to store for his grandchildren, as he expressed it. At the same time he wanted to take the opportunity to obtain copies of the *tempuun* included in Lemanius' book as well—these copies probably more for his own use than for his grandchildren's.[1] I will return briefly to these as well as other versions later, but first we shall enter Kakah Ramat's story, following Sempirang Laang (Sempirang of the Forest) as he walked the earth alone.[2] I have chosen not to retell Kakah Ramat's story in full, which, like other *tempuun*, includes long lists of names and titles of persons and spirits and places (cf. Hopes et al. 1997: 4). My purpose is not to provide a detailed analysis of the myth as such, but to present origins, and especially the origin of the relationship between spirits and human beings, as a theme and scheme in *belian* curing. However, even though I have shortened the story in places, I have, out of respect for Kakah Ramat's intentions and skills as a storyteller, chosen to retell it in his own words (translated by me), and allowed it to take up a fair amount of space.

> Sempirang Laang [Sempirang of the Forest] lived upon the earth, beneath the sky. All alone. It thus occurred to him: I am miserable being alone, with no other human being to be with. Every day he went walking with his blowpipe, looking for game, gathering greens. The days went by, one day after another. Suddenly, one day when he was walking about at random he heard the sound of a song. A beautiful song. Weak at his knees, elbows weary, he walked toward the sound. Reaching the spot from where it came he saw a human being, risen from the earth up to the throat. He saw that it was a person, a woman. A beautiful woman, lovely like a flower. "Where did you come from," Sempirang Laang asked the woman. "I am Ayang Lolang Longet [Noble Beautiful Longet]," she replied. "My origin is from Tonoi [a spirit of the earth], from below the surface of the earth." "Well, if that is so I will take you with me," Sempirang Laang answered her. "No, you cannot do that yet," she answered him, "I have not grown fully yet. I just reach up to my neck. But you can come back again after

eight days and eight nights. When this time has passed you return to this same spot. Then I will have grown ready." "Okay, so be it," Sempirang Laang answered. He left, heading for the house where he lived. There he stayed, waiting. But eight days had not yet passed when on the seventh day he set out for the same spot again. When he reached it he saw that the woman had now grown fully. Only the soles of her feet were still stuck to the ground. "I will take you with me now," said Sempirang Laang. "No, not yet," answered the woman, "my feet still stick to the ground." "I will take you anyway," Sempirang Laang insisted. Sempirang Laang thus cut off her feet from the surface of the earth (that is why there is still a hollow under our feet until this day). As soon as they were cut she came loose from the ground. Thus her title changed and she became Ape Bungen Tana [Ape Flower of the Earth].

Sempirang Laang returned home, the woman followed him. For a long time she lived with him, living a married life in the afternoons, making children during the nights. One, two, three, four months thus passed. Then one day Sempirang Laang announced: "I will go out to hunt with my blowpipe, to search for game. You stay at home and watch over the rice that I have outdoors drying. If it starts to rain, please bring it in." "Okay," Ape Bungen Tana answered. Thus Sempirang Laang went off blowpipe-hunting in the faraway woods.

Now the story of Sempirang Laang sinks, that of Ape Bungen Tana floats. She stayed in the house. Suddenly there was the sound of rain. She went out to collect the rice that Sempirang Laang had left out to dry in the sun. And thus she got caught in the rain. The rice was already collected and brought inside the house when Ape Bungen Tana dissolved into water. She dissolved because she was struck by the rain. Her new title thus became Kemang Rano [The Faded Flower]. Left of her was only a uterine sack.

Now the story of Kemang Rano sinks. She returned to earth. The story of Sempirang Laang floats. He came home from his blowpipe hunt. Approaching the house he saw that the rice that he had left to dry had been taken inside. But there was no human being around. Calling out, shouting for Ape Bungen Tana, he received no answer. Then he saw the uterine sack. There was water inside it. Glittering and glimmering water. Looking at the water he was at a loss. At that time Perejadi [the Creator] spoke out. "Do not mistrust. Fetch bark, bark from an old tree. Make it into a *tewilung* bowl. After that you bring some sour fruits: *munte, puai, petien, lepusu, semele*. Mash the fruit until it becomes soft. Then squeeze the fruit and pour it into the *tewilung* bowl, mixing it with the glittering and glimmering water. When you have done so you shall store the bowl and put a lid on it."

223

Sempirang Laang hence made a *tewilung* bowl and filled it with the water. He brought *puai, petien, munte, lepusu, semele* and squeezed the fruit, mixing it with the glittering and glimmering water. He put a lid on the bowl and stored it. Eight days and nights so passed. Then he heard the cry of a baby from inside the bowl. Looking inside he saw a child, a girl. He washed and powdered her. He then cooked gruel and fed it to the child. The gruel was made from rice; rice cooked until it became soft and watery. That gruel he fed to the child. For one day, two days, three, four, five days, ten days, for months the child was fed with the gruel. She grew and grew. Until she could eat porridge. Growing bigger and bigger. Until she could eat rice. Until she knew how to sit up. Until she knew how to crawl. Until she could stand up. Growing stronger and stronger, until she ate rice and meat. Bigger and bigger she became. Learning to descend to the ground, to bathe in the river. Learning how to dress. To cook for herself, to gather greens. To pound rice, to fetch water. To weed the fields, to harvest the rice. Until she became a beautiful woman.

"Beautiful, do you know what beautiful means?" Kakah Ramat jokingly asked us at this point of the story. The beauty that Kakah Ramat, with an amused and somewhat enigmatic smile, revealing the pleasure he always seemed to find in telling these stories, asked us if we recognized here was not only the physical beauty of Tewilung Uyung which aroused Sempirang Laang's desire, a beauty that will entice him to transgress proper and correct behavior for a second time (the first being when he took Ape Bungen Tana before the time was in, resulting in her extinguishment later on). It was also, and perhaps above all, I believe, the beauty of life itself, and of the process of coming of age, as it unfolds in all its simultaneous simplicity and complexity. The fascination with this beauty is expressed also by the attention in the myth to the everyday activities which are associated with this process, which exemplifies Luangan life as it unfolds through activities such as growing plants and cooking food, weeding, fetching water, bathing in the river. Such activities always seem to form an essential element of Luangan myths and stories in which, for example, the way Luangans enter a house, hanging up their jungle knives before sitting down, offering tobacco and betel quid ingredients before uttering greetings (see Howell 1989: 38 for similar conduct among the Chewong), is repeatedly pronounced and always caused amusement among members of the audience who recognized themselves through these acts. If interpreted in this way, Tewilung Uyung's beauty not only derives from her physical appearance, but also from the activities that define her as a fully grown human being, activities that make her recognizable as a fellow Luangan and make the myth into an account of what delineates human beings and human life conditions.

> Sempirang Laang now saw that the child had grown up. At this time he began to think of marrying her. But the child did not agree to his wishes. Sempirang Laang told her to search his head for lice. "From having wanted to do so, I do not want to any more," she answered. At that time her father used force attempting to make her do so. The child became angry. She hit him with the lice comb on his head. The blood flowed from where she had hit him with the comb on his forehead. "Well, if you do not agree there is nothing else for me to do than to leave for the village of *alang-alang* grasses at the edge of the earth and the sky," he told her. "I will leave some clothes with you, however: a shirt, a pair of trousers, a ring and a hat. If someone who wants to marry you comes along you shall give him these clothes and things of mine. If they suit him you shall marry him, he will be able to feed you. If not, you shall not do so, he cannot feed you." "Yes," the girl called Tewilung Uyung answered him.

As the reader might guess, after some time (in this version eight months, in some other versions of the myth, eight years) her father came back in disguise, asking for his daughter's hand. And as the clothes left by him fit him perfectly, she kept her promise and agreed to marry him.

> Thus the two of them got married. Living a married life during the day, making children during the night. One month, two, three, four, five months thus passed. At that time the woman, Tewilung Uyung, began to have cravings. She wanted to eat sour fruits: *munte, lepusu, semele, puai, petien.*[3] Before that her husband had not yet asked her to search his head for lice. But now that she already had cravings he asked her to do so. And so she did. She searched his head on the one side, and on the other side. And what did she see? She saw a scar.[4] "Oh, well indeed," she thought, "this is my father, the same one that I used to have before. But this has already gone too far. Now that I already have these cravings there is nothing else to do." Tewilung Uyung was already with child. Pregnant she was like the sugar palm in bloom on the hill.
>
> Nine months and ten days thus passed. Then a child was born. But the child had no arms and legs. It was round like a cucumber. With just the suggestion of a face. After that Tewilung Uyung soon became pregnant

again. And another child was born. Without legs this time, just with arms, eyes, ears, nose and mouth. The child grew a little and Tewilung Uyung became pregnant once more. Again a child was born. This time with legs, but without arms. As the child had become a little bigger Tewilung Uyung became pregnant again. And another child was born. With legs, but just one arm. That child grew and Tewilung became pregnant again. A child was born once more, a child with perfect arms and legs, but without eyes.

Thus it continued, one child after another being born, all malformed. One hundred and sixty children in all, Kakah Ramat rounds up, after giving quite a number of additional examples of such defective children.

> Well, there were enough of those children. The last ones were Punen and Melesia. Regarding some of the other ones: one had a bad temper and hit, smacked, kicked, struck, stuck, and cut the others. Another was a lecher who did not know the difference between his own kin and others'.

The malformations, the misbehavior, the excess of children: these were children of incest (*sahu sumbang*). The offspring of father and daughter, of Sempirang Laang's deceit (and, of course, the circumstances: there was not, after all, anyone else around for him to marry), they were bound to bring their parents misfortune. In some other versions of the origin story a *belian* ritual was called for at this moment, one of "whisking and waving" (*ngaper ngompas*), of "undoing and redoing" (*pejiak pejiau*), as Lemanius stated it in his version of the myth, aimed to rectify what went wrong. In Kakah Ramat's story there is just Perejadi intervening, sending down Silu Urai, Junjung Ayus Ngotus ("Silu the Originator," "Junjung Ayus the Instructor"). This does not necessarily exclude a *belian* ritual, though; I have heard Kakah Ramat tell the story with the ritual included, and I guess this element (the ritual) might just be so self-evident so as not to require mentioning (Kakah Ramat's style of telling a story was at times highly economical, consisting of one-word sentences).[5]

> Because of all this there was a confrontation. These children meant bad luck. Perejadi who looked down from the sky saw Sempirang Laang's and Tewilung Uyung's distress. He sent down Silu Urai and Junjung Ayus Ngotus. Silu Urai and Junjung Ayus so spoke: That child which is round, with no arms and legs, no eyes and ears, he shall be Tetung Galeng Bulan Langai. That child with no legs, but with eyes and ears and arms only shall be Tatau Galeng Gampai. The child with no arms, but legs, eyes and

ears shall be Pudong Seniang Pongong. The child with ears, eyes, and legs but only one arm shall be Seniang Sungkor. The child with arms and legs but no eyes shall be Seniang Posa. The child with arms and legs but only one eye shall be Seniang Piset. Make all these children ascend to heaven, to *Langit Balai Solai* [the Great Meeting Hall of the Heaven]. They shall become *seniang pali* and oversee the *pali* [taboos] of people who commit incest. They shall oversee the *pali* of people who commit theft and deceit. They shall oversee the *pali* of people who do not respect their in-laws. They shall oversee the *pali* of fires lighted in the wrong locations, of work inappropriately started in between. Of cane and rattan, house and forest. Of crops bent upside down.

And so it went on, the children becoming transformed into the different *seniang*, Kakah Ramat here describing, one by one, the locations and specific responsibilities of each of them. Because of the highly repetitious form of the presentation, I have here only included those that were mentioned first, the *seniang pali*, who together with the *seniang besarah,* who oversee *adat* (customary law) and *adat* negotiations, reside in the Great Meeting Hall of the Sky.

These *seniang* resemble the *petara* (*betara*), or so-called gods of the Iban, and like them form an example of "departmental deities" (Metcalf 1989: 69–71) common in some, but not all, Borneo societies. As such they perform, as a collectivity, the variety of roles attributed to a single God in some societies, and each acts within a fairly circumscribed sphere of influence. There is a great number of *seniang*, each of whom represents the "custodian" (*pengitung*) of some specific category of fundamental social or natural conditions, regulating sexual and social interaction and associated rules and taboos, personal fortune, fate, the solar, lunar, and other astral cycles, various natural cycles including the yearly seasons, the irregular fruiting of fruit trees, the seasonal occurrence of wild honey, and so on. These are conditions which are all in one way or another essential to Luangan subsistence, social life or personal well-being, and the sheer enumeration of the *seniang* represents powerful cosmological knowledge and gives a broad picture of what kind of things matter in Luangan lives. In a sense, the *seniang* are the ultimate powers in the universe, regulating the cosmos, nature, society, and human life.

Exerting a form of cosmic or global influence equally available to everyone and people in different localities, the *seniang* are indeed more god-like than most Luangan spirits, which typically exert a more or less localized influence. Being mostly celestial—with a few earth dwelling exceptions—and mainly contacted in major community rituals, and typically only as a last resort, they are also somewhat distant beings, who do not engage in direct personal interaction with people.[6] They are to some extent seen as "incarnations of morality" (Sillander 2004: 193), and unlike most spirits they do not occasionally succumb to such behavior as soul theft. Indicating their special status and aloofness, they notably accept only cooked food offerings. Nevertheless, the *seniang* are, as we shall see later, often interacted with in rituals in a rather informal and casual manner, and the predominantly benevolent influence over nature and people that they either may or may not exercise ultimately reflects human action and efforts to influence them, rather than inherent goodwill.[7]

But there were still plenty of children. So many that Sempirang Laang and Tewilung Uyung could not feed them all. Because of that Sempirang Laang went off to Paku Radek Puak Katar. There he found some *ramai bayan* mushrooms. Eight tree trunks covered. He gathered the mushrooms. One whole *temuyan* basket full. He took them with him and returned home. At home again he cooked the mushrooms. One large wok full. When they were cooked he distributed them to the children. They all ate, except for Punen and Melesia. And all the children became poisoned. But even if they were poisoned they did not die. Every one of the older children thus became poisoned.

Suddenly one child ran off and climbed a *putang* [*Shorea* sp.] tree. As he did so, he left a request. "Listen Punen, little sister. Here I Gerung become *naiyu*. Small rituals should be devoted to me. Grand rituals should be devoted to me as well. Some other day, some other night, when you cook the first sticky rice for a *kerewaiyu* [a harvest ritual for the first rice], when you cook the first rice for a harvest ritual, when you peel the ripening fruits, when you collect the honey amassing, then you shall give some to me, then you shall share it with me as well." "Okay," Punen, the little sister answered. And so Gerung ran off in the direction of the Door of the Skies, and became Naiyu Senkelewang Tatau, whose task it is to keep the door of the heavens clean. Another child ran off as well. A child named Bontik. He rushed up the *putang* tree. As he did so he also left a request. "Listen Punen, little sister. Here I, Bontik, become *timang*. Small rituals should be devoted to me. Grand rituals should be devoted to me as well. Some other day, some other night, when you cook the first sticky rice for a *kerewayu*, when you cook the first rice for a harvest ritual, when you peel the ripening fruits, when you collect the honey amassing, then you shall give some to me, then you shall share it with me as well."

So it continued, the children running off to different places and becoming *wok, tentuwaja, juata, tonoi*, as well as snakes, fish, mouse deer, wild boar, rhinos, all of them using the same words, making Punen promise to share her crop with them during rituals in the future.

> Of the children there were some who became animals. Others became *wok, bongai, bansi, buta, tontin*. Left were only Punen, the youngest sister, and Melesia. It is from Punen that the human beings trace their descent. Eight layers, eight generations leading back to Tanjung Ruang [a famous mythical ancestral village]. Eight layers, eight generations leading to Itak Ngurai, Kakah Ngurai ["Grandmother Originator," "Grandfather Originator"]. Leading to Ine Memea, Uma Mumayur ["Mother the Feeder," "Father the Provider"]. Ine Memea, Uma Mumayur originated us who come behind. Such is the story which leads here. Until us mankind of today, whose origin is from Punen, from Melesia.

Punen, mother of mankind, Melesia, mostly just figuring as an extension (*penyeleloi*) of Punen. Some people claimed that the meaning of Melesia (probably formed from *belesia*, "human being," as in the standard parallel expression *Punen senaring, tana belesia*, "Punen human being, land of human being") is the same as for "Malesia" (Malaysia), others that it simply means *manusia*, which is Indonesian for human being. With whom Punen begat her children is not clear either (was there, for example, another incestuous union here?). All this does not really seem to matter, however. Punen, Punen Senaring, *is* human being (*senaring* being the word for human being in the local language). It was with Punen that mankind as we know it today came into being. And Punen is of one origin, of one womb (*erai butung*), with various spirits, and some wild animals. She is their younger sister (*ani*). As we shall see shortly, *this*—the kinship, or more precisely, siblingship—does matter.[8] What also matters, however, is incest, described by Bloch (1971: 53) as "the conceptual antithesis of kinship," which defines, by way of opposition, the tradition-regulated field of productive and responsible moral relations of consanguinity and affinity.

Naiyu, timang, wok, bongai, tentuwaja, juata, tonoi: these are, together with their older siblings, the *seniang*, the most commonly invoked Luangan categories of spirits, and mention of them can metonymically be taken to stand for the rest.[9] Whether acting as guardian spirits or malevolent spirits, they all, as we have seen in the cases presented in this book, live in a reciprocal but highly ambiguous relationship with human beings. Inhabiting various parts of the Luangan environment they pervade the Luangan cosmos and circumscribe the existence of human beings. The spirits, as described in the myth of human origins, are a constitutive part of the environment inhabited by the Luangans and can be seen to represent both the limits and the potential of the predicament of human existence.

As among the Achuar Indians described by Philippe Descola (1994: 93), there is "a continuum between human beings and nature's beings" in the Luangan cosmography. As the origin myth tells us humans and non-humans share a common origin and, as Luangan ritual practice has shown us, the character of their relations is essentially social. Spirits (and animals, which, however, play a somewhat lesser role in Luangan myth and especially ritual practice than among many people with a similar "animistic" ontology) are like human beings, they are the siblings of human beings, demanding food and respect from their brothers and sisters (like close relatives do) and they are considered to have similar desires, habits and ways of life as human beings. It is this shared "subjecthood," which endows them with social characteristics, that forms the basis of what "siblingship" or "a common origin" signifies for Luangans. "The capacity to be with others, share a place with them, and responsively engage with them," which is what Bird-David (2006: 43), in her study of what she calls the "animistic epistemology" of the Nayaka foragers of South India, has described as "the critical attribute of the local sense of 'personhood,' ... extended to the non-human, the animate and the inanimate," is central for the Luangans' sense of "personhood" as well (blood-relatedness and descent being of little concern in defining Luangan kinship, not to mention "luanganness"). Through socialization of the natural environment, the Luangans—like other peoples with a similar "animistic" understanding of the world, as described by various scholars who have been revisiting the concept lately—open themselves to both the "mutualities" and "pluralities" that are in the world, "living jointly with the animated," rather than focusing on individual selves (Bird-David 2006: 44–45; cf. Descola 1992, 1994; Ingold 2000; Viveiros de Castro 1998, 2004).

At the same time as the Luangan spirits are fundamentally similar to human beings they are, however, as we have seen, also different from human beings. They tend to look more or less different and they have some qualities which human beings lack. Above all, they are what Luangans refer to as *gaib*, invisible, and they are, as I have pointed out on several occasions before, always to some extent evasive, enigmatic, and unpredictable. The Luangan spirits are needed and called for in times of sickness and adversity. They are negotiators and mediators, helping the *belian* with the curing, protecting human beings. But they are also the party negotiated with, the ones hurting people, causing them illness and punishing them for their wrong-doings. Spirits are summoned, called for, yet they are wanted at a distance, away from human being. This doubleness in approach reflects not only a role differentiation, dividing spirits into benevolent and malevolent ones (most spirits may, as said before, appear in both guises), but the fundamentally equivocal nature of spirit beings and their relations with human beings. In this respect they resemble the Wana spirits who are said to be "people like us here, but not" (Atkinson 1989: 37).

In a sense spirits are deficient human beings. Like the *bas* of the Chewong of peninsular Malaysia (Howell 1989: 104), they are "humans manqués, or humans gone wrong." As the *Tempuun Senaring* tells us, they are the outcome of a series of wrong-doings (Sempirang Laang taking Ape Bungen Tana before it is time, the incestuous union between father and daughter, the poisoning).[10] But this is not the whole story. Following the typical pattern of *pejiak pejiau*, there is also Perejadi, or Silu Ngintai and Ayus Ngokoi, interfering, and there is, in some versions of the story, a *belian* ritual turning things around. Sempirang Laang's and Tewilung Uyung's children are the children of incest—malformed, misbehaving, too numerous to rear—but upon ascending to the sky, or by climbing up the *putang* tree—acts which quite concretely symbolize their differentiation and dissociation from humankind—they become something else as well. Some of them become *seniang*: distant guardians over law and nature who have, if people fulfill their obligations toward them, the capacity to provide humans with a good life (*bolum buen*), a life in which there is, as it is often expressed in ritual contexts, "no sickness, plenty of rice, bountiful game, where you live happily, patients recover quickly, illnesses heal, dreams are auspicious, omens favorable" (*roten awe, mahan pare, mahan esa, bolum seneng, dongo golek, roten toke, upi buen, baya nado*). Others, in their turn, become *naiyu, timang, wok, bongai*: spirits who inhabit the village and forest environments of people and who are frequently called on for assistance or protection, but who also often turn malevolent, and thus should be kept at a certain distance, or in place, so to speak. Failing to become proper humans, the spirits thus become beings of a different kind: beings that ultimately evade attempts at control or seizure, but who at the same time retain an important connection to human beings, through which what is beyond human control can be negotiated. To be dependent on someone who is like, yet unlike, then, becomes an inescapable dilemma for human beings.

"Some other day, some other night, when you cook the first sticky rice for a *kerewaiyu*, when you cook the first rice for a harvest ritual, when you peel the ripening fruits, when you collect the amassing honey, then you shall give some to me, then you shall share it with me as well." This is the essence of kinship or relatedness: continuity, sharing, demands, dependency (an "if not …" can be read between the lines here) and responsibility, the dependency of younger siblings towards older siblings, of successors towards antecedents. This is also an important aspect of what origin stories are about. The word *tempuun* is derived from the word *puun*, meaning "tree trunk," "foundation," or "to own," a common metaphor in Austronesia for the relationship of dependency between successors and antecedents (see, for example, Fox 1996: 6–7). In a sense, the performance of origin stories creates and re-creates the foundation for the relationship between human beings and spirits, and the conditions for negotiation between them. Even when not spelled out, when not told or sung, but just alluded to, the idea of a common origin constitutes an obligation, and a possibility.

"Small rituals should be devoted to me, grand rituals should be devoted to me as well." This is what the spirits ask for from their younger siblings: rituals (the term used for ritual here is *awing*, a word which, as explained earlier, designates work in general, such as rice field work, but also "ritual work" such as a *belian* or a *gombok*). It is through rituals that the obligations of a common origin are fulfilled, and the possibilities created. It is through ritual that reciprocity is sustained, and the relatedness realized. As Bird-David (1999: 73) has observed for the relationship between the Nayaka and local *devaru* (superhuman beings): "*As and when* and *because* they engage in and maintain relationships with other beings, they constitute them as kinds of person: they make them 'relatives' by sharing with them and thus make them persons." And further: "devaru are relatives in the literal sense of being 'that or whom one interrelates with' (not in the reduced modern English sense of '*humans* connected with others by blood or affinity')."

Relating with Spirits

It is, as already mentioned, only in *nalin taun* rituals that the origin myth of heaven and the earth, *Tempuun Langit Tana*, along with that of human beings, *Tempuun Senaring*, may be chanted in full (whereas other *tempuun*, especially those of sacrificial animals and ritual paraphernalia, are chanted in, and are obligatory parts of, *buntang* and *gombok* rituals as well).[11] The *nalin taun* works to achieve its ends by inviting and presenting offerings to the *seniang* (something which, like the performance of the origin stories of heaven and the earth and human beings, may not be done during any other, lesser-ranking ritual).[12] As the origin myth reminds us, the *seniang* are the "guardians" (*pengitung*) of nature, meaning that it is they who determine whether and when good harvests will be obtained. Their inclinations in this respect can be influenced, however. In fact, human action is considered to be ultimately responsible for the condition of this relationship, and thus for conditions in nature. Hence, improper social conduct, which entails the transgression of rules and prohibitions whose observance is controlled by the *seniang*—and particularly illicit sexual relations (*sumbang*)—is usually identified as the cause of unfavorable natural conditions, whereas the remedy for such conditions, and the only measure sufficient to secure the benevolence of the *seniang*, is the performance of a *nalin taun* (or, at least, the promise of one, for example in the form of a *ngeraya*).

The *nalin taun* is, we should observe, a ritual attributed with special cosmological significance. Much more than expressing and invoking important aspects of Luangan cosmology, this ritual, on account of inviting and gathering all the *seniang*, and involving the enactment of *Tempuun Langit Tana* and *Tempuun Senaring*—and most other *tempuun* as well—recreates, as it were, the cosmos itself, and man's position in it. Conjuring the origins of the world and of elements in it essential to human existence, and renegotiating the (disturbed) relationship of human beings with spirits, the *nalin taun* revives an all-encompassing ontological order and man's moral commitment to it. Hence, this ritual, in an important sense, replicates and reinforces the myth. It works to define humanity and man's relation to the world—a vital aspect of which is the requirement of reciprocity associated with his relations to his spirit siblings.

Like the Sinhalese Suniyama rite described by Kapferer (1997: 177), the *nalin taun* is, in a sense, always "a first performance," which contains an "originating force," or "a capacity to bring forth."

> Reconfigured into the structure of rite, the myths become elements in a process of human (re)formation which unfolds the complexity of human sociality and the ways human beings must constantly create and recreate themselves and the orders of their worlds. (Kapferer 1997: 82)

Whereas the *nalin taun* to an important degree serves to effect "human (re)formation" through performance of the *tempuun*, and by presenting the numerous offerings that go with it, a *ngeraya* works indirectly, through allusion, one might say, invoking the promise of a *nalin taun*. Like the promise of *buntang* (see chapter 4), the promise of a *nalin taun* works as an attempt to influence the future. However, as is demonstrated in a dialogue performed between the human participants and the *seniang* during the *ngeraya* ritual held in Jelmu Sibak in September 1996, this is a promise that will be fulfilled only if the *seniang* keep their part of the deal. In initiating the negotiation, it is the humans who set its terms.

Taking a step back again to the *ngeraya* with which I initiated this chapter, we shall see how the *belian*—after having physically and verbally presented their offerings to the *seniang* as they climbed up the ladder—engage in a verbal negotiation and bartering with them. First naming and thus calling a great number of *seniang* from their various celestial locations, one of the *belian* then takes the role of a representative of the *seniang*, embodying him and speaking in his voice, and a negotiation is performed between him and the other *belian*, in which the latter state the people's requests and wishes. Some members of the audience are drawn into the negotiation as well, inserting claims, emphasizing and repeating those of the *belian*. Confirming that the *seniang* understands the requests, the *belian* embodying their representative inserts a "yes" (*oi*) every once in a while. It is well after midnight as we now enter the scene again and the *belian* are sitting on the floor under the *balei* in the rafters. The tone of the conversation is casual, reminiscent of everyday conversations between people as they plan how to go ahead with some work task, presenting requests (*pengake*) to each other:

"What we ask for is hot days," one of the *belian* declares.

"Oh?"

"We ask for ripening fruit, honey amassing, swarming fish, wild boar traveling in flocks," another *belian* inserts.

"*Oi,*" the *seniang* answers.

"Rice with clean seeds, sticky rice with clean kernels," the female ritual assistant continues.

"We ask for satisfaction and contentment," the first *belian* goes on.

"Health and safety," another *belian* adds.

"That widowers meet wives," someone in the audience inserts.

"*Oi!*"

"That women meet husbands."

"That's how it is. This is what we pay, and what we ask to happen from this day onwards," one of the *belian* continues. "This is what we offer, these are our requests. So that we can grow rice and obtain harvests. Rice with clean seeds, sticky rice with clean kernels."

"*Oi!*"

"We ask for refreshing coolness and renewed prosperity," the *belian* adds.

"So, if we will get that, we will have news to bring [i.e., of rituals that are promised to be implemented]. We are used to this, there is no way we would fail to announce news [i.e., of rituals]. As we people down here say: we follow [i.e., respond to] what withers. But if there is nothing that withers [i.e., the desired developments do not transpire], then you cannot expect that. If the grass doesn't wither, the earth doesn't crack [because of becoming parched], then this doesn't apply to us. It doesn't apply."

"Oh?"

"But enough of what would happen if it wouldn't apply. We ask that you protect and bless us."

"We ask for heat so that we can burn, so that we can make yearly swiddens. That we will be healthy and safe, do not suffer from headaches."

"That wild boars travel in flocks, fish swarm, honey amasses in heaps. This is it, this is what we ask for."

"Ok. So that's how it is!" the *seniang* replies. "Your requests are received! All your gifts are received! So they are received, and I will forward them to the master of ours. I will bring all of them along. And indeed

235

there's no end to it, there's not little that we have received, there's no end to our rewards. But be that as it may, you will have to wait until later. It is only later that you will obtain. If then, for example, the weather will become hot, and the felled tree trunks will all be burnt, that's thanks to us. If, for example, your honey will amass in heaps, that's thanks to us. If your fruits will ripen, it's thanks to us. This is the way it is. But what are the conditions under which this will apply? If this will not come true, is it you or us who are in debt? What is right, what is wrong?"

"If it does not come true, we do not owe you anything!" one of the *belian* declares.

"Oh, so that's how it is?!" the *seniang* replies, slightly surprised.

"It is you who owe us!" the *belian* claims.

"Oh, we are the ones in debt, so that's how it is!" the *seniang* affirms.

"Yes, you are the ones in debt."

"So, that's how it is!"

Thus it goes on, continuing along the same lines. The *seniang* reminds the people that they should keep to their side of the deal by offering water buffalo sacrifices and valued goods, and the *belian* and other members of the audience remind the *seniang* that more yet will be offered during the second day of the *ngeraya*. The shamans repeat the people's requests at length, in more or less the same formulaic expressions, stating, one by one, their visions of a good life, somewhat as if the very enunciation of them—and the received affirmation of the *seniang*—would already go halfway into bringing them into existence.

By embodying a representative of the *seniang*, the *belian* imposes a human perspective on them. The *seniang* are made to see—indeed somewhat tricked into seeing—the human point of view and to act accordingly as they are bound up in the negotiation. By thus engaging the *seniang* in dialogue the people of Jelmu Sibak, through their *belian* emissaries, act on the natural forces and conditions that are controlled by the *seniang* (e.g., the weather, luck, fate, etc., which are all regulated by particular *seniang*). It is most essentially through the promise of payment that the *belian* seek to persuade the *seniang* to provide what is included in a good life. Of importance in this context is not only the pledge of a possible future ritual but also the ritual performed and the offerings presented at this stage. Even though these offerings are not as extensive as those involved in the promised *nalin taun*, they are, together with the other aspects of ritual work, expected, or at least intended, to contribute to persuade the spirits to start acting as desired, by way of a balanced reciprocity, but also by sharing with them. To relate with spirits, to maintain relations with them (and especially the *seniang*), is an important incentive of the *ngeraya* in its own right, as of all *belian* rituals (and also one reason why rituals are so frequent among central Luangans, I think). By inviting them to join the people in eating the food served during the *ngeraya*, the *seniang* are drawn into a social event which manifests and reestablishes their relatedness with people (at the same time the opportunity is taken to attempt to please, coax, and manipulate them into doing what they are asked for). Thus the *ngeraya,* as a prelude, not only anticipates a certain course of events, but also contributes to create the prerequisites for it.

When the spirits in the myth of origin ask for rituals from their younger siblings, they ask for engagement and a share of their crops, which is precisely what they get in the *ngeraya*, not the least through the promise of further engagement that it constitutes. The dialogue between the *seniang* and the people points to how the "different points of view" from which spirits and humans "apprehend reality" (Viveiros de Castro 1998: 469) are made compatible through a process of listening to each voice from the perspective of the other (Bakhtin 1986). A "responsive understanding" (Bakhtin 1986: 69) is somewhat forced upon the *seniang* through the process of personification. The standardized formulations through which the people express their wishes as well as their insistence on how they are used to this, as they express it in the dialogue— how ritual is traditionally incorporated—also serves to oblige the *seniang* to respond actively to their requests. At the same time the dialogue remains unfinished and open-ended in the sense that it points beyond itself; promises will be fulfilled only in the future, both those of the people, and those of the *seniang*, as the representative of the *seniang* points out. Both parties are dependent on continued interaction to receive what they want. The promise thus constitutes what Bird-David, in discussing Nayaka trances and divination, has called "an enduring commitment to continue relating," or "a *prospective* commitment to continuing sharing and living together" (2004: 336, original italics) (as opposed to a retrospective search for causes).

How one practically should best go about achieving this is, as so often in dealings with spirits, a complex matter. The incessant rains in

September 1996 did not stop in time for everyone to be able to burn their fields, and for many people this meant that they did not obtain a rice harvest that year. The following year was even worse, with severe drought and forest fires, leading to a scarcity of rice, and even more of sticky rice—which is essential as an offering to spirits in ritual and could not be widely bought at downriver markets—resulting in an almost complete lack of larger rituals in many central Luangan villages in the swidden year of 1997–1998. In Sembulan it was whispered that someone in Jelmu Sibak had secretly wished for rain during the *ngeraya*, which was why it kept on raining. The quarrel between the *kepala adat* and his brother, and the discontent many people felt about the *kepala adat*'s position, were factors that were indirectly pointed to as disturbing the process. Elizabeth Coville (1989: 121) makes a similar observation for the Toraja of Sulawesi who also attribute poor yields to lack of agreement and unanimity in the village.

None of this made the *ngeraya* as such superfluous or ineffective in their view; immediate return is not, as the *seniang* notes in the dialogue, necessarily an expected result of ritual; individual rituals are not considered isolates but rather part of an ongoing negotiation between spirits and people. It should also be noted that the rivalry between Jelmu Sibak and Sembulan concerning Sembulan's lack of village autonomy might have made the people of Sembulan prone to blame the inhabitants of Jelmu Sibak for the lack of success (this rivalry was probably also one of the reasons that they did not participate in the *ngeraya* in the first place). In 2007, when Kenneth and I revisited Jelmu Sibak after a nine year-long break, another *ngeraya* ritual was under way, initiated by the same *kepala adat*, still in position, although now in quite poor health. The *nalin taun* promised in 1996 had not (yet) been implemented. The following year, 2008, turned out to be a very good agricultural year, with bountiful crops, and there was something of a *nalin taun* boom going on in the area, with rituals arranged in at least two of the nine villages in the district. There was talk about arranging one in Jelmu Sibak at this time as well but to my knowledge this has not yet been implemented (by this time the *kepala adat* had passed away).

The frequency of *nalin taun* rituals varies greatly between villages and different Luangan sub-groups, as does their length. Among Bentians and Teweh River Luangans they usually last sixteen or twenty-four days, whereas among the Benuaq they commonly last up to three months. As the largest ritual performed by the Luangans, the *nalin taun* requires huge material resources (which is one reason why it is seen as the only ritual where it is possible to "call down," *pedolui*, the *seniang*). These include food for all attendants, who include visitors from other villages, sometimes entire communities that are formally invited to participate and expected to reciprocate by inviting the village back to take part in a similar ritual at some point in the future, sacrifices of a large number of pigs, chicken, and one or preferably several water buffaloes, and wages for ritual experts as well as other people who help out. Besides these requirements, there is also a great demand for manpower to construct all the ritual decorations needed, including several *balei* (ritual shrines and plat-forms) built for different categories of spirits, and the construction of a *blontang*, a carved ironwood pole to which the water buffaloes are tied when killed, which afterwards remains as a monument commemorating the event.

Seen in this light, arranging a *ngeraya* is a much easier way to influence the *seniang*, and through them the natural conditions reg-ulated by them, than arranging a full-scale *nalin taun*. A *nalin taun* promised in a *ngeraya* can be postponed to some indeterminate point in the future—although a very good harvest is quite compelling in putting plans into practice, especially if it is followed by negative developments which might then be interpreted as expressing the discontentment of the *seniang*. In Jelmu Sibak the *kepala adat* who initiated the *ngeraya* rituals in 1996 and 2007 seemed, in fact, to favor this form of ritual over other forms of *belian* rituals (which he, as a Christian, did not regularly arrange). While involving relatively modest costs and only a short interruption of daily affairs and work, the *ngeraya*, as a community ritual, nevertheless worked to boost his authority and to integrate villagers, and it had the additional advan-tage of dealing with natural forces and godlike beings which from the point of view of his Christian identity made it somewhat less compromising than some other rituals. In general he condemned the performance of *belian* rituals and tried to prevent or at least influ-ence their scope (note that it was he who tried to stop people from arranging an extended death ritual with reference to government regulations as described in chapter 1). If the decision were left to him, he would likely have been quite happy never to implement the *nalin taun*, letting the *ngeraya* do the trick, so to speak.

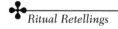

The *nalin taun*, which is mainly performed among East Kalimantan Luangans (the only exception probably being adjacent Teweh River Luangans), is a relatively new form of ritual among the central Luangans. It spread to the area largely as a result of tributary contacts with the Sultanate of Kutai, whose sphere of influence roughly extended to the present-day border between East and Central Kalimantan. Albeit indigenous, apparently originating with Benuaq Dayaks, the ritual was first performed by Dayaks in the downriver capital (Tenggarong) of the Kutai Sultanate during annual royal festivities (Erau) that were attended by central Luangan leaders who sought honorific titles from the Sultan, and it was as a result of influence from these visits that the ritual became adopted as a village ritual in upriver communities (see Sillander 2006). The *nalin taun* was introduced in the central Luangan area in the second half of the nineteenth century, at the time of settlement in nucleated villages and the development of communal leadership, both processes which were promoted by the ritual. It was the first local community ritual, arranged on the initiative of local leaders, who, like the Sultan, aspired to integrate the local population in villages (Sillander 2006: 319–320).[13] It was with motives comparable to those that the *kepala adat* initiated the *ngeraya* in Jelmu Sibak in 1996, even if the ritual served quite different purposes for most of its participants. For him the ritual principally served to legitimize his own authority and to integrate villagers. He was more than willing to leave the interaction with spirits in the hands of the *belian* and other ritual participants (tellingly, he only sporadically participated in the ritual, showing up at meals and during the bathing performed at its conclusion). For him the negotiation with the *seniang*, as well as the other activities of the *ngeraya*, was more a matter of formulating and constituting a collective identity than reformulating spirit relations.

Recalling Origins

Karena ka taun bayuh	Because you in past years
bulan alem	in foregone months
jaren panei erai lei	shared the same forefathers, the same foremothers
ika nyiwung erai butung	you originate from one womb
erai suut karung ipu	one bag of *ipu* bark

erai lombang kalung anyang	one box of ignition stones, one necklace[14]
tau butung ka lau uyat ka mole	your stomach might be hungry, your sinews tired
ye iro deo okan penyewaka	that's why there is plenty of food offerings
pengahan ka uli doyeng ehe	rewards to make you go back this evening

—Excerpt from a *belian sentiu* chant by Mancan

Origin myths, when performed during larger life rituals (*buntang, nalin taun*), are usually chanted by two or more *belian* who sit by the *longan*, a roughly two-meters tall ritual structure which serves as a focal point of the ritual activities. The chants are performed to the accompaniment of a slow-paced rhythm of drums which the *belian* beat while holding them in their laps, the leading *belian* first singing a line, which is then repeated by the other *belian* (usually at least two or three), the initiator joining in again halfway through the sentence. In comparison with narrated myths, the *tempuun* sung during rituals are chanted in a stylized and formal mode, and marked to a much higher degree by poetic attributes such as rhyme and parallelism, basic characteristics of Luangan ritual chanting. Since Kakah Ramat, in the version of the myth of mankind recounted above, was telling me and Kenneth the myth in a non-ritual setting, and since he primarily wanted to convey a story, he switched to "the language of everyday conversation," even though his "frame of reference" was still "the stylized mode," to deploy concepts used by Amin Sweeney (1987: 81) in analyzing Malay storytelling.[15] Chanting a *tempuun* is not something that can be done unpremeditatedly. It demands a ritual setting including decorations and offerings. Some ritual experts even insisted on burning incense and receiving token payments when presenting the myths in a narrative form. Furthermore, the chanting of one of the longer *tempuun* can already last over several days (with breaks for other programs in between), and the language of the *tempuun* is fairly archaic, both factors which, together with the style of chanting, render it difficult to catch the contents of chanted *tempuun* by just listening to them. However, this is something people seldom actively do anyway (save for *belian* novices who try to learn the chants), the *belian* often being left to themselves in the house during the phase of the rituals when the *tempuun* are chanted. The primary audience of ritually chanted *tempuun* consists of spirits.

241

When it comes to *Tempuun Langit Tana* and *Tempuun Senaring*, these myths are so seldom performed in ritual that it is mainly from narratives, rather than songs, that most people have gained access to their contents. Not many *belian* are able to perform these *tempuun* in ritual either; only a few senior *belian* can "lead" (*tonar*), the chants, while most other *belian* just know how to "follow" (*nuing*) these *belian*.[16] *Tempuun Senaring* is a popular myth though, and most people have heard it told as a narrative dozens of times and are able to retell it themselves, even if perhaps not with the amount of detail as in Kakah Ramat's version (variation between versions is also considerable; even Kakah Ramat told the myth in a number of different ways on different occasions, often being influenced by other versions he had recently heard).

However, even though *Tempuun Senaring* and *nalin taun* rituals are rarely performed, the theme of a common origin of spirits and human beings is important and figures frequently in other rituals and the chants included in them. Allusions to the myth of human creation were often made during "ordinary" *belian* rituals that were staged to cure individual patients and directed to "lesser" spirits than the *seniang*, such as *wok, bongai, naiyu, timang*, etc., which are called during almost every *belian* ritual. One such example is a *belian sentiu* chant that was performed by the *belian* Ma Sarakang when he was curing his chronically ill wife Nen Pare (cf. chapter 2). The chant was performed at the point in the curing process when offerings and respect were presented by the patient (*besemah be dongo*), an activity aimed to establish contact—as a prelude to further curing—with the spirits suspected of having made the patient ill. Holding a tray containing offerings (*okan penyewaka*) dedicated to these spirits in his hands, Ma Sarakang first summoned the spirits, calling them by name and place, then went on to describe the offerings, including a bowl filled with uncooked rice decorated with flowers, plaited coconut leaves, an egg, a betel nut, a beeswax candle, and a coin, all placed on a plate which was also filled with rice—a standard offering in *belian* rituals. Having done so he then pleaded to the spirits to receive the offerings and leave, reminding them of their shared origin with people:

toyak tuha bukun okan	these are the words the elders presented you
lingan kanen	
petulek lele uli	for all of you to return

petungkeng bala tubak	for the bad to be sent away
bote teriti lewi	don't try to make it worse
tolang sensei mon dasei	the bamboo rises above the floor
ala oon taun bayuh?	what did the olden days bring with them?
erai susur sensuren	it comes down to one origin
erai rarak derantai	one row lined up[17]
erai suut karung ipu	one bag of *ipu* bark
erai bangka sengkoi longan	one basket holding the *longan*
Nampe Ase erai ine	Nampe Ase, one mother
Tiong Goma erai uma	Tiong Goma, one father[18]
ala Bontik ngurai timang	Bontik originated *timang*
Gerung naan ngurai naiyu	Gerung originated *naiyu*
Kelos naan ngurai bongai	Kelos originated *bongai*
Demung ngurai tentuwaja	Demung originated *tentuwaja*
Hos ngurai nipe	Hos originated the snakes
erai susur sensuren	it comes down to one origin
Punen ngurai Malesia	Punen originated Malesia
iro susur taun bayuh	that is the origin from the olden days
serenaya tuning pita	the account from the first break of dawn
adi ka salung uli	to make all you guests return
kelua enken ehe	from here on
ka iya udo pita	you must not come in the morning
ka bote empet doyeng	you must not come in the afternoon
semah empe uyung unuk	the offering of respect encompasses the whole body
ampun empe puai bokang	the plea permeates the entire trunk
ampun ampen arang kami	the plea informs the movements of the hands
bongai uli lensangan walo	*bongai* return to the eight side roads
tentuwaja uli sopan	*tentuwaja* return to the puddle
naiyu uli buung langit	*naiyu* return to the vault of the heaven
timang uli unsok liang	*timang* return to the corner of the cave
juata uli danum	*juata* return to the waters
buta uli blai soya	*buta* return to the burnt down house
bansi uli etong batu	*bansi* return to in between the stones
tonoi uli baang bunge	*tonoi* return to the grove of flowers

This is a chant evoking the myth of human origins in the mind of the listener (human, spirit), a chant summoning the myth, bringing it alive. It is a chant presuming knowledge of a common history of both human and spirit listeners, replete with allusions to previous chants, myths, and rituals. In order to grasp this chant it is assumed that you know the myth, the tradition created by the recounting (*nempuun*) of the myth. Whereas *Tempuun Senaring* as chanted during a *nalin taun*—in full—serves to create and re-create the world of human beings through a detailed retelling of its origins, this song in a sense stays on a lower level (as Luangans would put it, differentiating rituals hierarchically according to the amount of work and the numbers of sacrifices they involve), limiting itself to hints and allusions. Ma Sarakang here attempts to invoke the reciprocal obligations of spirit and man by invoking their common origins, not word for word, but through what we might call intertextual references, conjuring the story behind the story, so to speak. Thus, it is by calling up a memory of common origins that Ma Sarakang recreates the relatedness and the reciprocity that it involves (which for some reason has been forgotten, with the patient consequently having fallen ill). Somewhat like the *ngeraya* which attempts to influence the future through a vow, the curing ritual here draws on the power of continuity, of mythmaking as an ongoing project of relatedness.

Reminding the spirits of "the olden days," Ma Sarakang conjures an image of the *longan*, the ultimate ancestral object, a storehouse of spiritual potency, the outward leaning legs of which are in some cases, as in his chant, held together at the base in a basket. Just as the legs of the *longan* are joined at the base, so are spirits and human beings born of "one mother," of "one father." Quoting from *Tempuun Senaring*—"Bontik originated *timang*, Gerung originated *naiyu*, Kelos originated *bongai*"—he brings the same point home in yet another way: it is from the siblings of Punen that the spirits originate (and Punen originated Man). This is what happened in the myth of origin. This is an "account from the first break of dawn." And this, too, is what Ma Sarakang wants to make happen now. Through his words, which recall the myth, he urges the spirits to fulfill their part of the deal, to behave as siblings. Presenting bountiful offerings to the spirits he fulfills his part of it, while asking them to withdraw to the places where they belong (to places assigned to them in the origin myth). Once again the concern here can be seen to be with actions aimed at invoking both sameness and difference, what Taussig (1993: 116) has called "the sort of action of becoming different while remaining the same," that is so central in Luangan social life (see also chapter 2).

To borrow an expression by Dennis Tedlock (1993: x), the myth alluded to in the chant should be read "not only for the past but for signs of a possible future." It is in order to recreate the relationship between spirit and man that Ma Sarakang evokes its origins. Repetition is a powerful means of recollection; through just a few words, a couple of well selected names—words and names his listeners have heard before, words and names closely tied up with the moment of creation—Ma Sarakang evokes a story of common origins. And he does it in a way that does not leave much room for argumentation. Reality is created almost furtively, between the lines, so to speak, or perhaps, one could say, in another story. Allusion brings forth what it aims to address, but leaves it unspoken, in an almost involuntary way, by the sheer power of tradition.

"The perfect narrative is," as Benjamin (1973c: 92) has stated it, "revealed through a variety of retellings." It is also as a retelling that Ma Sarakang's chant works. Reproduction is what brings forth the possibility of transformation. By evoking a history of relatedness, Ma Sarakang simultaneously brings it into being through ritual practice. In this sense the meaning *is* reproduction. Cosmology exists in motion: in ritual, in myth, in chants, in stories, and only in particular instantiations of each of these media. As Greg Urban (1996) argues, it is only when objectified in such instantiations that cosmology takes on a public character, and may be socially transmitted. In the Amerindian society studied by Urban it is "circulating discourse"— and narratives in particular—which enables the transmission of cosmological knowledge. This is true for the Luangans as well, although rituals, by way of both ritual chants and materially mediated and embodied ritual practices, may play an even more important role in this respect.[19] It is through allusion and evocation that myths are lived among Luangans, through ritual "retellings" that the relationship of similarity and difference that characterizes the relationship between humans and spirits is constituted. Through these "beginnings," in Lambek's (2007: 21) understanding of the concept, myth becomes, as Kapferer observes for Sinhalese sorcery myths: "a lived reality in which its existential force is discovered as a property of the unfolding dynamic of the complex of ritual practices of which it is a part" (1997: 82).

Sameness and Difference

> So these children of yours, who are of so many sorts, they will live well. Indeed they are other than Punen Senaring. Because those two with red body and fur, they are called the people of Naiyu. And those with dots and tail. They are called the people of Timang.
>
> The place of those two Naiyu is at the door of heaven. Those two live up there. But even if those two live up there, if you call them in the morning they will come in the morning, if you call them in the afternoon they will come in the afternoon, to you two, mother and father.
>
> —Excerpts from the origin myth of human beings (*Tempuun Senaring*) as written down by Lemanius (1996, my translation)

"You call them in the morning, they will come in the morning, you call them in the afternoon and they will come in the afternoon." This is Lemanius telling us the origin story, repeating the words of God who is instructing Sempirang Laang and Tewilung Uyung about the spirits' obligations to help their mother and father and, as an extension, humanity as a whole (who descend from Sempirang Laang and Tewilung Uyung). "From here on, you must not come in the morning, you must not come in the afternoon." This, in turn, is Ma Sarakang chanting, appealing to the spirits, trying to send them away—and keep them away—and so heal his patient. These two seemingly contradictory statements tell us something fundamental about human-spirit relations as we get to know them in Luangan song and myth.

As the philosopher Elizabeth Baeten (1996: 20) states, "the act of creation necessarily includes determination, delimitation, demarcation. Human creation (creation or constitution of the boundaries of the truly human) can be no different in this respect." Mythmaking (as creation) is "a giving shape," and giving shape is, as Baeten points out, "discovering and determining limits within the means provided by the creative context" (ibid.: 21). The Luangan myth of human origins (*Tempuun Senaring*) is no exception in this respect. In delineating the human being, in defining her shape and scope, it simultaneously explores her confines. Ultimately human existence is delimited in *Tempuun Senaring* by what could be called an envi-

246

ronment of unpredictability, an environment which is sometimes intimidating, and never totally controllable. Following philosophical naturalists like Baeten, this is something that might be termed nature, or natural processes. Nature here should not be understood as being opposed to culture—rather, culture is part of nature (cf. Descola 2006, 2009) just as human being is—but as standing for an "indefinitely plural environment," a world of "whatever is, in whatever way that it is" (Baeten 1996: 194). This is always, to some degree, a world of vicissitudes; a world where, to use Luangan vocabulary, crops might fail, game might keep away, illnesses may strike, wounds may not heal. It is a world beyond human control and purposive agency, the non-human backdrop of human existence. To the Luangans this is, as should be obvious by now, a world of spirits, both in the sense that the spirits are regarded as the agencies who control such unpredictable phenomena (e.g. illnesses, meteorological irregularities, fate, fortune) but also in the even more influential sense that it is through ritual contacts with spirits that the impact of such phenomena on man is mediated.[20] Spirits thus, in a sense, represent the non-human dominion to man, that which is beyond his reach but whose influence he may yet never escape.

The myth of origin explores the limits of human being, but it also presents kinship or "relatedness" (Carsten 1995; see also Bird-David 1999: 73) as a means of transcending boundaries (and incest and alterity as a way of representing what is "beyond"—alterity being a necessary condition for this ritually constituted enterprise as much as kinship). Myth, to cite Baeten again, "stakes out, as it were, the region of human being, not necessarily only in opposition to the non-human, but also in concert" (ibid.: 210). Like the Nayaka for whom "personifying something in the local terms directs inquisitive concerns to the being-together of oneself and the other and to learning mutualities within the *pluralities* that *are* in the world" (Bird-David 2006: 43, original italics), the Luangans get to know and act upon the world they inhabit by relating to it. Relatedness is what brings the other (whose motives and intentions can never be fully known) into the realm of familiarity, and thereby into some degree of predictability, or at least intelligibility (and this not only applies to the relationship between people and spirits, or people and animals, but also to relations between humans: non-kin have to be made kin, for example, through adoption or marriage, if you are going to entrust them with a more important role in your life).[21] Relatedness, and the requirements of reciprocity and sharing which constitutes it, is the common language, something which allows communication and negotiation by providing at least a minimal degree of commensurability. Differentiation, in fact, demands undifferentiation here; it is only by being like the other that you can work both with and against him.[22] Being like, as in the sense of sharing the same origin, enables you to obtain a certain, necessary distance from the spirits; it grants the power to influence, and keep the spirits away. In other words, it is by being like the other that you can resist his otherness (preventing him from harming you, for example), even while it is, at the same time, what enables you to make use of it in *belian* curing, for example (as the obligations associated with this identity are also what is assumed to make the spirits help you). Kinship, understood here as relatedness, thus constitutes a basis for collaboration as well as dissociation; it is what makes spirits come when you call them, and what makes them leave when you ask them to (or at least it should). It is the link between the world of spirits and the world of human beings, what gives human beings some amount of influence over what ultimately cannot be controlled (note that "fate" and "fortune" are dimensions of human life which are regulated by the *seniang*).[23]

It is not, however, something that can be taken for granted. Kinship or relatedness is not something stable, something that always will be, just because it once was there. In order for relatedness to be it has to be exercised, it has to be maintained: it is the relatives (and spirits) that you keep up your relations with that you can count on as true relatives, not those distant or "forgotten" ones that you know exist but seldom interact with. In order for kinship to really exist among the Luangans you have to engage in kin relations. This is why there have to be rituals, why spirits have to be called, fed and pleased. This is also why origins have to be told, again and again. In rituals, through invocations and through offerings, the siblingship between spirits and human beings is realized and made real. Only in singing origins, in full or through allusion, are origins made valid and compelling.

In this sense the relatedness between human beings and spirits is consistent with and an aspect of what Ingold calls an "animic ontology," according to which "beings do not propel themselves across a ready-made world but rather issue forth through a world-in-formation, along the lines of their relationships" (2006: 9). Animism, in Ingold's understanding, "is not a property of persons imaginatively projected onto the things with which they [people] perceive themselves to be surrounded. Rather ... it is the dynamic, transformative potential of the entire field of relations within which beings of all kinds ... continually and reciprocally bring one another into existence" (2006: 10).

* * *

Myth, in the diversity of its forms, is the medium through which human beings explore "the continuities" and "the discontinuities" between the human and the non-human spheres (Baeten 1996: 20). As such mythmaking is a living process, forever formed and re-formed in that "indefinitely complex environment we call our home" (ibid.: 21). This is why we should study myths in the varying contexts of their production: not as one story, but as several stories, together creating and re-creating the world for human beings. What all the different tellings or performances of the *Tempuun Senaring* do—through their differences as much as through their similarities—is to transmit the myth, and the notion of a common origin of spirits and people, as relevant and meaningful in a changing present. Conversely, it is by responding to the varying demands of the environment (be that incessant raining, illness, or state politics of religion)—by applying the myth as a constitutive and transformative force, capable not only of defining the world *of*, but also *for*, human beings—that the different performances succeed in passing it on. This is true for the incorporation of the myth in the *nalin taun* ritual, which serves not only cosmological purposes, but social ones as well, integrating villagers and promoting village leadership, and for the *ngeraya*, in which the origin myth is present only as part of a vow, as a promise to be fulfilled later.

Luangan mythmaking is not an activity which serves to seclude the past from the present; the myths do not depict "the past and the present as separate homogenities" (Seremetakis 1994b: 31). Mythmaking is a productive process, an act serving to renegotiate the present. The myths presented here are practices, they "say exactly what they do" (de Certeau 1984: 80). They conjure a relationship of reciprocity between spirits and people, for example, in order to transform (i.e., reestablish) this relationship. This clearly applies to myths chanted as part of rituals, or evoked through allusion in the curing process, but it also applies to myths told as stories (or made into written texts as in the case of Lemanius) in the sense that these tellings establish and help pass on the myths as authoritative tradition. The various instantiations of the myths open them up by constituting them not only as "origins," but as "beginnings," thus charging them with relevance. Among other things, and not least importantly, they confirm and perpetuate the relatedness between spirit and man as a plausible strategy for confronting the unpredictability of nature and the initial deformity of creation.

As with the *ngeraya* ritual, whose completion is always in some sense absent, there is no vanishing point in mythmaking. Bearing in mind that the *nalin taun* ritual is a relatively recent import in the Luangan ritual repertoire, the completion could even be interpreted as something imposed by leaders aspiring to promote their own leadership and village integration. In this respect, complete re-creation of the world and the order of the world, achieved through the recitation of all the *tempuun*, would then be subject to the development of an institution of village leadership and settlement. Be that as it may, it is not in a ready-made world, but in a world of "continual generation," "incipient, forever on the verge of the actual" (Ingold 2006: 10, 12) that the Luangans' myths are told and their rituals enacted. The relationship between spirits and human beings is "dialogic" rather than "essential" (Bird-David 2006: 47): born and re-born in the practice of negotiation and in the commitment to continued negotiation. To relate and keep relating with spirits is, as I have tried to show in this chapter, and the book as a whole, the basic entailment of "a common origin." A central aspect of repetition is thus commitment to relatedness. In this sense, the *ngeraya*, portrayed as a prelude in this chapter, also constitutes a simile for the endlessness of both mythmaking and *belian* curing.

Notes

1. Kakah Ramat could not read. He stored the photocopies that we gave him hidden even from his closest family and it seems that it was not only their contents that he was interested in, but their very material form or existence as well, the written text, which he saw as powerful in itself. Kakah Ramat frequently wanted us to read aloud Lemanius' *tempuun* and afterwards often integrated details from those into his own versions.

2. In *Tempuun Langit Tana*, the myth preceding *Tempuun Senaring*, Sempirang Laang was created from a small quantity of earth that was left over when the world was created—out of a piece of "original," preexisting earth—and he thus in a sense became the first human being (although Punen, his child, is often mentioned as the first true human being). As Fox (1987: 524) has noted for Insular Southeast Asian cosmologies, it is typical also for *tempuun* that "creation did not occur *ex nihilo*." As further indications of this, there are also spirits, animals and objects of different sorts featuring in many *tempuun*, whose origination is in fact only explained and understood to take place later, as recounted in other "younger" (*ure*) *tempuun*.

3. Sour fruit such as citrus fruit (*munte*) is often forbidden (*pali*) to eat by persons who have been ill and have undergone *belian* or by people who take Western medicines, as they are said to be dangerous to mix with these. In the myth of human origins the cravings for sour fruit during pregnancy and its role in the development of the fetus are explicitly connected, although I never received an explanation for the connection. Hopes et al. (1997: 32), in recounting a Benuaq version of the *tempuun*, claim that sour and bitter things are considered necessary for an unborn child to be properly formed, which is why pregnant women have cravings for such flavors.

4. This theme of an act of incest being detected by a scar discovered during delousing seems to be widespread in myths in Indonesia (for examples from Java, Banjar, and South Sulawesi, see Gibson 2005: 92–93).

5. As Hymes (1975: 47) has noted, "myth narrations do generally leave a good deal implicit." They do not state everything that would be needed to make the myth entirely clear. Indeed, he claims: "Full clarification, and especially explanations and asides, if present, are evidence that the narrative is *not* a native performance."

6. Reflecting the restricted importance of the *seniang* in ritual practice, the names and roles of the different *seniang* represent rather esoteric knowledge, and vary greatly between ritual experts and villages. Different ritual experts provided quite different listings of them than the one provided by Kakah Ramat here, and the total number of *seniang* recognized, if different sources were compiled, would be almost infinite.

7. The *seniang* also include some beings who have a more proximate human origin than those descending from the first man and woman, beings originating as particular ancestors who ascended to heaven and became immortal and deified. In addition there are also some *seniang* who "descended" (*dolui*) to earth in golden or iron palanquins to become the founding ancestors of particular descent lines and local groups. A group of famous early mythological heroes acting as the protagonists of many *tempuun*—Kilip, Nalau, Datu, Dara, etc.—notably also originate from a pair of *seniang*, and having turned invisible and "disappeared" (*gaib*) are not the actual genealogical ancestors of living people.

8. Siblingship is the basic idiom of relatedness among the Luangans. The word for sibling (*peyari*) may also be extended to mean "relative."

251

9. There is no general word for "spirits" among the Luangans. Instead they speak of individual categories of spirits such as *naiyu* or *timang* and often join two categories of spirits, such as *naiyu timang* or *wok bongai*, together, thus metonymically extending them to include other spirits as well. With the word "spirit," as I use it here, I do not intend to refer to some bodiless entity; spirits have bodies of different kinds, human-like or animal-like, even if they are mostly invisible to human beings (with the exception of *belian*, who may be able to see them on certain occasions).

10. In a Benuaq version of *Tempuun Senaring* a cannibalistic act is included as well, with the older siblings eating one of their younger siblings (Hopes et al. 1997: 37).

11. According to Michael Hopes et al. (1997: 13), who have compiled a collection of Benuaq *tempuun*, *Tempuun Langit Tana* is recited during "all large ceremonies" (a concept presumably including at least large death rituals) among the Benuaq, whereas *Tempuun Senaring* is chanted only during life rituals (*nalin taun*).

12. The *seniang* are offered food during ordinary *buntang* rituals as well. However, on such occasions they are usually not "descended" (*pedolui*), at least not all of them; the food is instead brought to their respective heavenly locations by the *belian*. Only the *nalin taun* is considered grand enough to host the *seniang*.

13. Today, the *Tempuun Langit Tana* and *Tempuun Senaring* myths are performed only during *nalin taun* rituals among the central Luangans. In which, if any, ritual context they were performed before the introduction of the *nalin taun*—which most informants insisted they were—is unclear. Presently, at least, they are not performed during the extended family *buntang* rituals of which the *nalin taun* represents a development. One possibility is that they were performed during so-called *nalin olo* (meaning "to treat the day") rituals, a particular kind of *buntang* rituals (or in some areas, a special form of one-day rituals) which are arranged specifically in order to treat incest.

14. These are objects of the past: a box in which ignition stones used to be stored and a necklace that was worn by the ancestors.

15. It was when recounting *Tempuun Langit Tana* (the origin myth of the sky and earth) that Kakah Ramat, and others telling us *tempuun*, stayed closest to the chanted mode, perhaps because this myth does not include much "action" in the usual understanding of the word, and thus is not easily translated into a story. The switching between everyday language and stylized mode was not always easily achieved for Kakah Ramat who sometimes had to go back to the chant, mumbling the lines for himself so as to remember names and genealogies. Even when dictating his story for writing, aiming at "completion," Kakah Ramat "forgot" things which had to be included afterwards.

16. Unfortunately, I never had the possibility to hear *Tempuun Senaring* being chanted during a *nalin taun* as there were no *nalin taun* rituals performed in the immediate area of my fieldwork during my time there. I did partic-

ipate for a few days in a couple of *nalin taun* rituals among the Benuaq, but this was towards the end of the rituals, not in the beginning when the *tempuun* are sung, as well as for a few days in the district capital of Bentian Besar in 1992, a year before I started my actual fieldwork, also at the end of the ritual. I have, however, attended the performance of other *tempuun* on multiple occasions, during *buntang* rituals and *gombok* mortuary rites.

17. This refers to the long rows of banana leaf packages containing rice which are customarily served to ritual participants during rituals.

18. Tiong Goma and Nampe Ase are names of mythological ancestors.

19. Urban (1996: 80, 96) makes the point that among the people that he studies, it is particularly "what lies beyond the realm of the senses" which is—and has to be—made known through circulating discourse (as this cannot be experienced directly).

20. Kirk Endicott (1979: 218) makes a similar point for the Batek of Peninsular Malaysia when he notes that "the use of anthropomorphic beings in explanations of the world opens up the possibility of ritually influencing those beings in order to manipulate the forces they are supposed to control."

21. Or, you could turn the argument around: people that you live in long-term relations with sooner or later become your kin. Non-kin, on the other hand, (*ulun*, "people"), are often treated with a great deal of suspicion and fear of poisoning (*ompan*) is widespread in relations with them.

22. Differentiation is thus not as unambiguous an outcome of myth here as Lévi-Strauss would have it: preceded by a state of undifferentiation, and achieved through a process of elimination (1969: 52; 1981). Undifferentiation is instead an inseparable part of the process of differentiation (see Girard 1978a, 1978b for a critique of Lévi-Strauss).

23. There seems to be a widespread notion of a kin relationship between spirits and humans among other Borneo peoples. The Iban say that they have a "sibling-like" relation to their spirits (Barrett 1993: 263) and that they share "a common ancestry" (Sather 2001: 65): "because of being kin, the shamans are free to challenge the spirts" (Sather 2001: 202). The Ngaju call the spirits their cousins (Jay 1993: 160), and the Kayan myth of origin states that humans are descended from spirits and that they thus share a common origin (Rousseau 1998: 98).

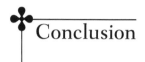

Conclusion

In fact, one can go on and ask oneself whether the relationship of the storyteller to his material, human life, is not in itself a craftsman's relationship, whether it is not his very task to fashion the raw material of experience, his own and that of others, in a solid, useful, and unique way.

—Walter Benjamin (1973c: 107)

In an influential new comparative treatise of what he calls the "largest remaining region of the world whose peoples have not yet been fully incorporated into nation-states," Scott examines the condition and roots of statelessness among the hill peoples of Zomia, the multinational cross-border highlands of mainland Southeast Asia (2009: ix). He argues that "virtually everything about … [the] livelihoods, social organization, ideologies, and … even [the] largely oral cultures" of these geographically marginal peoples, who live physically dispersed, have a flexible, egalitarian social structure, nebulous ethnic identities, and a mobile lifestyle based on swidden cultivation, "can be read as strategic positionings designed to keep the state at arm's length" (2009: x). Rather than representing, as "civilizational discourses" would claim, remnants of an ancestral culture, these peoples live the way they do by choice, because it allows them, at least in some respects, to stay out of state control. It is as "political adaptations of nonstate peoples to a world of states that are, at once, attractive and threatening" that Scott (2009: 9) argues we should understand these practices.

In this book I have explored how and why the Luangans of Kalimantan, a loosely integrated swidden-cultivating people who share many of the above-mentioned characteristics of the hill tribes studied by Scott, choose to maintain a tradition of curing practices, *belian*, even while it, along with other aspects of their social life,

254

marginalizes them in the eyes of both government officials and their downstream neighbors. Like Meratus shamanism described by Tsing (1993: 231), the practice of *belian* marks Luangans "as outside legitimate religion and thus possibly subversive (amoral) and certainly archaic (uncivilized)." This said, my primary research interest in this study has not been in the Luangans' relationship with the state, or in how their rituals, or other practices, help keep the state at bay. Nor has it been in how the *belian* rituals are influenced by state discourse, even though this influence is significant, and represents an important consideration in the book (especially in chapter 2). Again, as among the Meratus, shamanic discussion and ceremonial practice constitute a main forum through which the Luangans "accept, manipulate, and argue about their ethnic and political status" (Tsing 1993: 231).

Instead, I have in this study primarily been concerned with the positive qualities of some of the practices that define the Luangans' "statelessness." A principal purpose of the book has been to explore what motivates the Luangans to practice *belian* rituals, in spite of their marginalizing effect, to examine what it is that these rituals do for the Luangans—not only politically, but socially and existentially. The question of what the Luangans refuse, in Scott's sense, or why and how they refuse it, has thus been countered and complemented with what it is that they prefer—and why they do it.

These are questions, I have argued, that cannot be explored without consideration of how these rituals are organized and performed, or of the ontology and social reality that they reflect and reproduce. An unfixed and contingent quality marks not only Luangan socio-political life but also Luangan rituals, both exhibiting considerable flexibility and malleability, or a tendency for what Rosaldo (1993) calls "social grace," in the sense of an inclination for improvisation, reorientation and openness to contingency. Besides the great frequency of Luangan curing practices, what struck me when I started my fieldwork was their pervasive "indeterminacy" and "messiness." Ritual plans seemed to change constantly. Rituals succeeded, supplanted and overlapped each other. Multiple rituals were routinely performed for the same purpose, sometimes even simultaneously and in the same place. The same or very similar ritual activities were performed over and over again during the course of a ritual. Ends were not necessarily ends; rituals could be prolonged just as they seemed to be finished, or postponed and continued at a later point, sometimes in a different format. Analogously, people seemed to come and go somewhat as they pleased, and to switch between active and passive participation with apparent ease. In fact, the officiating *belian* themselves often switched between or—perhaps more to the point—maintained a simultaneous stance of absorption and distraction. They could be well on their way on a journey to search for the soul of a patient, for example, while simultaneously listening to the conversation going on around them and then suddenly join it in the midst of their chanting (see Rousseau 1998: 122 for a similar observation among the Kayan). In short, *belian* rituals did not correspond to a neatly bounded format, or closely follow a predetermined plan of action, but rather represented open-ended negotiations with spirits in which things happening while they proceeded affected their development.

A central argument of this book is that this unboundedness and contingency of *belian* curing are not expressions of a lack of structure, or order, as, for instance, members of the Hindu Kaharingan Council, founded in order to bring the local religions of South Borneo closer to the so-called world religions, would have it. Nor are they, at least not most of the time, expressions of a contest over authority, which would explain the indeterminacy or flexibility as a lack of consensus. Instead, they express something fundamental about the relationship between ritual representation and reality in *belian*, a relationship that has constituted a principal focus in this study. The world conjured in *belian* curing is not a ready-made world, but one constantly in the making. It is indeed, as I suggested in chapter 2, from the openness between representation and reality that much of the transformative potential of *belian* rituals derives. This is a two-way relationship; by evoking the world in its ambiguity and indeterminacy, rather than trying to contain it, the Luangans render their relationship to the world as complexly constituted and open-ended. By the same means, as ritual representation is subjected to the unpredictability and inconclusiveness of the reality represented, reality is portrayed as indeterminate and impressionable, and hence possible to influence through *belian*. To submit to the decrees of a world religion, as defined in state discourse or by the Hindu Kaharingan Council, would be to narrow down the scope of its potentiality. This is also why those Luangans who profess affiliation with Hindu Kaharingan often claim that they simultaneously practice both "Hindu Kaharingan" and "Kaharingan": these categories represent different aspects of their being-in-the-world, and their statements thus reject the closure imposed by the national discourse.

Influenced by studies of peoples with what variously has been called a "relational epistemology" (Bird-David 1999), or an "animic ontology" (Ingold 2006; cf. Descola 1992; Viveiros De Castro 1998)—according to which the boundaries between the human and the non-human realms are permeable, and sociality is extended to the non-human realm—I have analyzed *belian* rituals in terms of how they reflect and exemplify a way of relating to the world by "being alive" to it, in the sense of actively engaging with it from within, as participants in rather than as distanced observers of it (Ingold 2004: 51). Seen in this light, the *belian* rituals form platforms for an engagement with the spirit world which is open, or responsive, to its contingency even while they attempt to overcome it. This entails a stance whereby knowing and influencing something necessitates "reaching out to it," becoming alike by opening up to its plurality and stressing mutuality and relatedness (see especially chapter 6). The spirit world as represented in *belian* is unbounded and unpredictable, but it is also made, if not actually controllable, then at least companionable and negotiable through the evocation of a common origin between humans and spirits, and through sharing with the spirits, which in effect realizes this relatedness.

In an unpublished manuscript by the Luangan author Lemanius, to which I have referred on a number of occasions in this study, *belian* rituals are described as paths along which offerings of food and respect are brought to the spirits (*alan taka nganter segala semba sukep, segala ampun asi taka*). In my interpretation, the path should not here be conceived of as a site for a journey that stretches lineally from one point to another, as much as it should be regarded as constituting a bloc of "space-time," as in Bakhtin's (1981: 98) understanding of the "road" as a conventional literary "chronotope," in the sense of a locus of unforeseen chance encounters of multiple actors. It is as such a space-time of encounters between various parties in an ongoing negotiation of relationship that the typically meandering and diversifying path of *belian* curing is formed. Along the route new negotiation parties emerge: spirits arrive from both upstream and downstream realms, presenting differing requests, reflecting different aesthetic and dietary predilections, prompting different styles of curing to cater to them. Characteristically, the process of Luangan negotiation with spirits is hardly ever restricted to just one party singled out as being specifically responsible or relevant in a particular case but is extended to a variety of parties and performed not just to address the specific task at hand but aimed simultaneously to improve and maintain multiple relationships as a preventive measure or a goal in itself (cf. Atkinson 1987b: 125; Kuipers 1990: 42; Sillander 2004: 195).

In my study, the Luangan openness to a sociality that extends beyond the human domain to an ultimately uncontrollable spirit and natural world translates into an emphasis on "emergence," on "what happens by virtue of performance" (Schieffelin 1996: 64). I have tried to address this quality of *belian* rituals through a focus on concrete events which illuminate what the rituals do for particular participants in particular circumstances and how ritual action is affected by these events. Through this emphasis on the particular— which demonstrates the complex agendas of *belian*, ranging from the maintenance of tradition and the negotiation of identity, to the curing of illness and the coping with infant death—I have conveyed a picture of *belian* as a "space of possibilities," which contains the potential for negotiation of diverse concerns, realized through an adaptive medium of representation, attentive to the demands of the context and changing circumstances. This is perhaps exemplified most clearly in chapter 2, in the analysis of how the *belian* Tak Dinas struggled to maintain ritual plausibility in the face of political marginality and existential crisis through a montage-like ritual, in which the complexity of the Luangan world was allowed to enter the representation. In this particular ritual, improvisation and inspiration became exceptionally important aspects, even by Luangan standards, but a contextual orientation is more or less a characteristic of all *belian* rituals, which makes it impossible to grasp their full significance outside the actuality of performance. In the multifaceted and multi-styled *buntang* ritual analyzed in chapter 4, this was exemplified by the actions of the two *belian*, Mancan and Ma Putup, who, in between the segments of the *buntang* itself, acted on inspiration received during its course and, besides the official program of the *buntang*, performed their own agendas, bringing in new sources of empowerment (in Mancan's case a Javanese ancestor, in Ma Putup's a range of purportedly Arabic-speaking and other foreign spirit familiars). This attention to contextual circumstances was also reflected in the many revisions made regarding the length and format of this *buntang*, and in the reluctance that participants showed to pin down decisions in this regard.

It is as they are expressed in ritual practice that I have studied ritual representations, and as such, to borrow an expression of Keane's, "representations do not exist only in the abstract—as, for example, some disembodied 'discourse.' Rather, that they take concrete forms, situated in activities, is critical to their signifying, performative, and even casual capacities" (1997: xiv). In chapter 3, I described how figurines made out of wood or rice paste, representing human beings, were made into what Luangans call *ganti diri*, exchange objects given to spirits in return for human souls. In their very materiality, I argue, these objects sensuously bring forth reality for their human and spirit audiences. The concreteness of ritual representation is here an essential attribute of its evocative potential, and thus of its curative effect. A central element in this process is the all-important activity of "undoing and redoing," *pejiak pejiau*, the standardized two-phased ritual process of concretely presenting or enacting something, first in the wrong way, and then in the right way, which is performed in a number of ways in different phases of all *belian* rituals. The repetitive, pronounced process of representation and re-presentation as a precondition for transformation is predicated upon its tactile form of appropriation, I suggest, and as such is dependent on its instantiation in practice. The apparent distraction characteristic of the *belian* and the ritual participants in the particular ritual analyzed in that chapter, but also more commonly in *belian* rituals, testifies not so much to a lack of engagement on the part of the participants, as to the ongoingness of tradition, which confers a prominent quality of "everydayness" to rituals, a quality which forms an essential aspect both of their identity-shaping capacities and their ability to captivate and be experienced as taken-for-granted.

In the forests of Borneo lack of active use of a forest path causes it to fade away quickly as it becomes overgrown with tangled secondary growth; likewise the path of *belian* curing has been treaded through continuous interaction. On this path, the present is conjoined with the past by way of *mulung*, the *belian*'s spirit familiars, who are often their predecessors, and by way of ancestral words (*bukun tuha*), passed on through these predecessors, as well through the habituation of ritual participants to *belian* through lived tradition. As I lived among the Luangans during my fieldwork, I gradually came to expect *belian* when something out of the ordinary occurred, not only intellectually, so to speak, but often in an intuitive or embodied way, through a feeling of unease if a ritual for some reason did not materialize or was delayed. This, I propose, reflected a degree of habituation. I had become used to *belian* as the natural or appropriate way to deal with crisis and contingency. An expression of a similar unease was also evident among many Luangans who in a variety of circumstances conveyed a felt need for *belian*, including in instances when successful curing was considered highly unlikely and when shamans were reluctant or even refused to perform rituals. This may be interpreted as an expression of the compelling nature of *belian*, of how *belian* rituals formed part of their personal and collective history, to the extent of having become an embodied part of who they were, an aspect of their habitus. As Hanks (1987: 689) observes, summarizing a well-known argument of Bourdieu's: "part of the effectiveness of symbolic forms lies in their capacity to become natural and to naturalize what they represent." In the case of *belian*, ritualization is indissolubly associated with naturalization. *Belian*, to an important extent, constitutes the beaten "path" of relating-to-the-environment of the Luangans, it is an integral aspect of their way of being-in-the-world, in addition to being a central element of their "luanganness."

Belian rituals come in a number of styles or genres, of which three major varieties (all containing numerous sub-styles) are practiced by central Luangans. These genres address (at least partly) different spirit audiences, in different languages, and through different stylistic conventions. Certain illnesses tend to be dealt with through certain ritual styles and attributed to certain spirits who are considered to favor particular styles of contact. Thus, *belian* rituals are not infinitely open-ended but conform to particular conceptions of the addressees at the same time as they draw from a repertoire of situationally appropriate conduct established through previous experience. In chapter 4 I explored how all the major genres of *belian* curing performed by central Luangans (*belian luangan, belian bawo,* and *belian sentiu*) were juxtaposed within the same ritual, which was performed for a seriously ill community leader. Here the unpredictability and unboundedness of the spirit world, conceived to be ultimately beyond human control, was confronted through the means of genre diversification and condensation in a kind of stylistical heteroglossia in which the different genres complemented each other, forming concurrent strategies to influence the spirits, employing different "cultures" of representation to enhance ontological plausibility and operational success.

As Hanks argues for Mayan discourse genres expressed in official historical documents, *belian* ritual genres are "grounded in social practices of production and reception, rather than having an independent existence of their own" (1987: 676–677). In addition, individual *belian* rituals are historically contextualized in that they are directly and indirectly connected to other individual *belian* rituals, forming a tradition of *belian* curing. As I demonstrated in chapter 5, to regard individual *belian* performances as separate entities risks overlooking the significance that rituals hold for individual participants. Tradition is both an organic, living unity to which individual performances are constantly added and an embodied part of personal history that conditions how rituals are perceived. In chapter 5, I juxtaposed three bathing rituals that were performed in the same place, within a limited time period, in order to illustrate how they were connected to each other, not by intention or explicitly stated connection, but through the ritual participants' joint experiences, intertwined personal histories, and shared social predicament. In short, it is, in Bakhtin's vocabulary, in the "dialogic" relationship between ritual genres, history, improvisation, and extra-ritual events that individual rituals are shaped and gain plausibility as transformative devices. "Rituals," as Atkinson (1989: 13) observes, "have histories. Performances build on one another and are affected by, and in turn affect, what happens more generally in the world."

In broad outline, what *belian* rituals—and many other rituals for that matter—do for the people practicing them is determined situationally and always in some respects eludes fixation. Their outcomes are not predetermined, and their boundaries, even when they appear to be clearly marked, are in some respects imprecise or fuzzy. Hence, there is no finality when it comes to Luangan ritualization. *Belian* rituals, as this study has shown, are varied and emergent. However, they are also conventional and habitual. They follow a logic of their own, drawn from a repertoire of prescribed or habitually established exemplary activities, and gain their plausibility in relation to other performances. It is from the dialectic between what is perceived as given and what Jackson (2005: xxi), discussing life conditions more generally, has called a capacity "not only to reproduce what is given, but to reimagine and rework, even negate and confound, the given," that *belian* curers, like storytellers, "fashion the raw material of experience" (Benjamin 1973c: 107).

The potencies of *belian* curing are ultimately generated in practice. As Kapferer (1997: 177) observes for the practice of the Sinhalese Suniyama rite, "it is in the activities productive of the Suniyama—in the making of the rite—that the recreative energies of the rite become present and potent." Like Benjamin's storyteller, the *belian*'s relationship to the world is that of a craftsman. The *belian* does not just represent the world but in a sense creates it, or at least, conveys a particular vision, or version, of it. In this respect, *belian* may be seen as entailing a form of *poiesis*. Like the Suniyama, it transcends actual reality, and creates its own virtual reality, which, in Kapferer's terminology (1997: 180), is a "simulacrum"—not "a model of or for reality," in Clifford Geertz' (1966) sense. As such a "virtuality," it "does not simply dissolve into reality but brings it forth" (Kapferer 1997: 180).

In this study I have explored both the limits and the potentials of ritual representation. Unlike the Suniyama, *belian* rituals remain open to the indeterminacies of actuality, even in virtuality, in the sense that these rituals, even when they turn out to be highly conventional, form a sort of experiment through which the plurality of a bottomless and unbounded spirit world is engaged. Luangan spirits, like their Karo counterparts, provoke a way of reading experience as "uncertain, duplicitous, always open to revision" (Steedly 1993: 15). *Belian* curers act upon the world by trying out different possibilities at hand, by deploying different strategies of negotiation with a multitude of spirit beings. Sometimes this will work out as desired, sometimes not, but what is crucial is that the action of performing *belian* constitutes a condition for their way of "being alive" to the world in Ingold's sense. The fact that the Luangans, like the Nayaka, "persist in these practices despite their deficiencies" suggests that they are not only vital for addressing particular pressing problems which threaten well-being: "it behoves us to view them not only as a means of treating illness and misfortunes but also, more broadly, as authoritative, cultural practices regenerating deep-seated understandings about the world" (Bird-David 2004: 331). These understandings reflect historical and contemporary experiences of coming to terms with the exigencies and contingencies of a complex natural and socio-political environment through what might be called "a politics of spirits." Performing *belian* is a way of asserting and enacting an embodied, habitual cultural orientation of "luanganness," a tacit strategy of engaging with the world through ritual representations. It expresses commitment to a practice of relating to spirits, be they local or foreign, through which the Luangans fashion themselves as constitutive of their relations. In this respect the practice of *belian* constitutes a choice, a choice that is as much ontological as it is political.

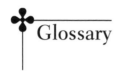

Glossary

Unless otherwise indicated, terms are in the Bentian dialect of the Luangan language. Indonesian terms are marked (I.).

abei	Category of heavenly spirits causing *sengkera-pei*, often depicted as animals.
adat (I.), *adet*	Customary law; tradition.
agama (I.)	Religion.
ansak	Suspended plaited tray containing offerings for spirits.
baang bunge	Village flower grove. Place for growing *samat* plants and plants used as ritual paraphernalia.
balei	A term for a variety of large, temporarily constructed outdoor or indoor shrines used for presenting offerings to spirits.
bansi	A category of predominantly malevolent female spirits with long nails originating as women dying in childbirth.
bantan	Ritual ship or swing used by the shaman to travel to the spirit realm.
bekawat	Shamanic treatment of patients during rituals.
belian	Generic designation for life as opposed to death rituals; the officiants of such rituals (also sometimes referred to as *pemelian*).
belian bawe	"Womens' *belian*"; distinct shamanic style associated with the Benuaq and the Tunjung; designation for an obsolete central Luangan style carried out solely by women.
belian bawo	Shamanic style said to originate in Pasir region. Chants partly in the Pasir language. Characterized by loud, rapid drumming, danc-

264

	ing, and heavy brass bracelets worn by the shaman.
belian dewa(-dewa)	A designation for several different shamanic styles associated with Malays, including the *sentiu*-like *belian dewa-dewa* of Tak Dinas (chapter 2), the *belian dewa* of Kakah Ramat (chapter 4), and a style associated with the Banjar Malays practiced by Central Kalimantan Luangans.
belian luangan	Shamanic tradition originating on the upper Teweh River. Considered the oldest style of curing practiced by the central Luangans. Based mainly on chants and ritual paraphernalia, does not include dancing or special ritual costume, except headcloth (*laung*). Includes *buntang* family rituals and *nalin taun* community rituals (although among some Benuaq Luangans these rituals are conducted in the *belian sentiu* style).
belian kenyong	Shamanic style associated with the Kutai sultanate. Sometimes regarded as subcategory of *belian sentiu*, although said to be much older.
belian sentiu	Shamanic style originating among the Benuaq, introduced to the central Luangan area in the 1970s. Characterized by elegant dancing and the use of ankle bracelets with ringing bells worn by the shaman. Employs downriver spirit familiars, and often addresses downriver Muslim *blis*, and hence does not usually include sacrifice of pigs. Partly performed in Kutai Malay.
bemueng	Incense wood (*Agathis* sp.) used in *belian luangan* and *belian bawo* rituals.
berejuus	"Soul search," basic ritual activity during which the shaman travels in search of patients' souls.
besemah	To present offerings and respect to spirits during rituals.
bidan	Midwife.

biyowo	*Cordyline terminalis*. Sharp-edged leaf which constitutes the shamans weapon, sometimes also described as a paddle.
blai	Single-family house; miniature spirit house, serving as a repository for minor offerings.
blai juus	Miniature house into which the souls of the sponsoring family/families enter at the conclusion of *buntang* rituals.
blis	Generic term for malevolent spirits.
bongai	Major category of malevolent spirits, associated with downriver locations and forests, often thought to cause diarrhea and epidemics.
buntang	Extended or multi-family ritual including both thanksgiving and curing, often performed in fulfillment of a vow given during curing rituals.
gaharu	*Aquilaria sp*. Incense wood used during *belian sentiu*. Collected for trade to the Middle East and Saudi Arabia.
ganti diri	Figurines or effigies made of rice paste or wood, etc., given to spirits in "exchange of the self" during rituals.
gombok	Secondary mortuary ritual performed after the funeral during which the souls of the deceased are escorted to the death realms.
jakat belian	"To stand up as *belian*"; to initiate or perform *belian* styles that include dancing such as *belian bawo* and *sentiu*.
jemu	Plate with burning incense.
jie	Leaf (unknown sp.) used by shamans together with *olung* to fan over offerings.
juata	Water spirit taking the form of a dragon, snake, leech, crab, etc.; often associated with downriver locations (sometimes considered to be Muslim).
junung	Ankle bracelets with bells worn by the *sentiu* shaman.
juus	The soul or animate principle of living human beings and animals. May occasionally wander off during dreams or be stolen by spirits.

kelelungan	The refined head souls of dead people which are escorted to Tenangkai during *gombok*. Important spirit familiar and protecting spirit.
kelentangen	Xylophone-like percussion instrument consisting of small gongs.
kerek keker	To call a lost soul with sounds similar to those made when one calls chickens.
kerewaiyu	Harvest ritual.
ketang	Heavy wrist bracelets made of brass worn in pairs to make a rattling sound by the shaman during *belian bawo*.
liau	Coarse body soul of dead human beings who are escorted to Mount Lumut during *gombok*. Common source of disturbance and soul theft.
longan	Designation for a variety of upright constructions serving as a place of congregation for spirits during rituals.
longan teluyen	A permanent *longan* made of ironwood serving as the ritual center of a *lou* and a place of storage for ancestral valuables.
lou	Extended family or multi-family house.
lou solai	Large extended family house; village longhouse serving as site of community rituals and gatherings.
Luing	The female spirit of rice; leading spirit familiar, different manifestations of which conduct negotiations with spirits during curing rituals, *buntang*, and *gombok*.
Lumut	Mountain in the upper Teweh area; location of village of the dead where the *liau* reside.
malik	To turn around, to transform.
mangir mulung	To summon spirit familiars.
manti	Community leader; extended family or house leader; adjudicator of *adat* law.
mulung	The spirit helpers of a *belian*. Often *belian* of the past, mythological as well as more or less recently deceased. Also include animal and other non-human spirits.

267

naiyu	Major category of personal and community protecting spirits and guardian spirits in nature taking human or animal form (as pythons, lizards, etc.). Associated with blood and potency. Animates the *longan* and other potent objects anointed with blood during rituals.
nakep juus	To catch the soul; basic ritual activity.
nalin taun	Community ritual performed in order to "treat the year," for purposes of purification and thanksgiving.
naper	To fan over a patient with leaves.
ngawat	To treat a patient.
ngebidan	Ritual performed after the birth of children for their welfare and to thank the midwife.
ngerangkau	Dance performed for the entertainment of the spirits of the dead during *gombok*.
ngeraya	Community ritual performed as a promise of a *nalin taun*, directed to the *seniang* who regulate yearly and natural cycles.
nyelolo	A ritual activity when the shaman wipes over patient's body with shredded banana leaves (*daon selolo*) in order to extract illness from it.
nyemah	To present offerings and respect to spirits.
okan penyewaka	Minor ritual food offerings presented to spirits as offerings or rewards.
olung	Leaf (unknown sp.) used by the shaman to fan over offerings.
pali	Taboo or restriction; category of spirits sanctioning the observance of *pali*.
panti penota	Chair used for ritual bathing.
pejiak pejiau	Standardized ritual process of doing or representing something first in the wrong way, and then in the right way, so as to enact a transformation, or ensure correct procedures, avert bad influence, etc.
pekuli	To make return or send back someone/something to its place or origin.
pengeruye	Persons assigned to collect and prepare ritual paraphernalia.

pengiring	Generic term for protecting spirits.
penyelenteng	Twined cloth vertically suspended from the ceiling together with an areca palm inflorescence serving as pathway between human and spirit realms during *belian* rituals.
penyempatung	Assistant of shaman, usually female.
pereau	"To seek the cause of an illness," diagnostic procedure in *belian*.
ringka jawa	Rattan basket tied to the stern of the *selewolo*, in which *liau* travels to Lumut during *gombok*.
roten	Illness (generic designation).
ruye	Ritual paraphernalia and decorations.
samat	Plants and trees planted in the flower grove or in a swidden after the birth of a child during *ngebidan*; invisible plant counterpart of human beings tended by the *seniang* in heaven.
sampan benawa	Soul search ship used during *buntang*.
sedediri	Small figurine representing human being made from rice paste, given in exchange for patients to spirits during rituals.
selewolo	Boat-like vessel used for transporting *kelelungan* (and the participating *wara*) to its afterworldly abode during *gombok*.
sempet	Decorated skirt worn by shamans in the *bawo* and *sentiu* tradition.
semur	Minor form of curing practice that in contrast to *belian* can be performed by almost anyone and which mainly consists of the recitation of spells and blowing on the patient.
sengkerapei	Illness or state of weakness associated with convulsions and the mimicking of the death throes of animals.
seniang	Category of mostly heavenly spirits who regulate fundamental conditions in nature and society.
sentous	Important ritual activity during which the soul of a sick person is bought back through exchange.

tapen	Failure to participate in social interaction; associated condition of soul weakness and susceptibility to spirit attack.
tempuun	Origin myth; corpus of myths chanted during major rituals recounting the origins of ritual paraphernalia, natural phenomena and cultural institutions.
Tenangkai	Village of the dead in heaven where the *kelelungan* reside.
tentuwaja	Forest spirit with pointed head associated with stagnant pools of water afflicting people with madness.
timang	Tiger or clouded leopard spirit; important category of *pengiring*, also often addressed in the capacity as *blis*.
tonoi	Spirits of the earth; guardian spirits of small children.
tota	Ritual bathing.
tuung	Drums played by shamans or members of the audience during rituals.
tuyang	Swing used by shamans to travel to the spirit realm.
tuwet (belian)	"To sit a *belian*"; to initiate or perform a *belian* in which the shaman mainly sits down during the performance (principally *belian luangan*).
utek tuha longan	Skulls of ancestors stored in a box above the *longan*.
wara	Death shaman, officiant of mortuary rituals.
wok	Major category of malevolent spirits, associated with graveyards, deep forests, often associated with illnesses involving coughing.

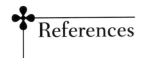

References

Acciaioli, Greg. 1985. "Culture as Art: From Practice to Spectacle in Indonesia." *Canberra Anthropology* 8(1&2): 148–172.

Adorno, Theodor W. 1991. *Notes to Literature*, vol. 1. Edited by Rolf Tiedemann. Translated by Shierry W. Nicholsen. New York: Columbia University Press.

Anderson, Benedict O'G. 1990. *Language and Power: Exploring Political Cultures in Indonesia*. Ithaca: Cornell University Press.

Appell, George N. and Laura W.R. 1993. "To do Battle with the Spirits: Bulusu' Spirit Mediums." In *The Seen and the Unseen: Shamanism, Mediumship and Possession in Borneo*, ed. Robert L. Winzeler. Borneo Research Council Monograph Series, vol. 2. Williamsburg: Borneo Research Council, pp. 55–99.

Aragon, Louis. 1994 [1926]. *Paris Peasant*. Translated by Simon Watson Taylor. Boston: Exact Change.

Arendt, Hannah. 1958. *The Human Condition*. Chicago: University of Chicago Press.

———. 1973. "Introduction: Walter Benjamin: 1892–1940." In *Illuminations*, ed. Hannah Arendt. London: Fontana Press, pp. 7–60.

Atkinson, Jane Monnig. 1987a. "Religions in Dialogue: The Construction of an Indonesian Minority Religion." In *Indonesian Religions in Transition*, ed. Rita Smith Kipp and Susan Rodgers. Tucson: University of Arizona Press, pp. 171–186.

———. 1987b. "The Effectiveness of Shamans in an Indonesian Ritual." *American Anthropologist* 89(2): 342–355.

———. 1989. *The Art and Politics of Wana Shamanship*. Berkeley: University of California Press.

Austin, John. L. 1962. *How to Do Things with Words*. Oxford: Oxford University Press.

Avé, Jan B. and Victor T. King. 1986. *People of the Weeping Forest: Tradition and Change in Borneo*. Leiden: The National Museum of Ethnology.

Babcock, Tim G. 1974. "Indigenous Ethnicity in Sarawak." *Sarawak Museum Journal* 22(43): 191–202.

Badan Koordinasi Penelitian Daerah. 1975. *Laporan Survey Kelompok Masyarakat Suku Bantian di Kecamatan Gunung Purei, Kabupaten Barito Utara, Kalimantan Tengah*. Direktorat Pembinaan Masyarakat Terasing, Direktorat Jenderal Bina Sosial, Departemen Sosial R.I.

Baeten, Elizabeth M. 1996. *The Magic Mirror: Myth's Abiding Power*. Albany: State University of New York Press.

Baier, Martin. 2007. "The Development of a New Religion in Central Kalimantan." *Borneo Research Bulletin* 38: 118–126.

Bakhtin, Mikhail M. 1981. *The Dialogic Imagination: Four Essays*. Edited by Michael Holquist. Translated by Caryl Emerson and Michael Holquist. Austin: University of Texas Press.

———. 1986. *Speech Genres and Other Late Essays*. Edited by Caryl Emerson and Michael Holquist. Translated by Vern W. McGee. Austin: University of Texas Press.

Barito Utara Dalam Angka. 2007. Badan Pusat Statistik, Kabupaten Barito Utara, Propinsi Kalimantan Tengah.

Barrett, Robert J. 1993. "Performance, Effectiveness and the Iban Manang." In *The Seen and the Unseen: Shamanism, Mediumship and Possession in Borneo*, ed. Robert Winzeler. Borneo Research Council Monograph Series, vol. 2. Williamsburg: Borneo Research Council, pp. 235–279.

Barrett, Robert J. and Rodney Lucas. 1993. "The Skulls are Cold, the House is Hot: Interpreting Depths of Meaning in Iban Therapy." *Man* 28(3): 573–596.

Barthes, Roland. 1977. "The Third Meaning." In *Image, Music, Text*. London: Fontana Press, pp. 52–68.

Bataille, Georges. 1985. "The Solar Anus." In *Visions of Excess, Selected Writings 1927–1939*. Minneapolis: University of Minnesota Press, pp. 5–9.

Bateson, Gregory. 1955. "A Theory of Play and Fantasy." *Psychiatric Research Reports* 2: 39–51.

Bauman, Richard. 1984. *Verbal Art as Performance*. Prospect Heights, Ill.: Waveland Press.

———. 1986. *Contextualization, Tradition and the Dialogue of Genres: Icelandic Legends of the Kraftaskáld*. Paper presented at the Annual Meeting of the American Anthropological Association, Philadelphia, PA.

Bauman, Richard and Charles L. Briggs. 1990. "Poetics and Performance as Critical Perspectives on Language and Social Life." *Annual Review of Anthropology* 19: 59–88.

Bell, Catherine. 1992. *Ritual Theory, Ritual Practice*. New York: Oxford University Press.

———. 1997. *Ritual: Perspectives and Dimensions*. New York: Oxford University Press.

Benjamin, Walter. 1973a. "The Work of Art in the Age of Mechanical Reproduction." In *Illuminations*, ed. Hannah Arendt. London: Fontana Press.

———. 1973b. "On Some Motifs in Baudelaire." In *Illuminations*, ed. Hannah Arendt. London: Fontana Press.

———. 1973c. "The Storyteller: Reflections on the Works of Nikolai Leskov." In *Illuminations*, ed. Hannah Arendt. London: Fontana Press.

Bernstein, Charles. 1998. "Introduction." In *Close Listening: Poetry and the Performed Word*, ed. Charles Bernstein. New York: Oxford University Press, p. 3–26.

Bernstein, Jay H. 1997. *Spirits Captured in Stone: Shamanism & Traditional Medicine among the Taman of Borneo*. London: Lynne Rienner Publishers.

Bird-David, Nurit. 1999. "'Animism' Revisited: Personhood, Environment, and Relational Epistemology." *Current Anthropology* 40: S67–S91.
———. 2004. "Illness-images and Joined Beings: A Critical/Nayaka Perspective on Intercorporeality." *Social Anthropology* 12(3): 325–339.
———. 2006. "Animistic Epistemology: Why Do Some Hunter-Gatherers Not Depict Animals?" *Ethnos* 71(I): 33–50.
Bloch, Maurice. 1971. *Placing the Dead: Tombs, Ancestral Villages, and Kinship Organization in Madagascar.* London: Seminar Press.
———. 1974. "Symbols, Song, Dance and Features of Articulation: Is Religion an Extreme Form of Traditional Authority?" *Archives Européenes de Sociologie* 15: 54–81.
Bock, Carl. 1988 [1881]. *The Headhunters of Borneo: A Narrative of Travel up the Mahakam and Down the Barito.* Singapore: Graham Brash Ltd.
Boddy, Janice. 1995. "Managing Tradition: 'Superstition' and the Making of National Identity among Sudanese Women Refugees." In *The Pursuit of Certainty: Religious and Cultural Formulations,* ed. Wendy James. London: Routledge, pp. 17–44.
Bourdieu, Pierre. 1977. *Outline of a Theory of Practice.* Cambridge: Cambridge University Press.
———. 1980. *The Logic of Practice.* Stanford: Stanford University Press.
———. 1994. "Structures, Habitus, Power: Basis for a Theory of Symbolic Power." In *Culture, Power, History: A Reader in Contemporary Social Theory,* ed. Nicholas B. Dirks, Geoff Eley and Sherry B. Ortner. Princeton: Princeton University Press, pp. 155–199.
Bowen, John R. 1991. *Sumatran Politics and Poetics: Gayo History 1900–1989.* New Haven: Yale University Press.
Brandon, James R. 1967. *Theatre in Southeast Asia.* Cambridge: Harvard University Press.
Briggs, Charles. L. 1996. "The Meaning of Nonsense, the Poetics of Embodiment, and the Production of Power in Warao Healing." In *The Performance of Healing,* ed. Carol Laderman and Marina Roseman. New York: Routledge, pp. 185–232.
Briggs, Charles L. and Richard Bauman. 1992. "Genre, Intertextuality, and Social Power." *Journal of Linguistic Anthropology* 2(2): 131–172.
Bruner, Jerome S. 1986. *Actual Minds, Possible Worlds.* Cambridge: Harvard University Press.
Buijs, Kees. 2006. *Powers of Blessing from the Wilderness and from Heaven: Structure and Transformation in the Religion of the Toraja in the Mamasa Area.* Leiden: KITLV Press.
Carsten, Janet. 1995. "The Substance of Kinship and the Heat of the Hearth: Feeding, Personhood, and Relatedness among Malays in Pulau Langkawi." *American Ethnologist* 22(2): 223–241.
Chalmers, Ian. 2006. *The Dynamics of Conversion: The Islamisation of the Dayak Peoples of Central Kalimantan.* Paper presented at the 16th Biennial Conference of the Asian Studies Association of Australia in Wollongong, 26–29 June 2006.

Clifford, James. 1997. *Routes: Travel and Translation in the Late Twentieth Century*. Cambridge: Harvard University Press.

Connerton, Paul. 1989. *How Societies Remember*. Cambridge: Cambridge University Press.

Coville, Elizabeth. 1989. "Centripetal Ritual in a Decentered World: Changing Maro Performances in Tana Toraja." In *Changing Lives, Changing Rites: Ritual and Social Dynamics in Philippine and Indonesian Uplands*, ed. Susan D. Russell and Clark E. Cunningham. Michigan: Center for South and Southeast Asian Studies, University of Michigan, pp. 103–132.

Csordas, Thomas J. 1996. "Imaginal Performance and Memory in Ritual Healing." In *The Performance of Healing*, ed. Carol Laderman and Marina Roseman. New York: Routledge, pp. 91–114.

Dalton, J. 1986 [1831]. "Mr Dalton's Journal of a Tour up the Coti River." In *Kutai, East Kalimantan: A Journal of Past and Present Glory*, ed. David Boyce. Kota Bangun. Originally published in the Singapore Chronicle, 12 May 1831.

Day, Tony. 2002. *Fluid Iron: State Formation in Southeast Asia*. Honolulu: University of Hawai'i Press.

de Certeau, Michel. 1984. *The Practice of Everyday Life*. Translated by Steven Rendall. Berkeley: University of California Press.

———. 1986. *Heterologies: Discourse on the Other*. Minneapolis: University of Minnesota Press.

Deren, Maya. 1965. "Notes on Ritual and Ordeal." *Film Culture* 39:10.

Derrida, Jacques. 1982 [1968]. "Différance." In *Margins of Philosophy*. Translated by Alan Bass. Chicago: University of Chicago Press, pp. 1–28.

Descola, Philippe. 1992. "Societies of Nature and the Nature of Society." In *Conceptualizing Society*, ed. A. Kuper. London: Routledge, pp. 107–126.

———. 1994. *In the Society of Nature: A Native Ecology in Amazonia*. Cambridge: Cambridge University Press.

———. 2006. "Beyond Nature and Culture: Radcliffe-Brown Lecture in Social Anthropology." *Proceedings of the British Academy* 139: 137–155.

———. 2009. "Human Natures." *Social Anthropology* 17(2): 145–157.

Dove, Michael R. 1988. "Introduction: Traditional Culture and Development in Contemporary Indonesia." In *The Real and Imagined Role of Culture in Development: Case Studies from Indonesia*, ed. Michael R. Dove. Honolulu: University of Hawaii Press, pp. 1–37.

———. 1993. "The Survival of Culture and the Culture of Survival: A Review Article." *Borneo Research Bulletin* 25: 168–181.

Drewal, Margaret T. 1992. *Yoruba Ritual: Performers, Play, Agency*. Bloomington: Indiana University Press.

Eliade, Mircea. 1964. *Shamanism: Archaic Techniques of Ecstasy*. Translated by William R. Trask. Princeton: Princeton University Press.

Endicott, Kirk. 1979. *Batek Negrito Religion: The World-View and Rituals of a Hunting and Gathering People of Peninsular Malaysia*. Oxford: Clarendon Press.

Errington, Shelly. 1989. *Meaning and Power in a Southeast Asian Realm*. Princeton: Princeton University Press.

Feldman, Jerome. 1985. "Ancestors in the Art of Indonesia and Southeast Asia." In *Ancestral Sculpture of Indonesia and Southeast Asia*, ed. Jerome Feldman. Los Angeles: UCLA Museum of Cultural History, pp. 35–44.

Fernandez, James. 1977. "The Performance of Ritual Metaphors." In *The Social Use of Metaphor: Essays on the Anthropology of Rhetoric*, ed. J.D. Sapir and J.C. Crocker. Philadelphia: University of Pennsylvania Press, pp. 100–131.

Feuilletau De Bruyn, W.K.H. 1934. "De Njoelibeweging in de Zuider- en Oosterafdeeling van Borneo." *Koloniaal Tijdschrift* 23: 41–65.

Firth, Raymond. 1967. *The Work of the Gods in Tikopia*. 2ⁿᵈ edn. London: Athlone Press.

Fox, James J. 1974. "Our Ancestors Spoke in Pairs: Rotinese Views of Language, Dialect, and Code." In *Explorations in the Ethnography of Speaking*, ed. Richard Bauman and Joel Sherzer. Cambridge: Cambridge University Press, pp. 65–85.

———. 1987. "Southeast Asian Religions: Insular Cultures." In *The Encyclopedia of Religion*, ed. M. Eliade. New York: Macmillan Publishing Company, vol. 13, pp. 520–530.

———. 1996. "Introduction." In *Origins, Ancestry and Alliance: Explorations in Austronesian Ethnography*, ed. James Fox and Clifford Sather. Canberra: The Australian National University, pp. 1–17.

Frazer, James G. 1922. *The Golden Bough. A Study in Magic and Religion*. Abridged edition. London: MacMillan.

Freeman, Derek. 1967. "Shaman and Incubus." *The Psychoanalytic Study of Society* 4: 315–343.

Fried, Stephanie G. 2001. "Shoot the Horse to Get the Rider: Religion and Forest Politics in Bentian Borneo." In *Indigenous Traditions and Ecology: The Interbeing of Cosmology and Community*, ed. John A. Grim. Cambridge: Harvard University Press, pp. 71–102.

———. 2003. "Writing for their Lives: Bentian Dayak Authors and Indonesian Development Discourse." In *Culture and the Question of Rights: Forests, Coasts, and Seas in Southeast Asia*, ed. Charles Zerner. Durham: Duke University Press, pp. 142–183.

Geertz, Clifford. 1966. "Religion as a Cultural System." In *Anthropological Approaches to the Study of Religion*, ed. M. Banton. Association of Social Anthropologists of the Commonwealth, Monograph 3. London: Tavistock Publications, pp. 1–46.

———. 1973a. "'Internal Conversion' in Contemporary Bali." In *The Interpretation of Cultures*. New York: Basic Books, pp. 170–189.

———. 1973b. "Ritual and Social Change: A Javanese Example." In *The Interpretation of Cultures*. New York: Basic Books, pp. 142–169.

———. 1980. *Negara: The Theater State in Nineteenth Century Bali*. Princeton: Princeton University Press.

George, Kenneth M. 1996. *Showing Signs of Violence: The Cultural Politics of a Twentieth-Century Headhunting Ritual*. Berkeley: University of California Press.

Geurts, Kathryn L. 2005. "Consciousness as 'Feeling in the Body': A West African Theory of Embodiment, Emotion and the Making of Mind." In *Empire of the Senses: the Sensual Culture Reader*, ed. David Howes. Oxford: Berg, pp. 164–178.

Gibson, Thomas. 2005. *And the Sun Pursued the Moon: Symbolic Knowledge and Traditional Authority among the Makassar*. Honolulu: University of Hawaii Press.

Girard, René. 1978a. "Differentiation and Reciprocity in Lévi-Strauss and Contemporary Theory." In *To Double Business Bound: Essays on Literature, Mimesis, and Anthropology*. Baltimore: The Johns Hopkins University Press, pp. 155–177.

———. 1978b. "Violence and Representation in Mythical Text." In *To Double Business Bound: Essays on Literature, Mimesis, and Anthropology*. Baltimore: The Johns Hopkins University Press, pp. 178–198.

Goffman, Erving. 1959. *The Presentation of Self in Everyday Life*. Garden City, NY: Doubleday Anchor.

———. 1974. *Frame Analysis. An Essay on the Organization of Experience*. Cambridge: Harvard University Press.

Golomb, Louis. 1985. *An Anthropology of Curing in Multiethnic Thailand*. Urbana: University of Illinois Press.

Gönner, Christian. 2002. *A Forest Tribe of Borneo: Resource Use among the Dayak Benuaq*. New Delhi: D. K. Printworld Ltd.

Grabowsky, F. 1888. "Die 'Olon Lawangan' in Südostborneo." *Ausland*, 581–585.

Grice, H.P. 1957. "Meaning." *Philosophical Review* 64: 377–388.

Handelman, Don. 1990. *Models and Mirrors: Towards an Anthropology of Public Events*. Cambridge: Cambridge University Press.

———. 2005. "Epilogue: Toing and Froing the Social." In *Ritual in its Own Right: Exploring the Dynamics of Transformation*, ed. Don Handelman and Galina Lindquist. New York: Berghahn Books, pp. 213–222.

———. 2006. "Framing." In *Theorizing Rituals: Issues, Topics, Approaches, Concepts*, ed. Jens Kreinath, Jan Snoek and Michael Strausberg. Leiden: Brill, pp. 571–582.

Hanks, William F. 1987. "Discourse Genres in a Theory of Practice." *American Ethnologist* 14(4): 668–692.

Haraway, Donna. 2003. *The Companion Species Manifesto: Dogs, People, and Significant Otherness*. Chicago: Prickly Paradigm Press.

Harris, Amanda. 2001. "Presence, Efficacy, and Politics in Healing among the Iban of Sarawak." In *Healing Powers and Modernity: Traditional Medicine, Shamanism, and Science in Asian Societies*, ed. Linda H. Connor and Geoffrey Samuel. Westport: Bergin & Garvey, pp. 130–151.

Hayles, N. Katherine. 1992. "The Materiality of Informatics." *Configurations* 1(1): 147–170.

Hefner, Robert W. 1985. *Hindu Javanese: Tengger Tradition and Islam*. Princeton: Princeton University Press.

———. 1990. *The Political Economy of Mountain Java: An Interpretative History*. Berkeley: University of California Press.

Hertz, Robert. 1960 [1907]. _Death and the Right Hand_. Translated by Rodney Needham and Claudia Needham. New York: Free Press.

Heryanto, Ariel. 1988. "The Development of 'Development.'" _Indonesia_ 46: 1–24.

Hopes, Michael, Madrah and Karaakng. 1997. _Temputn: Myths of the Benuaq and Tunjung Dayak_. Jakarta: Puspa Swara and Rio Tinto Foundation.

Hoskins, Janet. 1996. "From Diagnosis to Performance: Medical Practice and the Politics of Exchange in Kodi, West Sumba." In _The Performance of Healing_, ed. Carol Laderman and Marina Roseman. New York: Routledge, pp. 271–290.

Howe, Leo. 2000. "Risk, Ritual and Performance." _Journal of the Royal Anthropological Institute_ 6: 63–79.

Howell, Signe. 1989. _Society and Cosmos: Chewong of Peninsular Malaysia_. Chicago: The University of Chicago Press.

Hudson, Alfred. 1966. "Death Ceremonies of the Paju Epat Ma'anyan Dayaks." _Sarawak Museum Journal_, special monograph no. 1: "Borneo Writing and Related Matters."

———. 1967a. _The Barito Isolects of Borneo_. Data Paper No. 68, Department of Southeast Asian Studies. Ithaca: Cornell University Press.

———. 1967b. "The Padju Epat Ma'anjan Dayak in Historical Perspective." _Indonesia_ 4: 8–42.

Humphrey, Caroline and James Laidlaw. 1994. _The Archetypal Actions of Ritual. A Theory of Ritual Illustrated by the Jain Rite of Worship_. Oxford: Clarendon Press.

Hymes, Dell. 1975. "Breakthrough into Performance." In _Folklore: Performance and Communication_, ed. Dan Ben-Amos and Kenneth S. Goldstein. The Hague: Mouton, pp. 11–74.

Ingold, Tim. 2000. _The Perception of the Environment: Essays on Livelihood, Dwelling and Skill_. New York: Routledge.

———. 2004. "A Circumpolar Night's Dream." In _Figured Worlds: Ontological Obstacles in Intercultural Relations_, ed. J. Clammer, S. Poirier, and E. Schwimmer. Toronto: University of Toronto Press, pp. 25–57.

———. 2006. "Rethinking the Animate, Re-Animating Thought." _Ethnos_ 71(1): 9–20.

Jackson, Michael. 1998. _Minima Ethnographica: Intersubjectivity and the Anthropological Project_. Chicago: The University of Chicago Press.

———. 2005. _Existential Anthropology: Events, Exigencies and Effects_. Oxford: Berghahn Books.

———. 2007. _Excursions_. Durham: Duke University Press.

Jay, Sian. 1989. "The Basir and Tukang Sangiang: Two Kinds of Shaman among the Ngaju Dayak." _Indonesia Circle_ 49: 31–44.

———. 1993. "Canoes for the Spirits: Two Types of Spirit Mediumship in Central Kalimantan." In _The Seen and the Unseen: Shamanism, Mediumship and Possession in Borneo_, ed. Robert Winzeler. Borneo Research Council Monograph Series, vol. 2. Williamsburg: Borneo Research Council, pp. 151–170.

Kapferer, Bruce. 1991. *Celebration of Demons*. Washington/London: Smithsonian Institution Press/Berg.

———. 1997. *The Feast of the Sorcerer: Practices of Consciousness and Power*. Chicago: The University of Chicago Press.

———. 2005. "Ritual Dynamics and Virtual Practice: Beyond Representation and Meaning." In *Ritual in its Own Right*, ed. Don Handelman and Galina Lindquist. New York: Berghahn Books, pp. 35–54.

———. 2006. "Virtuality." In *Theorizing Rituals: Issues, Topics, Approaches, Concepts*, ed. Jens Kreinath, Jan Snoek and Michael Strausberg. Leiden: Brill, pp. 671–684.

———. 2008. "Beyond Symbolic Representation: Victor Turner and Variations on the Theme of Ritual Process and Liminality." *Journal of the Finnish Anthropological Society* 33(4): 5–25.

Keane, Webb. 1997. *Signs of Recognition: Powers and Hazards of Representation in an Indonesian Society*. Berkeley: University of California Press.

———. 2007. *Christian Moderns: Freedom and Fetish in the Mission Encounter*. Berkeley: University of California Press.

———. 2008. "The Evidence of the Senses and the Materiality of Religion." *Journal of the Royal Anthropological Institute* 14(1): 110–127.

———. 2010. "Marked, Absent, Habitual: Approaches to Neolitic Religion in Çatalhöyük." In *Religion in the Emergence of Civilization: Çatalhöyük as a Case Study*, ed. Ian Hodder. Cambridge: Cambridge University Press, pp. 47–76.

King, Victor T. 1979. *Ethnic Classification and Ethnic Relations: A Borneo Case Study*. Hull: University of Hull, Centre for Southeast Asian Studies, Occasional Papers no. 2.

———. 1993. *The Peoples of Borneo*. Oxford: Blackwell.

Kipp, Rita Smith. 1993. *Dissociated Identities: Ethnicity, Religion, and Class in an Indonesian Society*. Michigan: The University of Michigan Press.

Knapen, Han. 2001. *Forests of Fortune? The Environmental History of Southeast Borneo, 1600–1880*. Leiden: KITLV Press.

Knappert, S.C. 1905. "Beschrijving van de Onderafdeeling Koetai." *Bijdragen tot de Taal-, Land- en Volkenkunde* 58: 575–639.

Koblenzer, P.J. and N.H. Carrier. 1959–1960. "The Fertility, Mortality, and Nuptiality of the Rungus Dusun." *Population Studies* 13(3): 266–277.

Kondo, Dorinne K. 1990. *Crafting Selves: Power, Gender, and Discourses of Identity in a Japanese Workplace*. Chicago: University of Chicago Press.

Kotilainen, Eija-Maija. 1992. *When the Bones are Left: A Study of the Material Culture of Central Sulawesi*. Helsinki: The Finnish Anthropological Society.

Kuipers, Joel C. 1990. *Power in Performance: The Creation of Textual Authority in Weyewa Ritual Speech*. Philadelphia: University of Pennsylvania Press.

Laderman, Carol. 1983. *Wives & Midwives: Childbirth and Nutrition in Rural Malaysia*. Berkeley: University of California Press.

———. 1996. "The Poetics of Healing in Malay Shamanistic Performances." In *The Performance of Healing*, ed. Carol Laderman and Marina Roseman. New York: Routledge, pp. 115–142.

Lambek, Michael. 1981. *Human Spirits: A Cultural Account of Trance in Mayotte*. Cambridge: Cambridge University Press.

———. 2007. "Sacrifice and the Problem of Beginning: Meditations from Sakalava Mythopraxis." *Journal of the Royal Anthropological Institute* 13: 19–38.

Lawrence, A.E. and J. Hewitt. 1908. "Some Aspects on Spirit Worship amongst the Milano of Sarawak." *Journal of the Royal Anthropological Institute of GB and Ireland* 38: 388–408.

Lemanius. 1996. *Kitab Suci Sinar Mulia*. Unpublished manuscript.

Lévi-Strauss, Claude. 1963. "The Effectiveness of Symbols." In *Structural Anthropology*. New York: Anchor Books, pp. 181–201.

———. 1969. *The Raw and the Cooked: Introduction to a Science of Mythology*. Translated by John and Doreen Weightman. New York: Harper and Row.

———. 1981. "Finale." In *The Naked Man*. Translated by John and Doreen Weightman. New York: Harper and Row, pp. 625–695.

Lewis, Gilbert. 1980. *Day of Shining Red: An Essay on Understanding Ritual*. Cambridge: Cambridge University Press.

Li, Tania M. 1999. "Introduction." In *Transforming the Indonesian Uplands: Marginality, Power and Production*, ed. Tania Li. Amsterdam: Harwood Academic Publishers, pp. xiii–xxii.

Lindquist, Galina. 2008. "Loyalty and Command: Shamans, Lamas, and Spirits in a Siberian Ritual." *Social Analysis* 52(1): 111–126.

MacIntyre, Alasdair. 1988. *Whose Justice? Which Rationality?* Notre Dame: University of Notre Dame Press.

Magenda, Burhan. 1991. *East Kalimantan: The Decline of a Commercial Aristocracy*. Ithaca: Cornell Modern Indonesia Project, Monograph Series no. 70.

Mahin, Marko. 2009. *Kaharingan: Dinamika Agama Dayak di Kalimantan Tengah*. Ph.D. diss., Universitas Indonesia.

Maks, H.G. 1861. "Reis naar de Kapoeas en Kahajan in de Zuider- en Oosterafdeeling van Borneo. In de maanden maart, april en mai 1859." *Bijdragen tot de Taal-, Land- en Volkenkunde* 10(5/6): 466–558.

Mallinckrodt, Jacob. 1928. *Het Adatrecht van Borneo*, vol 1–2. Leiden: Dubbelman.

———. 1974 [1925]. *Gerakan Nyuli di Kalangan Suku Dayak Lawangan*. Jakarta: Bhratara.

Masing, James J. 1997. *The Coming of the Gods: An Iban Invocatory Chant (Timang Gawai) of the Balei River Region, Sarawak. Vol. 1: Description and Analysis*. Canberra: The Australian National University, Department of Anthropology, Research School of Pacific and Asian Studies.

Massing, Andreas W. 1982. "Where Medicine Fails: Belian Disease Prevention and Curing Rituals among the Lawangan Dayak of East Kalimantan." *Borneo Research Bulletin* 14(2): 56–84.

Mauss, Marcel. 1925. "Essai sur le don: Forme et raison de l'échange dans les sociétés archaïques." *L'Année sociologique*, new series 1.

Metcalf, Peter. 1989. *Where Are You Spirits: Style and Theme in Berawan Prayer.* Washington: Smithsonian Institution Press.

———. 1991 [1982]. *A Borneo Journey into Death: Berawan Eschatology from its Rituals.* Kuala Lumpur: S. Abdul Majeed & Co.

———. 2002. *They Lie, We Lie: Getting on with Anthropology.* London: Routledge.

———. 2010. *The Life of the Longhouse: An Archaeology of Ethnicity.* Cambridge: Cambridge University Press.

Metcalf, Peter and Richard Huntington. 1976. *Celebrations of Death: The Anthropology of Mortuary Ritual.* New York: Cambridge University Press.

Miles, Douglas. 1965. "Socio-Economic Aspects of Secondary Burial." *Oceania* XXXV: 161–174.

———. 1966. "Shamanism and the Conversion of Ngadju Dayaks." *Oceania* XXXVII 1: 1–12.

———. 1976. *Cutlass and Crescent Moon: A Case Study of Social and Political Change in Outer Indonesia.* Sydney: Centre for Asian Studies, University of Sydney.

Mitchell, Stanley. 1973. "Introduction." In *Understanding Brecht*, Walter Benjamin. London: New Left Books, pp. vii–xix.

Momberg, F., R. Puri and T. Jessup. 2000. "Exploitation of Gaharu, and Forest Conservation Efforts in the Kayan Mentarang National Park, East Kalimantan, Indonesia." In *People, Plants, and Justice: the Politics of Nature Conservation*, ed. Charles Zerner. New York: Columbia University Press, pp. 259–284.

Moore, Rachel O. 2000. *Savage Theory: Cinema as Modern Magic.* Durham: Duke University Press.

Morris, Harold S. 1993. "Shamanism among the Oya Melanau." In *The Seen and the Unseen*, ed. Robert Winzeler. Borneo Research Council Monograph Series, vol. 2. Williamsburg: Borneo Research Council, pp. 101–130.

———. 1997. "The Oya Melanau: Traditional Ritual and Belief with a Catalogue of Belum Carvings." *Sarawak Museum Journal* LII (73), special monograph no 9.

Müller, Salomon. 1857. *Reizen en Onderzoekingen in den Indischen Archipel*, vol. 1. Amsterdam: Frederik Muller.

Ortiz, Alfonso. 1969. *The Tewa World: Space, Time, Being, and Becoming in a Pueblo Society.* Chicago: Chicago University Press.

Ortner, Sherry B. 1978. *Sherpas through their Rituals.* Cambridge: Cambridge University Press.

———. 1989. *High Religion: A Cultural and Political History of Sherpa Buddhism.* Princeton: Princeton University Press.

Palmer, Gary B. and William R. Jankowiak. 1996. "Performance and Imagination: Toward an Anthropology of the Spectacular and the Mundane." *Cultural Anthropology* 11(2): 225–258.

Pedersen, Axel M. 2007. "Talismans of Thought: Shamanist Ontologies and Extended Cognition in Northern Mongolia." In *Thinking through Things: Theorising Artefacts Ethnographically*, ed. Amiria Henare, Martin Holbraad and Sari Wastell. London: Routledge, pp. 141–166.

Pedersen, Lene. 2006. *Ritual and World Change in a Balinese Princedom.* Durham: Carolina Academic Press.

Peluso, Nancy. 1992. *Rich Forests, Poor People: Resource Control and Resistance in Java.* Berkeley: University of California Press.

Pemberton, John. 1994. *On the Subject of "Java."* Ithaca: Cornell University Press.

Picard, Michel. 2004. "What's in a Name? Agama Hindu Bali in the Making." In *Hinduism in Modern Indonesia: A Minority Religion between Local, National, and Global Interests,* ed. Martin Ramstedt. London: RoutledgeCurzon, pp. 56–75.

Proust, Marcel. 1913. *A la recherche du temps perdu. Vol. 1: Du côté de chez Swann.* Paris: Grasset.

Radcliffe-Brown, Alfred. R. 1940. "On Social Structure." In *Structure and Function in Primitive Society.* London: Cohen and West.

Ramstedt, Martin. 2004a. "Introduction: Negotiating Identities – Indonesian 'Hindus' between Local, National, and Global Interests." In *Hinduism in Modern Indonesia: A Minority Religion between Local, National, and Global Interests,* ed. Martin Ramstedt. London: Routledge, pp. 1–34.

———. 2004b. "The Hinduization of Local Traditions in South Sulawesi." In *Hinduism in Modern Indonesia: A Minority Religion between Local, National, and Global Interests,* ed. Martin Ramstedt. London: Routledge, pp. 184–225.

Rao, Ursula. 2006. "Ritual in Society." In *Theorizing Rituals: Issues, Topics, Approaches, Concepts,* ed. Jens Kreinath, Jan Snoek and Michael Strausberg. Leiden: Brill, pp. 143–160.

Rappaport, Roy A. 1999. *Ritual and Religion in the Making of Humanity.* Cambridge: Cambridge University Press.

Reibel, G.J. 1976. *Landnutzung und Sozialstruktur im Hinterland von Sampit (Sudborneo).* Bonn: Rheinischen Friedrich-Wilhelms Universität.

Riwut, Tjilik. 1958. *Kalimantan Memanggil.* Jakarta: Endang.

Rosaldo, Renato. 1980. *Ilongot Headhunting 1883–1974: A Study in Society and History.* Stanford: Stanford University Press.

———. 1989. *Culture and Truth: The Remaking of Social Analysis.* London: Routledge.

———. 1993. "Ilongot Visiting: Social Grace and the Rhythms of Everyday Life." In *Creativity/Anthropology,* ed. S. Lavie, K. Narayan and R. Rosaldo. Ithaca: Cornell University Press, pp. 253–269.

Roseman, Marina. 1990. "Head, Heart, Odor, and Shadow: The Structure of the Self, the Emotional World, and Ritual Performance among Senoi Temiar." *Ethos* 18(3): 227–250.

———. 1991. *Healing Sounds from the Malaysian Rainforest: Temiar Music and Medicine.* Berkeley: University of California Press.

———. 1996. "'Pure Products Go Crazy': Rainforest Healing in a Nation-State." In *The Performance of Healing,* ed. Carol Laderman and Marina Roseman. New York: Routledge, pp. 233–270.

———. 2002. "Making Sense out of Modernity." In *New Horizons in Medical Anthropology: Essays in Honour of Charles Leslie,* ed. Mark Nichter and Margaret Lock. New York: Routledge, pp. 111–140.

Rousseau, Jérôme. 1990. *Central Borneo: Ethnic Identity and Social Life in a Stratified Society.* Oxford: Oxford University Press.

———. 1998. *Kayan Religion: Ritual Life and Religious Reform in Central Borneo.* Leiden: KITLV Press.

Rutherford, Danilyn. 1996. "Of Birds and Gifts: Reviving Tradition on an Indonesian Frontier." *Cultural Anthropology* 11(4): 577–616.

———. 2000. "The White Edge of the Margin: Textuality and Authority in Biak, Irian Jaya, Indonesia. *American Ethnologist* 27(2): 312–339.

Sather, Clifford. 1988. "Meri' Anak Mandi': The Ritual First Bathing of Infants among the Iban." *Contributions to Southeast Asian Ethnography* 7: 157–187.

———. 2001. *Seeds of Play, Words of Power: An Ethnographic Study of Iban Shamanic Chants.* Kuala Lumpur: The Tun Jugah Foundation.

Schärer, Hans. 1966. *Der Totenkult der Ngadju Dayak in Süd-Borneo.* 2 vols. Verhandelingen van het Koninklijk Instituut voor Taal-, Land-, en Volkenkunde 5 (1 & 2). The Hague: Martinus Nijhoff.

Schechner, Richard. 1985. *Between Theatre and Anthropology.* Philadelphia: University of Pennsylvania Press.

———. 2002. *Performance Studies: An Introduction.* London: Routledge.

Schepher-Hughes, Nancy. 1992. *Death without Weeping: The Violence of Everyday Life in Brazil.* Berkeley: University of California Press.

Schieffelin, Edward. 1985. "Performance and the Cultural Construction of Reality." *American Ethnologist* 12(4): 707–724.

———. 1996. "On Failure and Performance: Throwing the Medium Out of the Seance." In *The Performance of Healing,* ed. Carol Laderman and Marina Roseman. New York: Routledge, pp. 59–90.

Schiller, Anne. 1986. "A Ngaju Ritual Specialist and the Rationalization of Hindu-Kaharingan." *The Sarawak Museum Journal* 57: 231–241.

———. 1987. *Dynamics of Death: Ritual, Identity, and Religious Change among the Kalimantan Ngaju.* Ph.D. dissertation, Cornell University.

———. 1997. *Small Sacrifices: Religious Change and Cultural Identity among the Ngaju of Indonesia.* New York: Oxford University Press.

Schwaner, C.A.L.M. 1853. *Borneo. Vol. 1: Bescrijving van het Stroomgebied van den Borneo.* Amsterdam: P. N. van Kampen.

Scott, James. 2009. *The Art of Not Being Governed: An Anarchist History of Upland Southeast Asia.* New Haven: Yale University Press.

Searle, John. 1969. *Speech Acts.* Cambridge: Cambridge University Press.

Sellato, Bernard. 1989. *Hornbill and Dragon.* Jakarta: Elf Aquitaine Indonésie.

Seremetakis, Nadia C. 1991. *The Last Word: Women, Death, and Divination in Inner Mani.* Chicago: The University of Chicago Press.

———. 1994a. "The Memory of the Senses, Part I: Marks of the Transitory." In *The Senses Still: Perception and Memory as Material Culture in Modernity,* ed. Nadia Seremetakis. Chicago: University of Chicago Press, pp. 1–18.

————. 1994b. "The Memory of the Senses, Part II: Still Acts." In *The Senses Still: Perception and Memory as Material Culture in Modernity*, ed. Nadia Seremetakis. Chicago: University of Chicago Press, pp. 23–44.

Siegel, James T. 1983. "Images and Odors in Javanese Practices Surrounding Death." *Indonesia* 36: 1–14.

Sillander, Kenneth. 1995. "Local Identity and Regional Variation: Notes on the Lack of Significance of Ethnicity among the Bentian and the Luangan." *Borneo Research Bulletin* 26: 69–95.

————. 2004. *Acting Authoritatively: How Authority is Expressed among the Bentian of Indonesian Borneo*. Helsinki: University of Helsinki Press.

————. 2006. "Local Integration and Coastal Connections in Interior Kalimantan: the Case of the Nalin Taun Ritual among the Bentian." *Journal of Southeast Asian Studies* 37: 315–334.

————. 2010. "Teknonymy, Name-Avoidance, Solidarity and Individuation among the Bentian of Indonesian Borneo." In *Personal Names in Asia: History, Culture and Identity*, ed. Zheng Yangwen and Charles Macdonald. Singapore: NUS Press, pp. 101–127.

Silverstein, Michael and Greg Urban (eds). 1996. *Natural Histories of Discourse*. Chicago: University of Chicago Press.

Singer, Milton. 1958. "From the Guest Editor." *Journal of American Folklore* 71: 191–204.

Sjamsuddin, Helius. 1989. *Fighting Dutch Rule in the Nineteenth and Early Twentieth Centuries: The Social, Political, Ethnic and Dynastic Roots of Resistance in South and Central Kalimantan, 1859–1906*. Ph.D. dissertation, Monash University.

Spyer, Patricia. 1996. "Diversity with a Difference: *Adat* and the New Order in Aru (Eastern Indonesia)." *Cultural Anthropology* 11(1): 25–50.

————. 2000. *The Memory of Trade: Modernity's Entanglements on an Eastern Indonesian Island*. Durham: Duke University Press.

Steedly, Mary M. 1993. *Hanging without a Rope: Narrative Experience in Colonial and Postcolonial Karoland*. Princeton: Princeton University Press.

Stöhr, Waldemar. 1959. *Das Totenritual der Dajak*. Ethnologica, Neue Folge, band 1. Köln: Brill.

Stoller, Paul. 1997. *Sensuous Scholarship*. Philadelphia: University of Pennsylvania Press.

Struktur Bahasa Bawo. 1989. Jakarta: Pusat Pembinaan dan Pembangunan Bahasa, Departemen Pendidikan dan Kebudayaan.

Sweeney, Amin. 1987. *A Full Hearing: Orality and Literacy in the Malay World*. Berkeley: University of California Press.

Tambiah, Stanley J. 1985. *Culture, Thought, and Social Action: An Anthropological Perspective*. Cambridge: Harvard University Press.

Taussig, Michael. 1987. *Shamanism, Colonialism, and the Wild Man: A Study in Terror and Healing*. Chicago: The University of Chicago Press.

————. 1992. *The Nervous System*. New York: Routledge.

————. 1993. *Mimesis and Alterity: A Particular History of the Senses*. New York: Routledge.

————. 2009. *What Color is the Sacred?* Chicago: The University of Chicago Press.

Team Survey Suku Bawo. 1972. *Laporan Survey Suku Bawo, Kampung Bintang Ara, Kecamatan Gunung Bintang Awai, Kabupaten Barito Sealatan, Propinsi Kalimantan Tengah*. Jakarta: Direktorat Pembangunan Masyarakat Suku Terasing.

Tedlock, Dennis. 1993. *Breath on the Mirror: Mythic Voices*. San Francisco: Harper.

Tillema, H.F. 1939. "Jagerstammen op Borneo." *Onze aarde* 12.

Tromp, S.W. 1887. "Eenige Mededeelingen Omtrent de Boegineezen van Koetai." *Bijdragen tot de Taal-, Land- en Volkenkunde* 36: 167–198.

Tsing, Anna L. 1984. *Politics and Culture in the Meratus Mountains*. Ph.D. dissertation, Stanford University.

————. 1988. "Healing Boundaries in South Kalimantan." *Social Science Medicine* 27(8): 829–839.

————. 1990. "Gender and Performance in Meratus Dispute Settlement." In *Power and Difference: Gender in Island Southeast Asia*, ed. Jane Atkinson and Shelly Errington. Stanford: Stanford University Press, pp. 95–125.

————. 1993. *In the Realm of the Diamond Queen: Marginality in an Out-of-the-Way Place*. Princeton: Princeton University Press.

————. 1994. "From the Margins." *Cultural Anthropology* 9(3): 279–297.

Turner, Terence. 2006. "Structure, Process, Form." In *Theorizing Rituals: Issues, Topics, Approaches, Concepts*, ed. Jens Kreinath, Jan Snoek and Michael Strausberg. Leiden: Brill, pp. 207–246.

Turner, Victor. 1969. *The Ritual Process: Structure and Anti-Structure*. Harmondsworth: Penguin.

Tylor, Edward. B. 1871. *Religion in Primitive Society*. Gloucester: Peter Smith.

Urban, Greg. 1996. *Metaphysical Community: The Interplay between the Senses and the Intellect*. Austin: University of Texas Press.

Viveiros de Castro, Eduardo. 1998. "Cosmological Deixis and Amer-Indian Perspectivism." *Journal of the Royal Anthropological Institute* 4(3): 469–488.

————. 2004. "Exchanging Perspectives: The Transformation of Objects into Subjects in Amerindian Ontologies." *Common Knowledge* 10(3): 463–484.

Volkman, Toby A. 1985. *Feasts of Honor: Ritual and Change in the Toraja Highlands*. Urbana: University of Illinois Press.

de Vries, M.W. 1987. "Cry Babies, Culture, and Catastrophe: Infant Temperament among the Masai." In *Child Survival: Anthropological Perspectives on the Treatment and Maltreatment of Children*, ed. Nancy Scheper-Hughes. Dordrecht: D. Reidel Publishing Company, pp. 165–186.

Wadley, Reed L. 2000. "Reconsidering an Ethnic Label in Borneo: The 'Maloh' of West Kalimantan, Indonesia." *Bijdragen tot de Taal-, Land- en Volkenkunde* 156(1): 83–101.

Wechel, P. te. 1915. "Erinnerung an den Ost- und West-Dusun Ländern (Borneo)." *Internationales Archiv für Ethnographie* 22: 1–24, 43–58, 93–129.

Weinstock, Joseph. 1983. *Kaharingan and the Luangan Dayaks: Religion and Identity in Central-East Borneo*. Ph.D. dissertation, Cornell University.

Whittier, Herbert L. 1973. *Social Organization and Symbols of Social Differentiation: An Ethnographic Study of the Kenyah Dayak of East Kalimantan*. Ph.D. dissertation, Michigan State University.

Whyte, Susan Reynolds. 1997. *Questioning Misfortune: The Pragmatics of Uncertainty in Eastern Uganda*. Cambridge: Cambridge University Press.

Wikan, Unni. 1990. *Managing Turbulent Hearts: A Balinese Formula for Living*. Chicago: University of Chicago Press.

Wilder, William D. (ed.). 2003. *Journeys of the Soul: Anthropological Studies of Death, Burial, and Reburial Practices in Borneo*. Borneo Research Council Monograph Series, vol. 7. Maine: Borneo Research Council.

Wortmann, J.R. 1971. "The Sultanate of Kutai, Kalimantan-Timur, Borneo: A Sketch of the Traditional Political Structure." *Borneo Research Bulletin* 3(2): 51–55.

Index

Pahu: as religious center, 77; River, 77, 88n3
Palangkaraya, 65, 75, 76, 79–81, 110
pali (taboo), 133, 155, 173n6, 183, 202, 206, 211, 227, 251. *See also* taboo
Palmer, Gary B., 119
Pancasila (ideology), 62
parallelism, 56, 190, 193, 194, 241. *See also* ritual language
Pasir: language, 49, 56; region, 58, 117
Pedersen, Axel M., 119
Pedersen, Lene, 16
pejiak pejiau ("undoing and redoing"), 13, 54, 95, 186, 195, 213, 226, 231, 259
Peluso, Nancy, 66
Pemberton, John, 62
penyelenteng (ritual paraphernalia), 71, 94, 136
penyempatung (ritual assistant), 23n4, 90n13, 131, 146
pereau (divination), 53, 122n23, 131, 132, 133, 138, 139, 148, 149, 153, 159, 173n3, 176n23
performance theory, 15
personhood, 230
poiesis, 262
poisoning, 34, 231, 253n21
polyandry. *See* marriage
polygyny. *See* marriage
possession, 48, 72, 78, 164, 166, 168
power: discourse of, 60–62; foreign, 78, 157–158, 169; of the past, 118; political, 43–44, 60–62, 163; shamanistic, 82, 86, 92; spiritual, 6, 48, 75, 86, 92, 168, 169, 208; of tradition, 119, 245; of women, 87; of words, 72, 172, 193
practice theory, 9, 15, 18
Proust, Marcel, 116

Radcliffe-Brown, Alfred R., 210
rainforest, 37, 217
Ramstedt, Martin, 62, 63, 70n14
Rao, Ursula, 15
Rappaport, Roy, 20, 22n4

rattan, 25, 34, 37, 39, 47, 49, 133, 227; cultivation of, 61
Reibel, Günther J., 214n3
relatedness, 230, 232, 237, 244–245, 247–248, 250, 251n8, 257
relational epistemology, 257
religion: Austonesian, 13; Indonesian politics of, 60, 62, 80, 249; lack of, 62, 63, 81, 89n6, 255; and Luangan identity, 21, 25, 28–30, 63, 65; in opposition to tradition (*adat*), 22n3; world religion, 64, 111, 120n1, 256. *See also agama*; Hindu Kaharingan; Kaharingan
religious rationalization, 64, 80
representation: and reality, 2, 92, 103, 105, 112, 125–126, 150, 172, 256, 258; and ritual, 1, 9–13, 20, 85, 259
retelling: narrative, 222, 245; ritual, 244
ritual: audience, 14, 37, 49, 56, 69n9, 77, 80, 102, 113–115, 117, 145, 168, 194, 199, 202, 212, 224, 241, 259; and change, 6, 12, 16, 255; chants, 10–11, 17, 20, 48, 51, 56–57, 115, 117–118, 127, 184, 190, 193–194, 211, 220, 245; and emergence, 15–17, 19, 83–85, 258; and everydayness, 2, 7–11, 113–114, 118, 259; failure, 15, 23n5, 152–153, 172, 175n16, 195, 200; and finality, 261; framing, 11–12, 14; frequency of, 6–8, 11, 238, 255; genres, 14–15, 17–18, 48, 118–119, 128, 260–261; improvisation, 57, 258, 261; language, 56–57, 64, 193, 195; and performance theory, 14–15, 214, 258; promise of, 153, 161, 180, 233–234, 236–239; and risk, 15–16, 127, 150, 152–152, 158; and sensuousness, 12–13, 82, 87, 92, 102–103, 118–119, 178, 192–194, 211–213, 259; and virtuality, 10, 126, 262; as work (*awing*), 11, 22n4, 185, 232
ritual paraphernalia. *See ruye*